Total Knee Arthroplasty

Theofilos Karachalios

Editor

Total Knee Arthroplasty

Long Term Outcomes

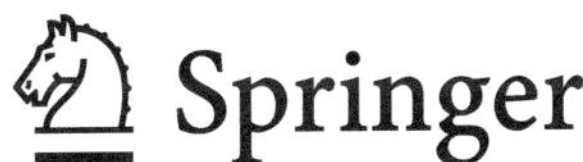

Editor
Theofilos Karachalios
Orthopaedic Department
University of Thessalia
Larissa
Greece

ISBN 978-1-4471-7111-9   ISBN 978-1-4471-6660-3   (eBook)
DOI 10.1007/978-1-4471-6660-3

Springer London Heidelberg New York Dordrecht

Springer-Verlag London Ltd. is part of Springer Science+Business Media (www.springer.com)

Preface

Up to the 1960s and early 1970s, it was common to see crippled women and men, with hip and knee joint deformities and serious restriction of movement, tottering very short distances using various walking aids. Patients often described how agonisingly painful their arthritic joints were. In November 1962, just over 50 years ago, the pioneer of hip reconstruction surgery, Sir John Charnley, made a modern breakthrough. Thanks to basic scientists, engineers, the industry and dedicated orthopaedic surgeons who have invested their scientific and professional lives to adult reconstructive surgery, we can now provide arthritic patients with painless joint movement and restoration of function.

The origins of total knee arthroplasty (TKA) can be traced back to 1889 in Berlin, where Themistocles Gluck gave a series of lectures describing a system of joint replacement using a unit made of ivory, using pumice and plaster of Paris. In the 1950s, the first surface replacement of the tibia was developed by McKeever. During the next decade, designers focused their efforts on constrained or hinged prostheses or on condylar replacement. Pioneering implant designs were problematic, mainly due to a high percentage of component loosening, breakages of the components and infection. Due to the complexity of knee joint biomechanics and kinematics, the clinical use of effective TKA designs was delayed by at least 15 years when compared with total hip arthroplasty (THA). The design phase of the 1970s and 1980s resulted in two different approaches, the anatomical and the functional, and this was the real advent of satisfactory clinical use of TKAs.

Total joint arthroplasty developed into one of the most important fields of surgery in the twentieth century [1]. However, the road to success for TKA has been neither easy nor without obstacles. Problems of surgical technique and soft tissue balancing arose; low-quality implants were used; patterns of failure were recognised; patellofemoral joint issues produced a high incidence of failure; surgeons have had to learn from devastating clinical failures, and patients have often been "fashion victims" in both TKA and THA [2].

During the early decades when the field arthroplasty was developing, surgeons were influenced by expert opinions and by studies undertaken by the designers of materials, which were sometimes biased. Industry-influenced data was neither filtered nor thoroughly assessed. We were led to believe that the implant is to blame for failures, and due to the lack of strong evidence to support the principles of our surgical techniques, we familiarised ourselves with both good and bad arthroplasty stratagems. Fortunately, we now have reliable educational and training programmes, we critically review high-quality literature and have evidence-based studies (Level I and II RCTs, meta-analysis and national registry data), and continental regulatory bodies inform and scrutinise industrial proposals. We also carefully record the complications that arise in our procedures and take preventive measures. It is now accepted that the long-term survival of a TKA is a multifactorial issue, since, other than the implant, factors related to diagnosis, the patient, the surgeon and surgical technique are also important. Added to these issues, there is the matter of finance. Health providers justifiably question the cost-effectiveness of arthroplasty procedures and especially the need for the introduction of newer, more expensive techniques and implants, which makes the need for systematic and credible research all the more important.

The knee joint functions as a type of biological transmission whose purpose is to accept and transfer a range of loads between and among the femur, patella, tibia and fibula without causing structural or metabolic damage. The purpose of a joint arthroplasty is to maximise the envelope of function for a given joint as safely as possible. It is a matter of optimised load transfer, the kinematics of the artificial joint, design issues and soft tissue metabolic and functional status. In the late 1990s, it was suggested that knees which had had joint arthroplasty surgery do not replicate the functional status of a healthy, uninjured adult joint. It has been also observed that patients with TKAs walk differently compared to normal controls. They show slower walking speed, shorter stride length, less time spent in the stance phase and stiff-legged gait. Many subjects also demonstrate an anterior sliding of the femur on the tibia, a phenomenon named paradoxical motion which has significant implications for the functional results of TKA. In the light of these observations, complications like irregular kinematics, abnormal patellar tracking, polyethylene wear and poor range of motion can be explained. Functional recovery in TKA is slow; a significant number of patients are not happy with the functional outcome of the procedure and feel that their surgery was not successful in enabling them to resume their regular physical activities or participate in age-appropriate recreational and sports activities.

For current practice and the future development of TKA, we need to be able to reply to the following questions: What is the optimal design and fixation of the implants we use for knee arthroplasty reconstruction? What are the gold standards? Can we do better? In an attempt to throw light on these questions, the present authors critically evaluate data from long-term clinical studies and assess various factors which may influence outcome. It is our opinion that even though much effort has been put into research, both by individual research centres and the implant industry, this has not always translated into the improvement of clinical outcome, and cost-effectiveness has not often been taken into account. It is also apparent that theoretical and laboratory studies do not always hold up in the cold morning light of long-term clinical studies and that there are few quality Level I and II clinical outcome studies.

In this book we focus on the long-term outcome of TKA, and we hope it will be useful both for the novice who seeks a quick introduction to this specific topic and for more experienced surgeons who seek an in-depth critical review of current practices.

References

1. Learmonth ID, Young C, Rorabeck C. The operation of the century: total hip replacement. Lancet. 2007;370(0597):1508–19.
2. Muirhead-Allwood SK. Lessons of a hip failure. BMJ. 1998;316(7132):644.
3. Blaha JD. The rationale for a total knee implant that confers anteroposterior stability throughout range of motion. J Arthroplasty. 2004;19:22–6.

Larissa, Hellenic Republic

Theofilos Karachalios

Contents

1   **A Brief History of Total Knee Arthroplasty**   1
Konstantinos Makridis and Theofilos Karachalios

2   **Kinematics of the Natural and Replaced Knee**   7
Lisa G. Coles, Subinu Gheduzzi, Anthony W. Miles,
and Harinderjit S. Gill

3   **Long Term Survival of Total Knee Arthroplasty.
Lessons Learned from the Clinical Outcome
of Old Designs.**   21
Konstantinos Makridis and Theofilos Karachalios

4   **Long Term Survival of Total Knee Arthroplasty.
Lessons Learn from the Clinical Outcome
of Old Designs. Second Generation of Implants
and the Total Condylar TKA**   29
Konstantinos Makridis and Theofilos Karachalios

5   **Total Knee Arthroplasty. Evaluating Outcomes**   39
Elias Palaiochorlidis and Theofilos Karachalios

6   **The Long Term Outcome of Total Knee Arthroplasty.
The Effect of Age and Diagnosis.**   49
Alexander Tsarouhas and Michael E. Hantes

7   **Long Term Outcome of Primary Total Knee Arthroplasty.
The Effect of Body Weight and Level of Activity**   55
Polykarpos I. Kiorpelidis, Zoe H. Dailiana,
and Sokratis E. Varitimidis

8   **Long Term Clinical Outcome of Total Knee
Arthroplasty. The Effect of the Severity
of Deformity**   69
Panagiotis Megas, Anna Konstantopoulou,
and Antonios Kouzelis

9   **Long Term Clinical Outcome of Total Knee
Arthroplasty. The Effect of Surgeon Training
and Experience**   79
Nikolaos Roidis, Gregory Avramidis,
and Petros Kalampounias

**10 Long Term Clinical Outcome of Total Knee
     Arthroplasty. The Effect of Limp Alignment,
     Implant Placement and Stability as Controlled
     by Surgical Technique**   85
     John Michos and Theofilos Karachalios

**11 Long Term Results of Total Knee Arthroplasty.
     The Effect of Surgical Approach**   101
     Dimitrios Giotikas and Theofilos Karachalios

**12 Long Term Outcome of Total Knee Arthroplasty.
     The Effect of Posterior Stabilized Designs.**   109
     George A. Macheras and Spyridon P. Galanakos

**13 Long Term Clinical Outcome of Total Knee
     Arthroplasty. The Effect Posterior Cruciate
     Retaining Design**   125
     Irini Tatani, Antonios Kouzelis, and Panagiotis Megas

**14 Rationale and Long Term Outcome of Rotating
     Platform Total Knee Replacement**   135
     Vasileios S. Nikolaou and George C. Babis

**15 Mid to Long Term Clinical Outcome of Medial
     Pivot Designs.**   143
     Nikolaos Roidis, Konstantinos Veltsistas,
     and Theofilos Karachalios

**16 Long Term Outcome of Total Knee Arthroplasty.
     The Effect of Implant Fixation (Cementless)**   155
     Theofilos Karachalios and Ioannis Antoniou

**17 Long Term Outcome of Total Knee Arthroplasty:
     The Effect of Polyethylene.**   163
     Eduardo García-Rey, Enrique Gómez-Barrena,
     and Eduardo García-Cimbrelo

**18 Long Term Outcome of Total Knee Arthroplasty.
     Condylar Constrained Prostheses**   169
     Konstantinos A. Bargiotas

**19 Long Term Outcome of Total Knee Arthroplasty
     Rotating Hinge Designs**   179
     Demetrios Kafidas and Theofilos Karachalios

**20 Clinical Outcome of Total Knee Megaprosthesis
     Replacement for Bone Tumors**   193
     Vasileios A. Kontogeorgakos

**21 Long Term Outcome of Total Knee Arthroplasty.
     The Effect of Patella Resurfacing.**   205
     Elias Palaiochorlidis and Theofilos Karachalios

**22 Infected Total Knee Arthroplasty. Basic Science,
Management and Outcome** 217
Theofilos Karachalios and George Komnos

**23 Short and Mid Term Outcome of Total Knee
Arthroplasty. The Effect of Rehabilitation** 227
Kyriakos Avramidis and Theofilos Karachalios

**24 Mid and Long Term Functional Outcome
of Total Knee Arthroplasty** 241
Nikolaos Rigopoulos and Theofilos Karachalios

**25 Long Term Outcome of Total Knee Arthroplasty.
The Effect of Navigation** 245
Aristides Zimbis and Theofilos Karachalios

**26 Quality of Life and Patient Satisfaction After Total
Knee Arthroplasty Using Contemporary Designs** 255
Zoe H. Dailiana, Ippolyti Papakostidou,
and Theofilos Karachalios

Index 267

Contributors

Ioannis Antoniou, MD Orthopaedic Department, Center of Biomedical Sciences (CERETETH), University of Thessalia, Larissa, Hellenic Republic

Orthopaedic Department, Center of Biomedical Sciences (CERETETH), University General Hospital of Larissa, Larissa, Hellenic Republic

Kyriakos Avramidis, MD, DSc Orthopaedic Department, General Hospital of Larissa, Larissa, Hellenic Republic

Gregory Avramidis, MD 3rd Orthopaedic Department, KAT Hospital, Athens, Hellenic Republic

George C. Babis, MD, DSc 2nd Orthopaedic Department, School of Medicine, Athens University, Konstantopouleio General Hospital Nea Ionia, Athens, Greece

Konstantinos A. Bargiotas, MD, DSc Orthopaedic Department, University General Hospital of Larissa, Larissa, Hellenic Republic

Lisa G. Coles, PhD Department of Mechanical Engineering, University of Bath, Bath, UK

Zoe H. Dailiana, MD, DSc Department of Orthopaedic Surgery, Faculty of Medicine, School of Health Sciences, University of Thessalia, Larissa, Hellenic Republic

Spyridon Galanakos, MD, DSc 4th Orthopedic Department, KAT Hospital, Athens, Greece

Eduardo García-Cimbrelo, MD, PhD Orthopaedics Department, Hospital La Paz-Idi Paz, Madrid, Spain

Sabina Gheduzzi, PhD Department of Mechanical Engineering, University of Bath, Bath, UK

Harinderjit S. Gill, PhD Department of Mechanical Engineering, University of Bath, Bath, UK

Dimitrios Giotikas, MD, DSc Department of Trauma and Orthopaedics, Addenbrookes Hospital–Cambridge, University Hospitals NHS Foundation Trust, Cambridge, UK

Enrique Gómez-Barrena, MD, PhD Orthopaedics Department,
Hospital La Paz-Idi Paz, Madrid, Spain

Michael E. Hantes, MD, DSc, PhD Department of Orthopaedic Surgery,
University Hospital of Larissa, Larissa, Greece

Faculty of Medicine, School of Health Sciences, University of Thessaly,
Larissa, Greece

Demetrios Kafidas, MD Orthopaedic Department, University of Thessalia,
Larissa, Hellenic Republic

Petros Kalampounias, MD 3rd Orthopaedic Department, KAT Hospital,
Athens, Hellenic Republic

Theofilos Karachalios, MD, DSc Orthopaedic Department,
Faculty of Medicine, School of Health Sciences,
Center of Biomedical Sciences (CERETETH), University of Thessalia,
University General Hospital of Larissa, Larissa, Hellenic Republic

Polykarpos I. Kiorpelidis, MD Department of Orthopaedic Surgery
and Musculoskeletal Trauma, Faculty of Medicine,
School of Health Sciences, University of Thessalia, Larissa,
Hellenic Republic

George Komnos, MD Orthopaedic Department,
Center of Biomedical Sciences (CERETETH), University of Thessalia,
Larissa, Hellenic Republic

Orthopaedic Department, General Hospital of Karditsa,
Karditsa, Hellenic Republic

Anna Konstantopoulou, MD Department of Orthopaedics
and Traumatology, University Hospital of Patras, Rion, Greece

Vasileios Kontogeorgakos, MD, DSc Department of Orthopaedic Surgery,
ATTIKON University General Hospital, Athens, Hellenic Republic, Greece

Medical School, University of Athens, Athens, Hellenic Republic, Greece

Antonios Kouzelis, MD, DSc Department of Orthopaedics
and Traumatology, University Hospital of Patras, Rion, Greece

George A. Macheras, MD, DSc 4th Orthopedic Department,
KAT Hospital, Athens, Greece

Konstantinos Makridis, MD Orthopaedic Department,
Center of Biomedical Sciences (CERETETH),
University of Thessalia Hellenic Republic, Larissa, Hellenic Republic

Panagiotis Megas, MD, DSc Department of Orthopaedics
and Traumatology, University Hospital of Patras, Rion, Greece

John Michos, MD, DSc Senior Consultant Orthopaedic Surgeon,
D' Orthopaedic Department, Asklepieion General Hospital, Boula, Athens

Anthony W. Miles, PhD Department of Mechanical Engineering,
University of Bath, Bath, UK

Vasileios S. Nikolaou, MD, PhD, MSc 2nd Orthopaedic Department,
School of Medicine, Athens University, Konstantopouleio General Hospital
Nea Ionia, Athens, Greece

Elias Palaiochorlidis, MD, DSc Orthopaedic Department,
Center of Biomedical Sciences (CERETETH), University of Thessalia,
Larissa, Hellenic Republic

Ippolyti Papakostidou, RN, DSc Department of Orthopaedic Surgery,
Faculty of Medicine, School of Health Sciences, University of Thessalia,
Larissa, Hellenic Republic

Eduardo García-Rey, MD, PhD, EBOT Orthopaedics Department,
Hospital La Paz-Idi Paz, Madrid, Spain

Nikolaos Rigopoulos, MD Orthopaedic Department,
Center of Biomedical Sciences (CERETETH), University of Thessalia,
Larissa, Hellenic Republic

Nikolaos Roidis, MD, DSc 3rd Orthopaedic Department, KAT Hospital,
Athens, Hellenic Republic

Alexander Tsarouhas, MD, DSc Private Orthopedic Surgeon, Kalambaka,
Thessaly, Greece

Sokratis E. Varitimidis, MD, DSc Department of Orthopaedic
Surgery and Musculoskeletal Trauma, Faculty of Medicine,
School of Health Sciences, University of Thessalia, Biopolis, Larissa,
Republic Hellenic

Konstantinos Veltsistas, MD 3rd Orthopaedic Department, KAT Hospital,
Athens, Hellenic Republic

Aristides Zimbis, MD, DSc Orthopaedic Department,
Center of Biomedical Sciences (CERETETH), University of Thessalia,
Larissa, Hellenic Republic

School of Health Sciences, Faculty of Medicine, University of Thessalia,
Larissa, Hellenic Republic

Irini Tatani, MD Department of Orthopaedics and Traumatology,
University Hospital of Patras, Rion, Greece

A Brief History of Total Knee Arthroplasty

Konstantinos Makridis and Theofilos Karachalios

Introduction

The development of total knee arthroplasty (TKA) is characterized by the manufacturing of appropriate interposition materials, clinical application of knee biomechanics and the use of secure and reliable methods of component fixation. Since the introduction of resection and interposition arthroplasty procedures and the introduction of polycentric and geometric knees, significant improvements and important innovations have been made. The design of the total Condylar knee set the standard for modern TKA in combination with the surgical techniques of flat bone cuts, symmetrical flexion/extension gaps and careful ligament release. TKA has thus become one of the most successful orthopaedic surgical procedures. Recent innovative ideas such as patient specific instrumentation and computer-assisted surgery have the potential to further improve the effectiveness, durability and longevity of TKA designs.

The main indication for surgery, in patients with an arthritic knee, is constant pain and disability which negatively affect the quality of life and functional status of the patient, in activities such as standing, walking and climbing stairs. The aim of surgery is to restore damaged cartilage and underlying bone, creating an artificial joint which will function as a normal knee. Restoration of limb alignment and joint kinematics are crucial, since malalignment of knee prostheses has been implicated in long term complications, including stiffness, patello-femoral instability, accelerated polyethylene wear, and implant loosening [1].

The evolution of TKA has passed through various steps and stages. The initial trials to reconstruct a degenerative joint included the procedures of resection and interposition arthroplasty, but the results were disappointing. Following these primitive techniques, first generation implants were manufactured and introduced including polycentric and geometric knees. While short term results were promising, time has revealed many disadvantages and complications. It can be said that the modern era began during the decade of 1970, where the basic concepts and principles of TKA were set and most of the modern designs were developed [2].

K. Makridis, MD
Orthopaedic Department, Center of Biomedical Sciences (CERETETH), University of Thessalia, Larissa, Hellenic Republic

T. Karachalios, MD, DSc (✉)
Orthopaedic Department, Faculty of Medicine, School of Health Sciences, Center of Biomedical Sciences (CERETETH), University of Thessalia, University General Hospital of Larissa, Mezourlo region, 41110 Larissa, Hellenic Republic
e-mail: kar@med.uth.gr

The purpose of this chapter is to provide a brief review of the historical development of TKA (Table 1.1) and to present the step by step evolution from the initial surgical techniques through the primitive and first generation knee implants up until the current designs.

History of the TKA

The first attempts to reconstruct a damaged or degenerated knee joint were reported at the end of nineteenth and the beginning of twentieth century. Resection arthroplasty of the knee was first reported by Fergusson in 1861, a procedure in which an incision was made and excess bone was removed to improve motion and stability [3]. Verneuil et al. [4] in 1863 tried to prevent bone growth between the resected joint surfaces by inserting a flap of joint capsule between them. In an attempt to simplify the mechanics of the knee, Gluck proposed the complete resection of articulating surfaces and cruciate ligaments and used a hinged prosthesis made of ivory to recreate the joint. The beginning of 1900 was the era of interposition arthroplasty and several substances were used, like fat (Lexer in 1917), chromatized pig's bladder (Baer in 1918), fat and fascia lata (Murphy in 1913, Putti in 1921 and Albee in 1928), cellophane (Sampson in 1949), sheets of nylon (Kuhns in 1950) and skin (Brown in 1958). Campbell popularized the use of free fascial transplants as an interposition material. Some of these techniques had limited success in ankylosed knees, but in general the mid and long-term results were disappointing [5–13].

Between 1950 and 1960 several authors used different types of metallic molds in the form of femoral or tibial hemiarthroplasties [14, 15], while other surgeons designed and developed specific hinged implants for cases of severe arthritis and instability. The application of intramedullary stems improved the function of these prostheses which was an extra motivation for further development. Judet presented the first hinged prosthesis made of acrylic [16], while Magnoni, Waldius and Shiers reported similar devices which also used medullary stems to provide stability and restore limb alignment [17–19]. To

Table 1.1 History of the TKA

1800
1861 → Ferguson resection arthroplasty
1863 → Verneuil resection arthroplasty
1891 → Gluck ivory hinged prosthesis
1900
1913 → Murphy fat and fascia lata
1917 → Lexer fat
1918 → Baer chromatized pig's bladder
1921 → Putti fat and fascia lata
1924 → Campbell free fascial transplants
1928 → Albee fat and fascia lata
1947 → Judet acrylic hinge
1949 → Sampson cellophane, Magnoni acrylic hinge
1950 → Kuhns sheets of nylon
1951–1958 → Brown skin interposition, Walldius/ Shiers metallic hinges,
1960 → McKeever metal tibial components
1966 → MacIntosh metal tibial components
1969 → Gunston Polycentric knee, Eftekhar Mark I
1970 → Kodama – Yamamoto Mark I, Freeman-Swanson knee
1971 → Geomedic knee, Duocondylar knee, Sheehan hinged prosthesis
1972 → UCI knee, Anatomic knee, Leeds knee
1973 → Attenborough hinged prosthesis, Geometric II, ICLH, Eftekhar Mark II
1974 → Total Condylar knee, Duopatella knee
1975 → Ewald, Kodama Mark II, Cloutier, Anametric, Posterior Cruciate Condylar
1976 → Guepar hinged, Oxford Meniscal knee, Total Condylar II, New Jersey knee
1977 → Buechel-Pappas, Bringham, Gustilo knees
1978 → Install-Burstein Posterior Stabilized, Kinematic Posterior Stabilized & Cruciate Sparing
1979 → Gliding Meniscal Knee, Freeman-Samuelson
1980 → LCS mobile bearing, PCA
1983 → AGC
1980 → PFC Sigma, Miller-Gallante, Stanmore hinged
1987 → Natural knee
1989 → Install-Burstein Posterior Stabilized II, Kinemax
1990 → Duracon
1992 → Interax
1993 → Profix
1995 → Nex-Gen, Advance
1996 → Scorpio
1997 → Wright Medical medial pivot
2000s
Genesis I, Genesis II, Legion and Journey II, Natural knee Flex and LPS-Flex Mobile, Triathlon and Scorpio NRG, Vanguard, patient specific techniques and computer-assisted surgery

deal with the problems of patellofemoral pain and loosening, McKeever [20] and MacIntosh [21] introduced the concept of patellar prostheses and the use of metal tibial components. However, biomechanical issues, poor metallurgy, improper fixation and frequent infection resulted in high failure rates.

Innovations such as the use of bone cement as a fixation material and the introduction of high density polyethylene plastic as a bearing surface gave great impetus to the further development of TKA. The polycentric and geometric designs launched the era of first generation knee replacements and Gunston was one of the first surgeons to experiment on these prostheses [22]. The Gunston polycentric knee was a minimally constrained implant and consisted of two separate high density polyethylene surfaces. Mimicking the low friction concept used earlier by Charnley in THA, minimizing bone cuts and preserving both cruciate ligaments, Gunston tried to reproduce the polycentric motion of the normal knee.

During the same year, Eftekhar presented his design using a metal-backed tibial component with modular polyethylene inserts [23]. Implants were fixed with cement and the use of long intramedullary stems would secure fixation. The Eftekhar Mark I knee would evolve into a condylar TKA design later, the Eftekhar Mark II. The first geometric knee arthroplasty (Geomedic or Geometric I Knee) was presented by Coventry, Riley, Finerman, Turner and Upshaw [24]. The preservation of both cruciate ligaments, high conformity, improved fixation of the tibial component with the use of small pegs and nonresurfacing of the patella were the main concepts of this design. The evolution of this implant was the Geometric II knee. The concept of geometric design was applied to another two implants manufactured by Zimmer in 1975. The Geotibial knee had a tibial peg to improve fixation and the Geopatellar knee had a femoral flange to improve patellar tracking. The evolution of these implants was the Multi-Radius, Miller Galante, Miller Galante II, and Nexgen knees. In the same year, Howmedica presented a similar but more anatomical design, the Anametric knee which would evolved into the porous coated anatomical knee (PCA) and eventually the Duracon knee.

Simultaneously with the development of first generation arthroplasties, several hinged prostheses were developed, like the Sheehan, Attenborough, Stanmore and the most popular Guepar prosthesis. Despite the initial enthusiasm, however, these prostheses failed because of a high rate of patellofemoral complications, breakage of the implant, early wear and loss of fixation. Nowadays, hinged arthroplasties are used in revision, tumour and cases with a high risk of instability.

Alongside with the development of the polycentric and geometric knees the idea of creating total condylar TKA evolved. Aiming to reconstruct normal joint surfaces, these designs consisted of a single piece femoral component covering both medial and lateral condyles, a single piece tibial component resurfacing both the medial and lateral plateaus, and bone cement was used for fixation. The patella femoral joint was not necessarily included in the design; some types had a femoral flange, but patellar buttons had not yet come into use. Surgical techniques were based on two philosophies: the anatomic and functional approaches. According to the first approach, only the articular surfaces were replaced or resurfaced, both cruciate ligaments and most of the soft tissue constraints were preserved and the implant surfaces were designed in such a way as to minimize the risk of soft tissue impingement. According to the functional approach, the mechanics of the knee were simplified by resection of the condyles and the cruciate ligaments and the main concern was to create parallel and equal gaps in flexion and extension.

In 1970, Kodama and Yamamoto introduced the first anatomical total condylar knee [25]. The single piece polyethylene tibial component had a central cut out for preservation of both cruciate ligaments and fixation was based on press-fit enhanced by fins and staples. This knee later evolved as Mark I, II, III and finally the New Yamamoto Micro-Fit knee manufactured by Corin. At the same time, Waugh and Smith presented the UCI knee which had no femoral flange. This implant later evolved into the Gustillo-Ram and Genesis I and II knees [26].

Patellar buttons were probably first used in the Anatomical knee designed by Townley.

Patellofemoral tracking was assisted by the construction of a femoral flange, while range of motion was improved with the design of different sagittal and medio-lateral radii of curvatures [27]. The Total Knee Original was the evolution of this implant. Another development, the Leeds knee, was more complex than the Anatomic knee [28]. Unfortunately, the concept of creating curved bone surfaces to fit the femoral component and the complexity of tibial component design led to significant difficulties in its manufacturing and usage. In a similar way, the Ewald knee became less popular due to its high conformity design which restricted the motion of the joint.

The Hospital of Special Surgery (HSS) was the major center where the manufacturing and development of TKA was flourished. In 1971, Ranawat implanted the first Duocondylar knee which was symmetrical, anatomical and cemented [29]. An improved design was presented some years later (the Duopatella knee), having an additional anterior femoral flange and a single tibial insert with a posterior cut out for preservation of the PCL. The Duopatella knee would evolve into the PFC Modular and PFC Sigma knee design (Depuy) as well as the Kinematic, Kinematic II, Kinemax and Kinemax Plus systems (Howmedica).

The functional approach to knee design was applied in the use of the Freeman Swanson knee [30]. Both cruciate ligaments were sacrificed to simplify the kinematics of the knee, while the femoral cuts were made to be flat, preserving the bone. The introduction of specific instrumentation, spacers and intramedullary guides were very innovative for those years. The Imperial College London Hospital knee (ICLH) (Protek and Howmedica) and the Freeman Samuelson knee were the descendants of this implant.

The Total Condylar knee (TC) was the most substantial design that has influenced all modern implants. This knee combined the advantages of the anatomical bicondylar and the conforming surface design. Its sagittal radius mimicked the natural knee and patellar tracking was improved by the anterior femoral flange and a patellar button made of polyethylene. The bearing surfaces were double dished to provide better stability.

The surgical technique, which included flat bone cuts, symmetrical flexion/extension gaps and careful ligament release led to a high success rate [31]. The evolution of the Total Condylar knee included the Total Condylar II and the Insall-Burstein Posterior Stabilized knee systems.

During 1975–1980, several mobile bearing arthroplasties were presented. Unrestricted rotational movements, low constraint forces and minimal loosening were proposed as the main advantages of these prostheses. O'Connor and Goodfellow presented the Oxford Meniscal Knee arthroplasty [32], while Buechel and Pappas described the bicruciate-retaining and rotating platform designs which would be named as the New Jersey Knee System which would later evolve as the Low Contact Stress (LCS) and the LCS Rotating Patellar Replacement knee (DePuy) [33]. In 1977, Polyzoides and Tsakonas presented another mobile meniscal bearing knee named the Gliding Meniscal knee (Zimmer) which would later evolve into the Rotaglide knee (Corin) [34].

During the decades of 1980 and 1990 only small changes and modifications were made to existing prostheses. The main issues needing further clarification and research were fixation with or without cement, polyethylene wear, use of fixed or mobile bearings, achievement of good alignment, and patella replacement. In 1980, DePuy introduced the LCS mobile bearing knee and Howmedica the PCA total knee system. In 1983, Biomet presented the AGC knee, and 1 year later Johnson & Johnson promoted the PFC Sigma knee and Zimmer introduced the Miller-Galante knee. In 1987, the Natural knee was manufactured by Intermedics and in 1989 the Insall-Burstein II posterior stabilized knee was available on the market. The same year Howmedica introduced the Kinemax knee and 1 year later the same company presented the Duracon implant. In 1992 Howmedica introduced the Interax total knee system and in 1993 Smith & Nephew manufactured the Profix knee. Three years later Zimmer introduced the NexGen and Wright Medical the Advance knee system. In 1996, Osteonics promoted the Scorpio knee and in 1997 Wright Medical presented the medial pivot knee.

Newer implants were manufactured over the following years, the most popular ones including: Genesis I, Genesis II, Legion and Journey II by Smith & Nephew, Natural knee Flex and LPS-Flex Mobile by Zimmer, Triathlon and Scorpio NRG by Stryker and Vanguard knee by Biomet. Furthermore, recent innovations have been promoted by several companies based on the concepts of patient specific knee solutions and computer-assisted knee surgery. Visionaire system (Smith & Nephew), Tru-Match protocol (DePuy), Persona knee (Zimmer) and Signature knee (Biomet) consist the most popular patient specific knee systems. Navigation surgery systems are available by Stryker, DePuy and B-Braun Aesculap companies.

Conclusions

The reconstruction of the knee joint has passed through various steps and stages. Over the years and following resection and interposition arthroplasties, significant improvements were made in the field of knee biomechanics, surgical approach, fixation techniques and implant design. Introduction of the Total Condylar knee proved to be the keystone in the modern development of TKA. By preserving the main principles of this knee design and adding some new elements to later developments of knee implants, TKA has became one of the most successful surgical procedures in Orthopaedic science.

References

1. Luyckx T, Vanhoorebeeck F, Bellemans J. Should we aim at undercorrection when doing a total knee arthroplasty? Knee Surg Sports Traumatol Arthrosc. 2014. [Epub ahead of print].
2. Laskin RS. New techniques and concepts in total knee replacement. Clin Orthop. 2003;416:151–3.
3. Fergusson W. Excision of the knee joint. Recovery with a false joint and a useful limb. Med Times Gaz. 1861;1:60.
4. Verneuil A. De la creation d'une fausse articulation par section ou resection partielle de los maxillaire inférieur, comme moyen de remedier a lankylose vraie ou fausse de la mâchoire inférieure. Arch Gen Med. 1860;15:174–284. 5e serie.
5. Murphy JB. Ankylosis. Arthroplasty, clinical and experimental. J Am Med Arthroplast. 1905;44:1573.
6. Baer WS. Arthroplasty with the aid of animal membrane. Am J Orthop Surg. 1918;16:1–29.
7. Campbell WC. Arthroplasty of the knee. Ann Surg. 1924;80:88–102.
8. Lexer E. Joint transplantation and arthroplasty. Surg Gynecol and Obstet. 1925;40:782–809.
9. Albee FH. Original features in arthroplasty of the knee with improved prognosis. Surg Gynecol Obstet. 1928;47:312–28.
10. Samson JE. Arthroplasty of the knee joint. J Bone Joint Surg Br. 1949;31B:50–2.
11. Kuhns JG, Potter TA. Nylon arthroplasty of the knee joint in chronic arthritis. Surg Gynecol Obstet. 1950;91:351–62.
12. Brown JE, McGaw WH, Shaw DT. Use of cutis as an interposing membrane in arthroplasty of the knee. J Bone Joint Surg Am. 1958;40A:1003–18.
13. Potter TA, Weinfeld MS, Thomas WH. Arthroplasty of the knee in rheumatoid arthritis and osteoarthritis. J Bone Joint Surg Am. 1972;54A:1–23.
14. Campbell WC. Interposition of vitallium plates in arthroplasties of the knee. Preliminary report. Am J Surg. 1940;47:639–41.
15. Townley CO. Articular-plate replacement arthroplasty for the knee joint. Clin Orthop. 1964;36:77–85.
16. Judet J, Judet H. Presentation of an instrument. Mechanical study of a knee prosthesis. Chirurgie. 1975;101:294–5.
17. Majnoni dTntignano JM. Articulation totales en resine acrylique. Rev Orthop. 1950;36:535–7.
18. Shiers LGP. Arthroplasty of the knee. Preliminary report of a new method. J Bone Joint Surg Br. 1954;36B:55360.
19. Walldius B. Arthroplasty of the knee using an endoprosthesis. Acta Orthop Scand. 1957;S24:1–12.
20. McKeever DC. Patellar prosthesis. J Bone Joint Surg Am. 1955;37A:1074–84.
21. Macintosh DL. Hemiarthroplasty of the knee using a space-occupying prosthesis for painful varus and valgus deformities. J Bone Joint Surg Am. 1958;40A:1431.
22. Gunston FH. Polycentric knee arthroplasty. J Bone Joint Surg Br. 1971;53B:272–5.
23. Eftekhar NS. Total knee-replacement arthroplasty. Results with the intramedullary adjustable total knee prosthesis. J Bone Joint Surg Am. 1983;65A:293–309.
24. Coventry MB, Finerman GA, Riley LH, Turner RH, Upshaw JE. A new geometric knee for total knee arthroplasty. Clin Orthop. 1972;83:157–62.
25. Yamamoto S. Total knee replacement with the Kodama-Yamamoto knee prosthesis. Clin Orthop. 1979;145:60–7.
26. Waugh TR, Smith RC, Orofino CF, Anzel SM. Total knee replacement: operative technic and preliminary results. Clin Orthop. 1973;94:196–201.
27. Townley CO. The classic: articular-plate replacement arthroplasty for the knee joint.1964. Clin Orthop. 2005;440:9–12.
28. Seedhom BB, Longton EB, Dowson D, Wright V. Biomechanics background in the design of a total replacement knee prosthesis. Acta Orthop Belg. 1973;39:164–80.

29. Ranawat CS, Shine JJ. Duo-condylar total knee arthroplasty. Clin Orthop. 1973;94:185–95.
30. Freeman MA, Swanson SA, Todd RC. Total replacement of the knee using the Freeman-Swanson knee prosthesis. 1973. Clin Orthop. 2003;416:4–21.
31. Insall J, Ranawat CS, Scott WN, Walker P. Total condylar knee replacement: preliminary report. 1976. Clin Orthop. 2001;388:3–6.
32. Murray DW, Goodfellow JW, O'Connor JJ. The Oxford medial unicompartmental arthroplasty: a ten-year survival study. J Bone Joint Surg Br. 1998;80B:983–9.
33. Buechel Sr FF, Buechel Jr FF, Pappas MJ, D'Alessio J. Twenty-year evaluation of meniscal bearing and rotating platform knee replacements. Clin Orthop. 2001;388:41–50.
34. Polyzoides AJ, Dendrinos GK, Tsakonas H. The Rotaglide total knee arthroplasty. Prosthesis design and early results. J Arthroplasty. 1996;11:453–9.

Lisa G. Coles, Sabina Gheduzzi, Anthony W. Miles, and Harinderjit S. Gill

Introduction

The human knee comprises two articulating joints: the tibiofemoral joint and the patellofemoral joint, and a complex soft tissue envelope (Fig. 2.1). It has evolved to meet our current locomotion needs over millions of years, and is relatively unique within the mammalian world [1–4]. Few mammals can stand fully extended on their hind legs and even fewer can walk in a bipedal stance allowing the body to rotate around the extended knee [5]. In contrast to other mammals, the human knee has, therefore, evolved to withstand the large lateral quadriceps forces required to achieve this motion. This, alongside many other evolutionary developments, has resulted in the complex structure we term the human knee.

This chapter discusses the historical and contemporary understanding of natural knee kinematics and the effect of total knee arthroplasty (TKA) on the kinematics of the joint. Initially, the issues associated with understanding the kinematics of a joint comprising three rigid bodies, which can each move in six degrees of freedom, will be discussed. The methods that have been used to assess knee kinematics will be highlighted and the issues involved in the analysis and interpretation of kinematic data considered. The main body of the chapter will then detail the historical development of the modern understanding of human knee kinematics, and finish with a discussion of the kinematics of the replaced joint.

Rigid Body Kinematics

The human knee comprises four bones: the tibia, the fibula, the femur and the patella; and two articulating joints: the tibiofemoral joint and the patellofemoral joint. The fibula provides no articulating surface at the knee joint and is, therefore, omitted from discussions of kinematics. Each of

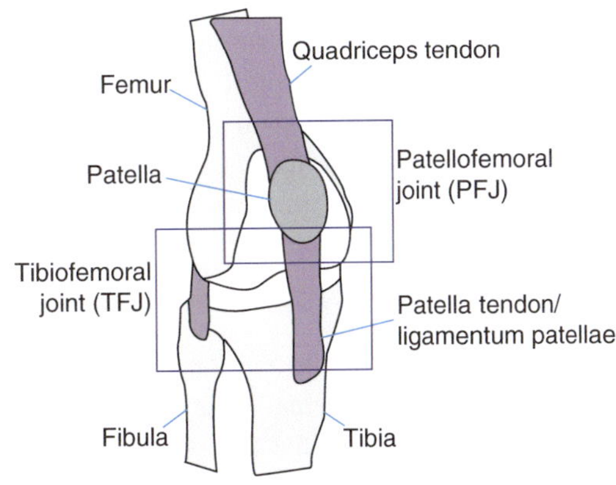

Fig. 2.1 The joints of the human knee

L.G. Coles, PhD • S. Gheduzzi, PhD • A.W. Miles, PhD
H.S. Gill, PhD (✉)
Department of Mechanical Engineering,
University of Bath, Bath, UK
e-mail: richie.gill@ndorms.ox.ac.uk

© Springer-Verlag London 2015
T. Karachalios (ed.), *Total Knee Arthroplasty: Long Term Outcomes*,
DOI 10.1007/978-1-4471-6660-3_2

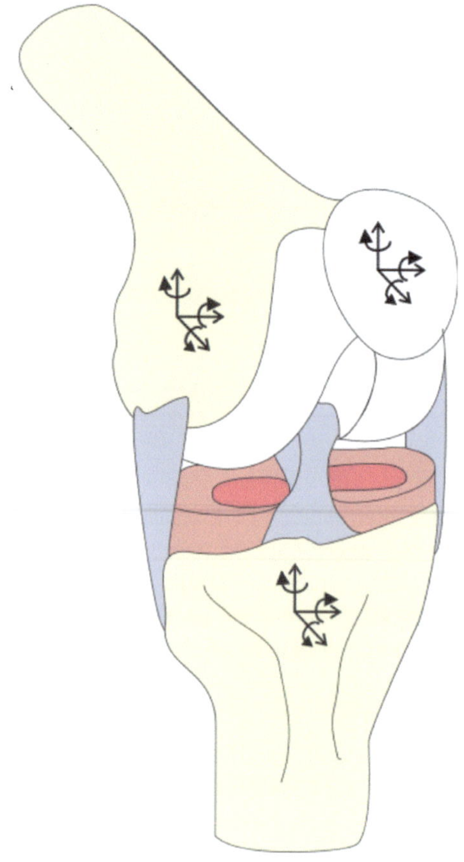

Fig. 2.2 Rigid body

these bones, which are generally considered as rigid bodies, is free to move in six degrees of freedom: three rotations and three translations (Fig. 2.2). The knee is also constrained by a multitude of passive and active soft tissue structures. Most notable are the collateral and cruciate ligaments, and the extensor and flexor mechanisms [6]. Knee motion is governed by bone geometry and the soft tissue envelope. Assessing and describing the overall motion of the knee is, therefore, a complex task.

The assessment of the motion of the bones within the knee, the kinematics, is normally considered individually for the two separate joints. This simplifies the situation to some extent, by limiting the problem to the description of the movement of one rigid body, e.g. the tibia, relative to a second rigid body, e.g. the femur.

The measurement of the movement of a rigid body can be a highly erroneous process. There are many methods to assess the movement of a rigid body, each with associated limitations. However, perhaps more significant, but less well understood, are the errors and uncertainties commonly introduced as a result of the methods used to combine, transform, and represent the kinematics of two bodies moving relative to one and other.

The methods used presently and historically to assess human knee kinematics are discussed in detail by Freeman and Pinskerova [7] and Pinskerova et al. [8], and summarised in this chapter. Before the advent of imaging techniques, such as X-rays, the movement of the bones within the knee joint was assessed through anatomical dissections of cadaveric samples [8]. Cadaveric bone samples were sliced and the shapes of the articulating surfaces assessed [9]. The influence of soft tissue structures has also been studied through sequential anatomical dissection of individual soft tissue structures [10–12]. These methods are destructive and invasive, and do not allow the assessment of the joint throughout the full range of motion [7].

As X-ray technology became more widely available and improved, surgeons and scientists were able to assess the joint articulating surfaces of both cadaveric and *in vivo* subjects in different static positions. However, X-rays only give a 2D view of what is a 3D joint and are generally taken in anatomic, but ultimately arbitrary, planes. They commonly led to a narrow and non-physiological view of knee motion, and the development of complex theories of motion which, although still prominent today, often led to an imperfect understanding of joint movement [8].

More recently, a variety of methods using a combination of X-rays, fluoroscopy, RSA, CT, MRI, and image matching methods have been developed to allow the assessment, in 3D, of the relative motions of the articulating surfaces, or the motion of the contact points between the bones during passive and active motions [7]. It is important to note that the relative motions of the articulating surfaces and the motion of the contact point between the bones are not equivalent measurements, and cannot be used interchangeably.

An assessment of the relative motion of the articulating surfaces is usually achieved by tracking the displacement of the bones directly using anatomical reference landmarks and 3D image registration. An assessment of the motion of the contact point between two surfaces is achieved by tracking the point where the distance between the bone surfaces is smallest. This does not correspond to the motion of the bones [7]. It is also important to note the difference between a passive and an active situation. During an active kinematic assessment, when the muscles are loaded, the knee joint soft tissues will be under tension. The soft tissues will, therefore, guide and limit knee motion to a greater extent than during passive motion. This has been demonstrated to affect joint kinematics [13, 14].

Medical imaging techniques are often limited to static, quasi-static, or, at most, very controlled dynamic situations. Conversely, movement analysis methods can be used to assess joint kinematics during a wide variety of daily living activities. Markers located on the skin of the subject are tracked using optical sensors. A minimum of three non-orthogonal markers can be used to calculate the instantaneous position and attitude (rotational position) of a bone segment. Such calculations assume the segment is a rigid body and that minimal slip of skin and soft tissues occurred [15].

Mathematical methods, based on the model of the human body as a kinematic chain, comprising multiple links or bone segments, can then be used to estimate the kinematics of a joint, such as the knee. This estimation requires the reliable and consistent selection of a global reference system, repeatable anatomical landmark registration, and appropriate manipulation of position vectors and attitude matrices [16]. There are many ways to interpret position and attitude matrices: based on Cardan angles, helical axes, geometrical assumptions or anatomical locations [1, 17]. Some methods are at risk of gimbal-lock at certain degrees of flexion, and all of the methods are complicated by the coupled relationship between the different rotational degrees of freedom [17, 18]. Analysis has demonstrated that in degrees of freedom with relatively little motion, i.e. external/internal rotation of the knee, different methods can result in the calculation of angles which vary by more than 30° [17]. Issues associated with anatomical landmark registration and the discussion of whole joint kinematics in a consistent manner can also occur when imaging methods are used to assess joint motion. This complex subject is discussed in greater detail by Cappozzo et al. [17] and Woltring [18].

The assessment and description of the six degrees of freedom motion of rigid bodies, such as the bones within the knee, is complex, associated with a number of errors, and open to misinterpretation. These issues have to be borne in mind when assessing kinematic studies. However, as will be discussed in the following sections, consistent theories can be constructed, when the results of multiple studies are combined and compared in light of these limitations.

Normal Knee Kinematics[1]

The kinematics of the human knee has been investigated for over 150 years (Fig. 2.3). The periods of development that lead up to the current understanding can be broadly split into three: early understanding, classical theory and modern theory (Fig. 2.3).

Early Understanding

In 1836, the Weber brothers [9] dissected a human cadaver and examined the shapes and relative movements of the bones within various lower limb joints. They demonstrated the circular nature of the posterior femoral condyles, and that longitudinal rotation, around a medial pivot, occurs alongside flexion. Further early work, using an early form of motion capture systems, supported the assertion that the knee joint experiences longitudinal rotation coupled to any flexion movement [8].

The first radiographic study to be carried out on the knee led to the suggestion that it could be modelled as a linkage mechanism. Zuppinger

[1] Elements of this section are taken from the first author's PhD thesis (Thesis copy-write retained by author).

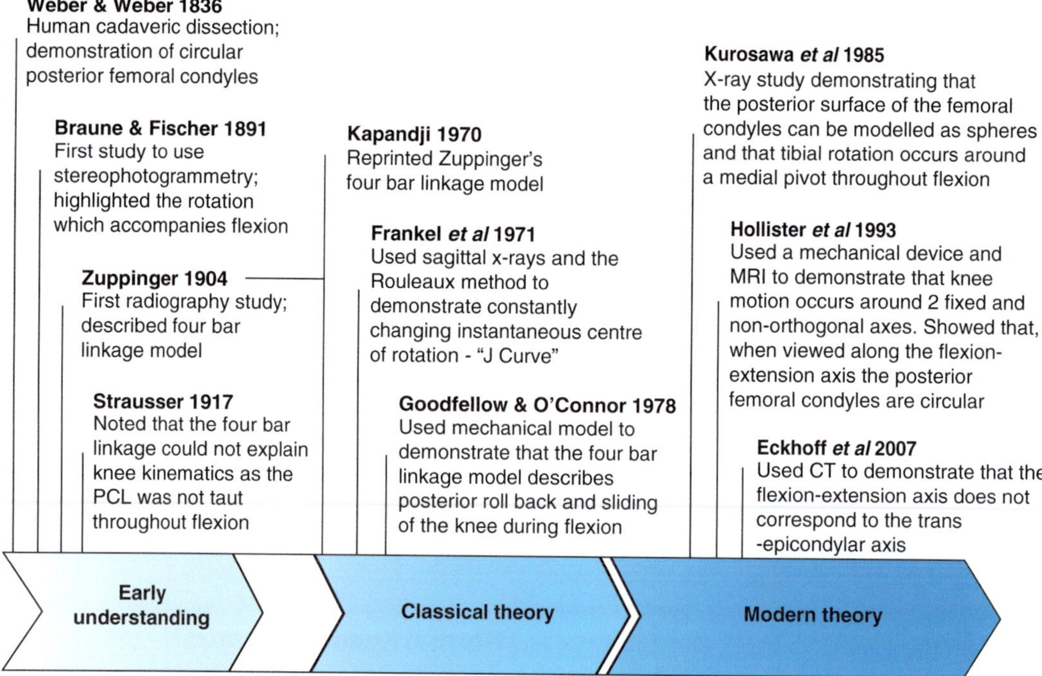

Fig. 2.3 Timeline depicting the development of the modern knee kinematic theories [2–4, 8, 19, 20]

assumed that the cruciate ligaments remain taut throughout the flexion range and, along with the tibia and femur, formed a rigid four bar linkage. Other early work disputed the assumption that the posterior cruciate ligament (PCL) was taut throughout the range of flexion. However, it was only the four bar linkage image that was remembered and incorporated into classical theory in the 1970s. Many of the other early studies, carried out largely by anatomists, were in German and largely forgotten as English became the primary language of science [8].

Classical Theory

Little work to develop understanding of knee joint kinematics was carried out in the period from 1917 to 1970. However, in the 1970s, scientists and engineers, mostly unaware of much of the early work published in German and French, began using X-rays and other imaging techniques to attempt to describe knee kinematics [8]. Sagittal plane X-rays were taken of cadaveric and *in vivo* knees. The axis of tibiofemoral flexion was assessed using the Rouleaux method, making the assumption that the two axes of the joint are planar. Such analyses, which are subject to significant errors if images are not taken in the plane of motion, demonstrated that the instantaneous centre of rotation of the knee, when viewed in the sagittal plane, moves in a semi-circle or a J shaped curve [2, 21–23]. The four bar linkage mechanism, originally proposed by Zuppinger and reprinted by Kapandji has classically been used to describe the complex motion inferred by the moving centre of rotation. This model was considered to describe not only flexion-extension of the knee joint, but also the femoral posterior translation and rotation known to occur with flexion. The four bar linkage mechanism does not take into account the axial rotation of the tibia relative to the femur previously reported to occur alongside flexion [2, 3].

Modern Theory

In the 1980s there was renewed interest in the anatomy of the distal femur, and how this may inform understanding of knee kinematics.

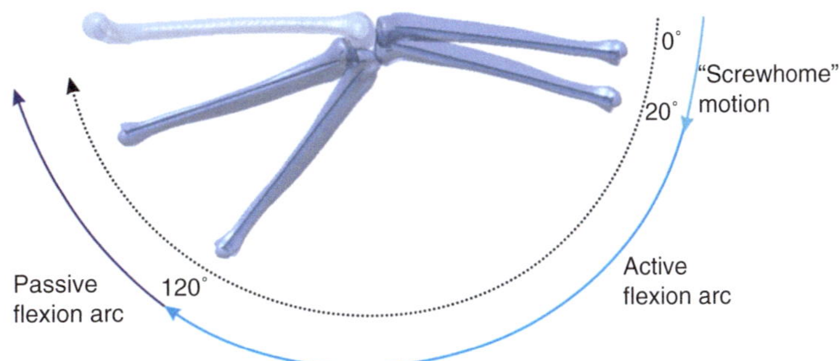

Fig. 2.4 Phases of knee motion (After: Freeman and Pinskerova [1])

Kurosawa et al. [4], used X-ray images and calliper measurements of cadaveric knees to demonstrate that the posterior femoral condyles can be modelled as spheres. The circularity of the distal femoral condyle was further demonstrated by Elias et al. [24], who indicated that the centre of the lateral and medial spheres corresponded with the insertion points of the collateral ligaments.

In 1993, Hollister et al. [20] demonstrated, using cadaveric specimens, that knee motion can be simply described as rotations around two non-orthogonal axes. These axes are not related to normal planes of motion and can, therefore, be difficult to interpret anatomically and surgically. Hollister was also able to demonstrate that the flexion axis, which coincides with the circular centres described by Elias et al. [24], does not move relative to the femur during the majority of the flexion range. The longitudinal axis of the knee passes though the medial plateau of the tibia and is not in the same plane as the flexion axis.

Using MRI scans Hollister also confirmed that, when viewed along the flexion axis, the posterior femoral condyles have a constant radius [20]. This work was taken further by Freeman, Eckhoff, and others [25–29], who demonstrated, using 3D imaging techniques such as MR, CT, and fluoroscopy, that the posterior section of the femoral condyles can be modelled as cylinders with coincident axes. This coincident axis is the flexion axis of the knee and does not correspond with the surgical transepicondylar axis [19].

The work of Hollister, Freeman, and others has led to the formulation of modern knee kinematic theory [1, 7, 20]. Modern theory is based around the notion that knee motion occurs in three distinct phases, as depicted by Fig. 2.4.

The "Screwhome" arc of motion describes tibiofemoral flexion/extension from full extension to approximately 20° of flexion. In full extension both the collateral and cruciate ligaments are taut [12]. During a passive extension motion, at approximately 20° of flexion, the knee appears to rock as the femoral condyles shift from the flexion to the extension facets. The medial condyle rolls up on to the tibial extension facet causing its centre to move approximately 1.2 mm posteriorly, whereas the lateral condyle rolls down the tibial anterior horn moving up to 2 mm distally as the lateral collateral ligament (LCL) relaxes. This results in posterior roll back and a net internal tibial rotation, relative to the femur, in the order of 1° axial rotation for every 2° of flexion [1, 7, 12, 30, 31].

At, and near, full extension of the tibiofemoral joint, the patella is located proximal to the trochlear groove of the femur [32]. During this phase of motion, there is little femoral geometry to constrain the patella movement. It is, therefore, restricted largely by soft tissues, namely the retinaculum and quadriceps mechanism [33].

During the active flexion arc, approximately 20–120° of flexion, the femur rotates about the flexion axis [1, 7, 20]. During passive motion, in this range of flexion, the femoral medial condyle moves very little anteriposteriorly, whereas the lateral condyle moves posteriorly. This equates to a small amount of posterior roll back, and tibial internal rotation around a medial pivot of approximately 10–20° [1, 7, 13, 30, 34–37]. There are

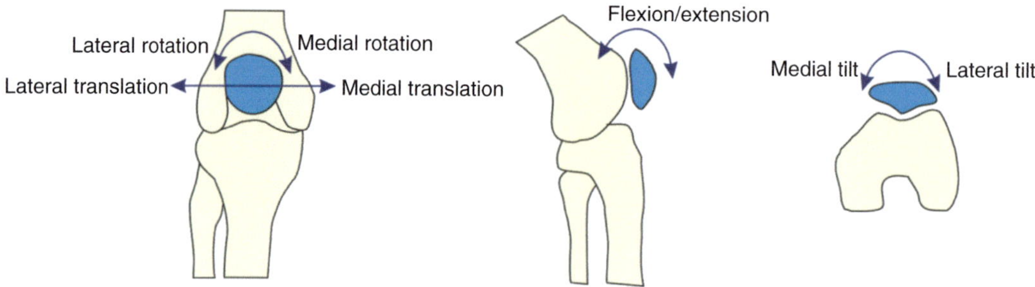

Fig. 2.5 Patella degrees of freedom

multiple theories as to the cause of this tibial rotation, which is reduced when muscle forces are present [13]. It has been suggested that tibial rotation may be a result of the lack of symmetry in the collateral ligaments; throughout flexion the medial collateral ligament (MCL) remains isometric, but the LCL slackens slightly with flexion [12, 38]. The posterior distal insertion point of the LCL also acts to force the lateral femoral condyle posteriorly and hence induce rotation [38]. Alternatively, it may be due to the difference in constraint and conformity provided by the lateral and medial menisci [1, 39].

Tibial rotation is undoubtedly necessary in deeper flexion to facilitate the femur and tibia moving in relation to each other [40]. However, its role in early flexion is less clear. Although tibial rotation is passively coupled to flexion, it can be reversed or prevented when muscle loading is applied, and may be an evolutionary hangover [7, 13, 28, 35, 40]. Posterior rollback in the natural knee is largely driven by the action of the cruciate ligaments and stabilised by the MCL [12, 41, 42].

During active flexion, the patella rotates around the femoral condyles with an axis of rotation that is parallel to the femoral flexion axis [43–47]. Patella flexion is proportional to tibiofemoral flexion but lags by approximately 30 % [48]. The patella contacts the trochlear groove at approximately 10–20° of femoral flexion [32, 33]. From this point until approximately 90° of tibiofemoral flexion, the patella runs deep within the congruent trochlear grove. Throughout this range of motion, femoral geometry forms the primary constraint to patella subluxation [33].

The patella initially translates medially and then laterally from approximately 30° of tibiofemoral flexion onwards (Fig. 2.5) [32, 43–45, 49–52]. With increased tibiofemoral flexion, the patella also rotates medially to a maximum of approximately 15° at 50° of tibiofemoral flexion [32]. This pattern is highly variable, even within the healthy population, and is greatly affected by foot orientation [43, 49, 53]. Similarly, the reported patterns of patella tilt vary widely. Many studies report a medial tilt in early tibiofemoral flexion, which becomes lateral from approximately 30° to 90° of tibiofemoral flexion [43, 49, 53]. Conversely, other studies have indicated an entirely lateral tilt, often demonstrating a medial lean in tibiofemoral deep flexion [43–45, 52, 54, 55]. The high variability in reported patella kinematics may be a result of the inherent instability in the joint, which is a result of limited bony constraints. However, the high variability may also be due to the wide range of assessment methods and the assumptions that have to be made when assessing bone kinematics [52, 53].

Tibiofemoral flexion in excess of approximately 120° is called passive flexion as the muscles have insufficient moment arms to actively move the limb. It is, therefore, only possible with additional external forces, such as body weight [1]. During the passive flexion arc of motion the tibia ceases to axially rotate and the femur as a whole begins to move posteriorly as the femoral condyles articulate with the tibial posterior horns [1]. There is some evidence that tibial rotation continues in Asian subjects [37]. During this range of motion the patella sits deeply within the intercondylar notch [56].

Knee Kinematics After Total Knee Arthroplasty

Early TKA designs aimed to facilitate load transfer at the knee via a planar hinge. Although still in use for patients with severe deformities and soft tissue insufficiencies, hinge designs have largely been replaced by total condylar designs. Total condylar implants replace both the tibial and femoral surfaces, and sometimes the patella articulating surface, with components that are not mechanically linked. Significant development has occurred in recent decades in terms of the design of the implants and the tools used to implant them [57].

The design of the femoral prosthetic component is not consistent across replacement systems [58]. Older implant systems are designed based on the traditional J curve or instantaneous centres of rotation theory of tibiofemoral kinematics. They, therefore, exhibit a range of sagittal radii in the functional range of motion and have been reported to suffer from mid-range instability as the collateral ligaments suddenly slacken when the centre of rotation changes [59, 60]. More recent designs are based on modern kinematic theory and only have one sagittal condylar radius in the functional range of motion. The centre of rotation of single radius knees is designed to coincide with the insertion points of the collateral ligaments. This maintains the natural ligament isometry in early and mid-flexion, preventing the issues of mid-range instability. Femoral component designs also vary in terms of frontal plane radii and trochlear groove design [61].

In the majority of commercially available designs, the tibial implant is split into base plate and bearing components to allow ease of manufacture, flexibility within surgery, and, if required, the ability to replace the bearing without requiring a full revision [62]. The bearing can be permanently locked to the base plate using wires or pins, in what is known as a fixed bearing configuration. Alternatively, it may be allowed to rotate and/or translate with respect to the tibial base plate. This is known as a mobile bearing [63]. Modern implant systems are supplied with a variety of bearings, which provide varying degrees of constraint to the tibiofemoral joint. The most common systems are defined as Cruciate Retaining (CR), Cruciate Sacrificing (CS) or Posterior Stabilised (PS).

Early CR designs were based on the retention of both cruciate ligaments and provided little tibial constraint. However, the retention of both cruciates added a significant amount of complexity to the procedure and prevented effective reconstruction of significant joint surface deformities. Most modern total condylar implants, therefore, require the removal of the anterior cruciate ligament (ACL) to enable placement of the prosthesis [64]. CR bearings have anterior cut outs to allow retention of the PCL, which is relied on to guide joint motion. The conformity, with respect to the femoral component, of CR bearings varies with manufacturer and model. Some designs use relatively shallow tibial plateaus and rely on the PCL to provide constraint, while others use conforming surfaces, which closely match the femoral geometry [58, 64, 65].

The retention of the PCL is thought to enhance the physiological relevance of the joint motion as it prevents anterior motion of the femur in the natural knee [12]. However, studies have indicated that the PCL may be unable to provide sufficient constraint without the ACL [66]. Some surgeons, therefore, routinely resect it. It may also be necessary to resect the PCL due to damage or degeneration. In these cases the surgeon may choose to use a CS or PS bearing. CS bearings are similar in design to CR bearings, but are all highly conforming [58], often with high anterior lips to prevent excessive anterior motion [63]. PS bearings have a cam-post system, which provides additional anterioposterior, but not mediolateral constraint, especially in deeper flexion [63]. The interaction of the post and cam guides the joint motion [65].

As Fig. 2.6 highlights, the percentage of patellae resurfaced during primary TKA procedures varies across the developed world [67–69]. Many papers and reports agree that the patellofemoral joint is one of the primary reasons for revision following TKA [70], but there is no consensus as to whether resurfacing is or is not beneficial [71]. Recent reviews and

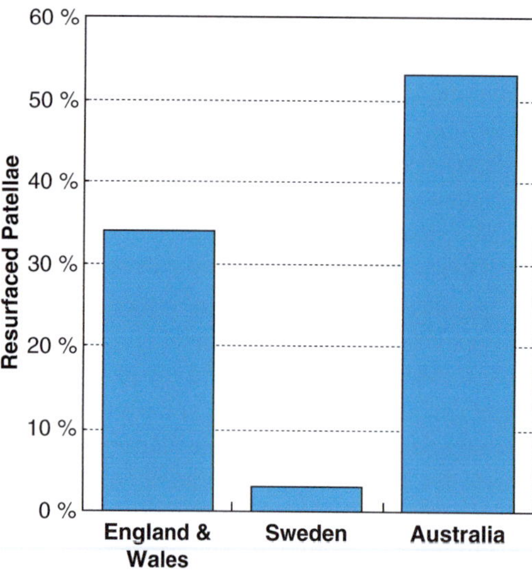

Fig. 2.6 Percentage of primary total condylar

retrospective registry studies have highlighted the increased risk of failure in non-resurfaced joints but note the lack of reliable evidence to support or explain this, and disagree as to its significance [68, 72–76].

There are a variety of patella implant designs used in modern TKA [77, 78]. The majority of implants are designed to sit on the surface of the cut bone, but some are intended to be inset into the bone. Most modern systems include a dome patella button option [79–86]. Some commonly used systems are also provided with asymmetric, medialised dome buttons [81, 84], or an anatomical, asymmetrical design [85]. Dome shaped designs are intended to be relatively forgiving to malplacement and soft tissue changes within the joint. Conversely, asymmetrical designs are intended to facilitate more anatomical and congruent tracking, and to increase the contact area within the patello-femoral joint [77].

Significant developments have taken place since early knee replacement designs were introduced in the 1970s. Despite this, as the following sub-sections will detail, in many ways modern TKA systems are not able to fully replicate natural tibiofemoral and patellofemoral kinematics.

Tibiofemoral Kinematics

Various *in vivo* and cadaveric studies have been carried out using motion analysis and fluoroscopic methods to assess the 3D kinematics of the tibiofemoral joint after TKA. There is limited evidence that some implant designs result in a reversal of the natural pattern of tibial internal rotation with knee flexion [50]. However, the majority of studies indicate that, following TKA, irrespective of design or constraint, tibial rotation is maintained, but significantly reduced [16, 34, 87–92]. In contrast, evidence suggests that tibial rotation is maintained at pre-surgery levels following uni-condylar knee replacement [91]. Uni-condylar knee replacement involves the resurfacing of only one set of femoral and tibial condylar surfaces. There is, therefore, no need to remove any soft tissue structures. The cruciate ligaments are able to continue to guide knee motion in a natural manner [12].

Reports are inconsistent with respect to how retaining the PCL after TKA affects the pattern of tibial femoral rotation [34, 50, 93]. However, resection of the PCL does appear to limit tibial rotation, unless the posterior constraint provided by the PCL is replaced in some way [12, 34]. The amount of tibial rotation induced by a PS system is partly dependent on the design of the post-cam mechanism and the amount of joint flexion, which is allowed before the post and cam engage [34, 87–89]. The majority of systems use a posterior cam system but recent developments have involved the addition of an anterior cam system, in an attempt to replicate the constraint provided by the ACL. Such highly constrained systems, often termed bi-cruciate systems demonstrate tibial rotational patterns approaching those of the native knee, but still do not reliably replicate natural joint mechanics [94–96]. The amount of tibial rotation, which occurs after TKA, can also be influenced by tibial bearing design. Bearing surfaces can be designed to guide the femoral rotation and hence induce rotation with or without the presence of a post-cam system [88].

Little is known about the effect of slight variations in the design of the femoral component on tibial rotation, but the addition of relative motion

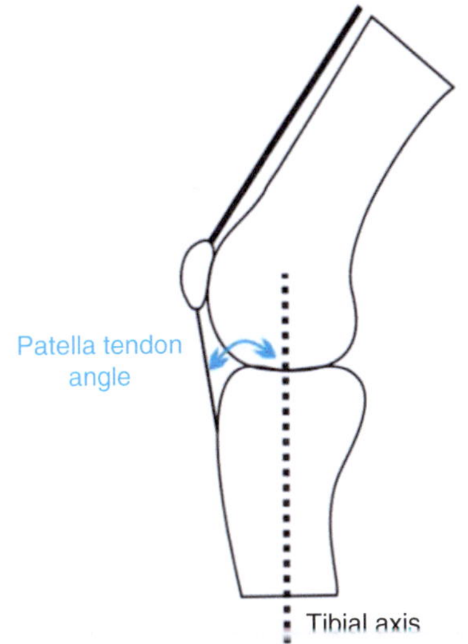

Fig. 2.7 Patella tendon angle

between the tibial base plate and bearing does not appear to affect tibial rotation [16]. It has been shown that, after TKA, the axis of tibial longitudinal rotation is more varied and more central than in the natural knee, especially with CR bearings [88, 93, 97]. The use of an anterior cam mechanism may improve this [95], as may the use of a medial pivot design instead of a post-cam system. In a medial pivot design, the tibial bearing geometry provides significantly greater constraint to the medial rather than lateral compartment [96].

In vivo and cadaveric studies of overall joint kinematics have also demonstrated that TKA affects the amount of femoral roll back experienced during flexion. In the most part, modern PS systems appear to fulfil their design aims and reliably induce femoral posterior roll back [88, 90], as do medial pivot designs [96]. However, the use of mobile bearings or CR systems has been demonstrated to result in consistent anterior femoral motion [16, 45, 50, 93]. This is likely because resection of the ACL, and in some cases the PCL, has altered the anterioposterior stability of the joint [12].

The anterioposterior position of the femur can also be inferred from the patella tendon angle (Fig. 2.7). A negative patella tendon angle implies a posterior position of the femur; whereas an increasingly positive angle suggests anterior movement. The patella tendon angle may also be altered by tibiofemoral rotations and patella movements and is therefore only an indicator, not a direct measure, of sagittal plane knee kinematics.

In the natural knee the patella tendon angle reduces linearly with increasing flexion as the femur rolls back. The degree to which this is replicated after TKA is highly design dependent [96, 98]. However, modern, single radius and bi-cruciate stabilised designs appear to induce more natural kinematics [96, 99, 100]. Only unicondylar replacements have been shown to reliably replicate a natural patella tendon angle throughout the range of motion [96, 101].

Patellofemoral Kinematics

In contrast to studies concentrating on the tibiofemoral joint, those investigating the patellofemoral joint use largely cadaveric methods. TKA has generally been shown to cause an increase in patella flexion [46, 51]. However, modern single radius designs may replicate more natural flexion patterns [44, 102]. Modern implant systems have also been reported to result in more superior patella positions after TKA. Other reported patella variables such as, mediolateral shift, mediolateral tilt, and rotations are inconsistent after TKA [44].

The tilt of the patella following TKA has been reported to be both more medial, and more lateral than the natural knee [44, 45, 50, 51, 103, 104]. Changes in this degree of freedom appear to be very design specific and may be less significant with PS and mobile bearing designs [102, 105, 106]. Similarly, both lateral and medial shifts of the patella after TKA, and internal and external rotational changes, have been reported using a variety of implants, with a range of constraints [50, 51, 102, 103, 105, 106].

TKA clearly affects the kinematics of the patellofemoral joint. This may suggest that implant trochlear groove geometry does not reproduce the conformity with the natural patella or a replaced patella button, which would be expected in the healthy knee. In terms of the non-resurfaced condition, this has been supported by computational measurements of trochlear groove geometries [107].

Conclusion

A multitude of contemporary and historical studies have helped to explain and describe natural knee kinematics. There are undoubtedly variations among even the healthy population, especially in terms of patella kinematics, but common patterns are clear. Modern implant designs do not replicate natural or consistent kinematics in the replaced knee. If this ultimate aim is to be achieved, greater effort needs to be concentrated on understanding precisely how modern design philosophies affect knee kinematics, as currently this is not clear. It may be necessary to return to the drawing board and reconsider how best to incorporate the modern understanding of natural knee kinematics into an artificial joint.

References

1. Freeman MA, Pinskerova V. The movement of the knee studied by mri. Clin Orthop Relat Res. 2003;410:35–43.
2. Frankel VH, Burstein AH, Brooks DB. Biomechanics of internal derangement of the knee pathomechanics as determined by analysis of the instant centers of motion. J Bone Joint Surg. 1971;53(5):945–77.
3. Goodfellow J, O'Connor J. The mechanics of the knee and prosthesis design. J Bone Joint Surg Br Vol. 1978;60-B(3):358–69.
4. Kurosawa H, Walker PS, Abe S, Garg A, Hunter T. Geometry and motion of the knee for implant and orthotic design. J Biomech. 1985;18(7): 487–99.
5. Lovejoy CO. Evolution of human walking. Sci Am. 1988;259(5):118–25.
6. Palastanga N, Field D, Soames R. Anatomy & human movement. 4th ed. Oxford: Butterworth-Heinemann; 2002.
7. Freeman MR, Pinskerova V. The movement of the normal tibio-femoral joint. J Biomech. 2005;38(2):197–208.
8. Pinskerova V, Maquet P, Freeman M. Writings on the knee between 1836 and 1917. J Bone Joint Surg Br Vol. 2000;82-B(8):1100–2.
9. Weber W, Weber E (trans: Maquet P, Furlong R). Mechanics of the human walking apparatus. Berlin: Springer; 1992.
10. Chun YM, Kim SJ, Kim HS. Evaluation of the mechanical properties of posterolateral structures and supporting posterolateral instability of the knee. J Orthop Res. 2008;26(10):1371–6.
11. Pasque C, Noyes FR, Gibbons M, Levy M, Grood E. The role of the popliteofibular ligament and the tendon of popliteus in providing stability in the human knee. J Bone Joint Surg. 2003;85(2):292–8.
12. Brantigan OC, Voshell AF. The mechanics of the ligaments and menisci of the knee joint. J Bone Joint Surg. 1941;23(1):44–66.
13. Hill PF. Tibialfemoral movement 2: the loaded and unloaded living knee studied by mri. J Bone Joint Surg. 2000;82:1196.
14. Victor J, Labey L, Wong P, Innocenti B, Bellemans J. The influence of muscle load on tibiofemoral knee kinematics. J Orthop Res. 2010;28(4):419–28.
15. Gill H, Biden E, Cooke P, O'connor J. Gait analysis. In: Pysent PB, Carr AJ, Fairbank J, editors. Gait analysis. Edinburgh/New York: Butterworth-Heinemann; 1997.
16. Wolterbeek N, Garling EH, Mertens BJ, Nelissen RGHH, Valstar ER. Kinematics and early migration in single-radius mobile- and fixed-bearing total knee prostheses. Clin Biomech. 2012;27(4):398–402.
17. Cappozzo A, Della Croce U, Leardini A, Chiari L. Human movement analysis using stereophotogrammetry. Part 1: theoretical background. Gait Posture. 2005;21(2):186–96.
18. Woltring HJ. Representation and calculation of 3-d joint movement. Hum Mov Sci. 1991;10(5):603–16.
19. Eckhoff D, Hogan C, Dimatteo L, Robinson M, Bach J. ABJS best papers. Clin Orthop Relat Res. 2007;261:238–44.
20. Hollister AM, Jatana S, Singh AK, Sullivan WW, Lupichuk AG. The axes of rotation of the knee. Clin Orthop Relat Res. 1993;290:259–68.
21. Churchill DJ, Incavo SJ, Johnson CC, Beynnon BD. The transepicondylar axis approximates the optimal flexion axis of the knee. Clin Orthop Relat Res. 1998;356:111–8.
22. Soudan K, Van Audekercke R, Martens M. Methods, difficulties and inaccuracies in the study of human joint kinematics and pathokinematics by the instant axis concept. Example: the knee joint. J Biomech. 1979;12(1):27–33.
23. Smidt GL. Biomechanical analysis of knee flexion and extension. J Biomech. 1973;6(1):79–92.
24. Elias SG, Freeman MA, Gokcay EI. A correlative study of the geometry and anatomy of the distal femur. Clin Orthop Relat Res. 1990;260:98.
25. Eckhoff DG, Bach JM, Spitzer VM, Reinig KD, Baqur MM, Baldini TH, Flannery NM. Three-dimensional mechanics, kinematics, and morphology of the knee viewed in virtual reality. J Bone Joint Surg Am. 2005;87(Supplement 2):71–80.
26. Eckhoff DG, Dwyer TF, Bach JM, Spitzer VM, Reinig KD. 3D morphology of the distal part of the femur viewed in virtual reality. J Bone Joint Surg. 2001;83(S2P1):43–5.
27. Eckhoff DG, Dwyer TF, Bach JM, Spitzer VM, Reining KD. 3D morphology and kinematics of the distal part of the femur viewed in virtual reality part 2. J Bone Joint Surg. 2003;85:97–104.
28. Iwaki H, Piskerova V, Freeman MA. Tibiofemoral movement 1: the shapes and relative movements of

the femur and tibia in the unloaded cadaver knee. J Bone Joint Surg. 2000;82:1189–95.

29. Asano T, Akagi M, Tanaka K, Tamura J, Nakamura T. In vivo 3D knee kinematics using a biplanar imaging technique. Clin Orthop Relat Res. 2001;388:157–66.

30. Komistek RD. In vivo fluroscopic analysis of the normal human knee. Clin Orthop Relat Res. 2003; 410:69–81.

31. Leszko F, Hovinga KR, Lerner AL, Komistek RD, Mahfouz MR. In vivo normal knee kinematics: is ethnicity or gender an influencing factor? Clin Orthop Relat Res. 2010;469(1):95–106.

32. Schindler OS, Scott WN. Basic kinematics and biomechanics of the patello-femoral joint. Acta Orthop Belg. 2011;77:421–31.

33. Barink M, Meijerink H, Verdonschot N, Kampen A, Waal Malefijt M. Asymmetrical total knee arthroplasty does not improve patella tracking: a study without patella resurfacing. Knee Surg Sports Traumatol Arthrosc. 2006;15(2):184–91.

34. Komistek RD, Mahfouz MR, Bertin KC, Rosenberg A, Kennedy W. In vivo determination of total knee arthroplasty kinematics. J Arthroplast. 2008;23(1):41–50.

35. Karrholm J, Brandsson S, Freeman MA. Tibialfemoral movement 4: changes of axial tibial rotation caused by forced rotation at the weight bearing knee studied by RSA. J Bone Joint Surg. 2000; 82:1201–3.

36. Massin P, Boyer P, Hajage D, Kilian P, Tubach F. Intra-operative navigation of knee kinematics and the influence of osteoarthritis. Knee. 2011;18(4):259–64.

37. Nakagawa S, Kadoya Y, Todo S, Kobayashi A, Sakamoto H, Freeman MA, Yamano Y. Tibiofemoral movement 3: full flexion in the living knee studied by mri. J Bone Joint Surg. 2000;82:1199–2000.

38. Victor J, Wong P, Witvrouw E, Sloten JV, Bellemans J. How isometric are the medial patellofemoral, superficial medial collateral, and lateral collateral ligaments of the knee? Am J Sports Med. 2009; 37(10):2028–36.

39. Wyss U, Kim IY, Cooke D, Amiri S. Mechanics of the passive knee joint. Part 2: interaction between the ligaments and the articular surfaces in guiding the joint motion. Proc IMechE Part H J Eng Med. 2007;221(8):821–32.

40. Wilson DR, Feikes JD, Zavatsky AB, O'connor JJ. The components of passive knee movement are coupled to flexion angle. J Biomech. 2000;33(4):465–73.

41. Heller MO, Konig C, Graichen H, Hinterwimmer S, Ehrig RM, Duda GN, Taylor WR. A new model to predict in vivo human knee kinematics under physiological-like muscle activation. J Biomech. 2007;40 Suppl 1:S45–53.

42. Robinson JR, Bull AMJ, Thomas RRD, Amis AA. The role of the medial collateral ligament and posteromedial capsule in controlling knee laxity. Am J Sports Med. 2006;34(11):1815–23.

43. Belvedere C, Leardini A, Ensini A, Bianchi L, Catani F, Giannini S. Three-dimensional patellar motion at the natural knee during passive flexion/extension. An in vitro study. J Orthop Res. 2009; 27(11):1426–31.

44. Belvedere C, Catani F, Ensini A, Moctezuma De La Barrera JL, Leardini A. Patellar tracking during total knee arthroplasty: an in vitro feasibility study. Knee Surg Sports Traumatol Arthrosc. 2007;15(8): 985–93.

45. Von Eisenhart-Rothe R, Vogl T, Englmeier KH, Graichen H. A new in vivo technique for determination of femoro-tibial and femoro-patellar 3D kinematics in total knee arthroplasty. J Biomech. 2007; 40(14):3079–88.

46. Stiehl J. Kinematics of the patellofemoral joint in total knee arthroplasty. J Arthroplast. 2001;16(6): 706–14.

47. Iranpour F, Merican AM, Baena FRY, Cobb JP, Amis AA. Patellofemoral joint kinematics: the circular path of the patella around the trochlear axis. J Orthop Res. 2010;28(5):589–94.

48. Amis AA, Senavongse W, Bull AMJ. Patellofemoral kinematics during knee flexion-extension: an in vitro study. J Orthop Res. 2006;24(12):2201–11.

49. Katchburian MV, Bull A, Shih YF, Heatley FW, Amis A. Measurement of patella tracking: assessment and analysis of the literature. Clin Orthop Relat Res. 2003;412:241–59.

50. Merican AM, Ghosh KM, Iranpour F, Deehan DJ, Amis AA. The effect of femoral component rotation on the kinematics of the tibiofemoral and patellofemoral joints after total knee arthroplasty. Knee Surg Sports Traumatol Arthrosc. 2011;19(9): 1479–87.

51. Hsu HC, Luo ZP, Rand JA, An KN. Influence of patellar thickness on patellar tracking and patellofemoral contact characteristics after total knee arthroplasty. J Arthroplast. 1996;11(1):69–80.

52. Sheehan FT, Zajac FE, Drace JE. In vivo tracking of the human patella using cine phase contrast magnetic resonance imaging. J Biomech Eng. 1999; 121(6):650–6.

53. Suzuki T, Hosseini A, Li JS, Gill TJT, Li G. In vivo patellar tracking and patellofemoral cartilage contacts during dynamic stair ascending. J Biomech. 2012;45(14):2432–7.

54. Heinert G, Kendoff D, Preiss S, Gehrke T, Sussmann P. Patellofemoral kinematics in mobile-bearing and fixed-bearing posterior stabilised total knee replacements: a cadaveric study. Knee Surg Sports Traumatol Arthrosc. 2010;19(6):967–72.

55. Baldwin MA, Clary C, Maletsky LP, Rullkoetter PJ. Verification of predicted specimen-specific natural and implanted patellofemoral kinematics during simulated deep knee bend. J Biomech. 2009;42(14): 2341–8.

56. Stiehl JB. A clinical overview patellofemoral joint and application to total knee arthroplasty. J Biomech. 2005;38:209–14.

57. Ranawat CS. History of total knee replacement. J South Orthop Assoc. 2002;11(4):218–26.

58. Callaghan JJ, Rosenberg AG, Rubash HE, Simonian PT, Wickiewicz TL. The adult knee. Philadelphia: Lippincott Williams & Wilkins; 2003.

59. Ostermeier S, Stukenborg-Colsman C. Quadriceps force after TKA with femoral single radius. Acta Orthop. 2011;82(3):339–43.

60. Ward TR, Pandit H, Hollinghurst D, Moolgavkar P, Zavatsky AB, Gill HS, Thomas NP, Murray DW. Improved quadriceps mechanical advantage in single radius tkrs is not due to increased patella tendon moment arm. The Knee. 2012;19(5):564–70.

61. Fitzpatrick CK, Rullkoetter PJ. Influence of patellofemoral articular geometry and materials on mechanics of the unresurfaced patella. J Biomech. 2012;45(11):1909–15.

62. Robinson RP. The early innovators of today's resurfacing condylar knees. J Arthroplast. 2005;20(1 S1): 2–26.

63. Mow V. Basic orthopaedic biomechanics and mechano-biology. 3rd ed. Philadelphia: Lippincott Williams & Wilkins; 2005.

64. Sathasivam S, Walker PS. Design forms of total knee replacement. Proc IMechE Part H J Eng Med. 2000;214(1):101–19.

65. Morrey B. Total joint arthroplasty. 3rd ed. Philadelphia: Churchill-Livingstone; 2003.

66. Shelburne KB, Pandy MG, Torry MR. Comparison of shear forces and ligament loading in the healthy and ACL-deficient knee during gait. J Biomech. 2004;37(3):313–9.

67. National Joint Registry, 2012. 9th annual report.

68. Swedish Joint Registry, 2011. Annual report 2011. Registry, S. N. J.

69. Australian Joint Regestry, 2012. 2012 annual report.

70. Sharkey PF, Hozack W, Rothman RH, Shastri S, Jacoby SM. Why are total knee arthroplasties failing today? Clin Orthop Relat Res. 2002;404:7–13.

71. Breeman S, Campbell M, Dakin H, Fiddian N, Fitzpatrick R, Grant A, Gray A, Johnston L, Maclennan G, Morris R, Murray D. Patellar resurfacing in total knee replacement: five-year clinical and economic results of a large randomized controlled trial. J Bone Joint Surg Am. 2011;93(16): 1473–81.

72. Lygre SHL, Espehaug B, Havelin LI, Vollset SE, Furnes O. Failure of total knee arthroplasty with or without patella resurfacing. Acta Orthop. 2011;82(3): 282–92.

73. Clements WJ, Miller L, Whitehouse SL, Graves SE, Ryan P, Crawford RW. Early outcomes of patella resurfacing in total knee arthroplasty. Acta Orthop. 2010;81(1):108–13.

74. Calvisi V, Camillieri G, Lupparelli S. Resurfacing versus nonresurfacing the patella in total knee arthroplasty: a critical appraisal of the available evidence. Arch Orthop Trauma Surg. 2009;129(9):1261–70.

75. Pavlou G, Meyer C, Leonidou A, As-Sultany M, West R, Tsiridis E. Patellar resurfacing in total knee arthroplasty: does design matter? J Bone Joint Surg. 2011;93(14):1301.

76. Forster MC. Patellar resurfacing in total knee arthroplasty for osteoarthritis: a systematic review. Knee. 2004;11:427–30.

77. Schindler OS. Basic kinematics and biomechanics of the patellofemoral joint part 2: the patella in total knee arthroplasty. Acta Orthop Belg. 2012;78: 11–29.

78. Brick GW, Scott RD. The patellofemoral component of total knee arthroplasty. Clin Orthop Relat Res. 1988;231:163–78.

79. Sigma cr 150 fixed reference surgical technique with high performance instruments [online]. DePuy. Available from: http://www.depuy.com/sites/default/ files/products/files/Sigma%20CR150%20 Final%20ST.pdf. Accessed 25 July 2013.

80. Nexgen legacy ® knee lps – flex [online]. Zimmer. Available from: http://www.zimmer.co.uk/content/ pdf/en-US/NexGen_LPS_Flex-Fixed_Brochure_ (97-5964-101).pdf. Accessed 25 July 2013.

81. Triathlon knee system surgical protocol. Montreux; 2006

82. Agc premier instrumentation cr or ps surgical technique [online]. Biomet. Available from: http:// www.biomet.co.uk/userfiles/files/Knees/AGC/ FLK214%20AGC%20Premier%20ST.pdf. Accessed 25 July 2013.

83. Vanguard instrumentation options [online]. Biomet. Available from: http://www.biomet.co.uk/resource/1848/ System%20Summary.pdf. Accessed 25 July 2013.

84. Scorpio NRG CR & PS surgical protocol. Montreux; 2009,

85. Lcs® rps flexion product rationale [online]. DePuy. Available from: http://www.depuy.com/sites/default/ files/products/files/9075-16-000-v1-LCS-RPS-PR_ EN.pdf. Accessed 25 July 2013.

86. Knee arthroplasty [online]. B Braun. Available from: http://www.bbraun.com/cps/rde/xchg/bbraun-com/ hs.xsl/knee-arthroplasty.html. Accessed 25 July 2013.

87. Mahoney OM, Kinsey TL, Banks AZ, Banks SA. Rotational kinematics of a modern fixed-bearing posterior stabilized total knee arthroplasty. J Arthroplast. 2009;24(4):641–5.

88. Catani F, Belvedere C, Ensini A, Feliciangeli A, Giannini S, Leardini A. In-vivo knee kinematics in rotationally unconstrained total knee arthroplasty. J Orthop Res. 2011;29(10):1484–90.

89. Klein GR, Parvizi J, Rapuri VR, Austin MS, Hozack WJ. The effect of tibial polyethylene insert design on range of motion – evaluation of in vivo knee kinematics by a computerized navigation system during total knee arthroplasty. J Arthroplast. 2004;19(8): 986–91.

90. Browne C, Hermida J, Bergula A, Colwelljr C, Dlima D. Patellofemoral forces after total knee arthroplasty: effect of extensor moment arm. Knee. 2005;12(2):81–8.

91. Casino D, Martelli S, Zaffagnini S, Lopomo N, Iacono F, Bignozzi S, Visani A, Marcacci M. Knee stability before and after total and unicondylar knee replacement: in vivo kinematic evaluation utilizing navigation. J Orthop Res. 2009;27(2):202–7.

92. Nagamine R, Whiteside LA, White SE, Mccarthy DS. Patella tracking after total knee arthroplasty. Clin Orthop Relat Res. 1994;304:263–71.

93. Victor J, Banks S, Bellemans J. Kinematics of posterior cruciate ligament-retaining and -substituting total knee arthroplasty: a prospective randomised outcome study. J Bone Joint Surg Br Vol. 2005;87-B(5):646–55.

94. Innocenti B, Labey L, Victor J, Wong P, Bellemans J. An in-vitro study of human knee kinematics: natural vs. replaced joint. In: Sloten J, Verdonck P, Nyssen M, Haueisen J, editors. An in-vitro study of human knee kinematics: natural vs. replaced joint. Berlin/Heidelberg: Springer; 2009.

95. Catani F, Ensini A, Belvedere C, Feliciangeli A, Benedetti MG, Leardini A, Giannini S. In vivo kinematics and kinetics of a bi-cruciate substituting total knee arthroplasty: a combined fluoroscopic and gait analysis study. J Orthop Res. 2009;27(12):1569–75.

96. Van Duren BH, Pandit H, Beard DJ, Zavatsky AB, Gallagher JA, Thomas NP, Shakespeare DT, Murray DW, Gill HS. How effective are added constraints in improving TKR kinematics? J Biomech. 2007;40 Suppl 1:S31–7.

97. Gamada K, Jayasekera N, Kashif F, Fennema P, Schmotzer H, Banks SA. Does ligament balancing technique affect kinematics in rotating platform, PCL retaining knee arthroplasties? Knee Surg Sports Traumatol Arthrosc. 2008;16(2):160–6.

98. Pandit H, Duren B, Price M, Tilley S, Gill H, Thomas N, Murray D. Constraints in posterior-stabilised TKA kinematics: a comparison of two generations of an implant. Knee Surg Sports Traumatol Arthrosc. 2013;21(12):2800–9.

99. Pandit H, Ward T, Hollinghurst D, Beard DJ, Gill HS, Thomas NP, Murray DW. Influence of surface geometry and the cam-post mechanism on the kinematics of total knee replacement. J Bone Joint Surg Br Vol. 2005;87-B(7):940–5.

100. Duren BH, Pandit H, Price M, Tilley S, Gill HS, Murray DW, Thomas NP. Bicruciate substituting total knee replacement: how effective are the added kinematic constraints in vivo? Knee Surg Sports Traumatol Arthrosc. 2012;20(10):2002–10.

101. Hollinghurst D, Stoney J, Ward T, Robinson BJ, Price AJ, Gill HS, Beard DJ, Dodd C a F, Newman J, Ackroyd CE, Murray DW. Kinematics of compartmental knee replacement – in vivo comparison of four different devices. J Bone Joint Surg Br Vol. 2005;87-B(SUPP III):344.

102. Belvedere C, Ensini A, Leardini A, Dedda V, Feliciangeli A, Cenni F, Timoncini A, Barbadoro P, Giannini S. Tibio-femoral and patello-femoral joint kinematics during navigated total knee arthroplasty with patellar resurfacing. Knee Surg Sports Traumatol Arthrosc. 2014;22(8):1719–27.

103. Heinert G, Kendoff D, Preiss S, Gehrke T, Sussmann P. Patellofemoral kinematics in mobile-bearing and fixed-bearing posterior stabilised total knee replacements: a cadaveric study. Knee Surg Sports Traumatol Arthrosc. 2011;19(6):967–72

104. Tanzer M, Mclean CA, Laxer E, Casey J, Ahmed AM. Effect of femoral component designs on the contact and tracking characteristics of the unresurfaced patella in total knee arthroplasty. Can J Surg. 2001;44(2):127–33.

105. Armstrong AD, Brien HJC, Dunning CE, King GJW, Johnson JA, Chess DG. Patellar position after total knee arthroplasty. J Arthroplast. 2003;18(4):458–65.

106. Sawaguchi N, Majima T, Ishigaki T, Mori N, Terashima T, Minami A. Mobile-bearing total knee arthroplasty improves patellar tracking and patello-femoral contact stress in vivo measurements in the same patients. J Arthroplast. 2010;25(6):920–5.

107. Varadarajan KM, Rubash HE, Li G. Are current total knee arthroplasty implants designed to restore normal trochlear groove anatomy? J Arthroplast. 2011;26(2):274–81.

Long Term Survival of Total Knee Arthroplasty. Lessons Learned from the Clinical Outcome of Old Designs

Konstantinos Makridis and Theofilos Karachalios

Introduction

Total knee arthroplasty (TKA) is one of the most innovative surgical interventions, replacing the weight bearing surfaces of the knee joint in order relieve pain and improve function. It is commonly performed in people with advanced osteoarthritis and also for other knee diseases such as rheumatoid, psoriatic and post-traumatic arthritis. Restoration of limb alignment and joint kinematics are crucial, since TKA malalingment has been implicated in long term complications, including stiffness, patellofemoral instability, accelerated polyethylene wear and implant loosening. Thus, following the basic principles of TKA surgery and understanding the technical aspects inherent in the specific instruments used are of great importance in the pursuit of a satisfactory outcome [1]. Developments in surgical expertise and technology have provided orthopedic surgeons with a plethora of options during surgery. Materials of advanced quality, high versatility of the instrumentation and an increasingly detailed understanding of knee biomechanics have established TKA as one of the most successful orthopaedic procedures [2]. Additionally, the advent of patient specific implants, along with computer-assisted and robotic surgery has given orthopaedic surgeons the option of performing femoral and tibial cuts, enabled correction of the mechanical axis and implant insertion with high accuracy and minimum error rate [3].

Similarly, in the years preceding the rapid development of TKA, surgeons had to overcome serious technical difficulties and complications using the first generation of implants and techniques. In this chapter we provide an overview of early clinical outcomes, complications and lessons learned from the use of the first generation of TKAs.

First Generation (Polycentric and Geometric) TKAs

The modern era of TKAs started at the end of 1960s and at the beginning of 1970s. The main concepts and proposed techniques included minimal bone cuts (resurfacing implants), use of single piece femoral components covering both medial and lateral condyles and the use of single piece tibial components covering both tibial condyles. Bone cement (PMMA) was used for fixation.

K. Makridis, MD
Orthopaedic Department, Center of Biomedical Sciences (CERETETH), University of Thessalia, Larissa, Hellenic Republic

T. Karachalios, MD, DSc (✉)
Orthopaedic Department, Faculty of Medicine, School of Health Sciences, Center of Biomedical Sciences (CERETETH), University of Thessalia, University General Hospital of Larissa, Mezourlo region, Larissa 41110, Hellenic Republic
e-mail: kar@med.uth.gr

© Springer-Verlag London 2015
T. Karachalios (ed.), *Total Knee Arthroplasty: Long Term Outcomes*,
DOI 10.1007/978-1-4471-6660-3_3

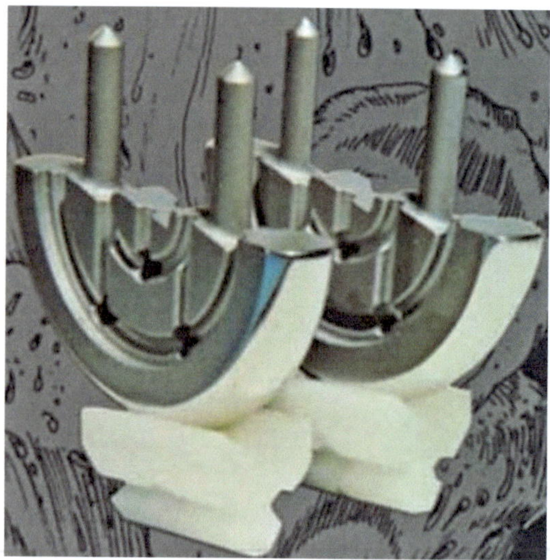

Fig. 3.1 The polycentric total knee arthroplasty is shown

Although some implants had a femoral flange, patellofemoral articulation was not necessarily a design feature and patellar implants – buttons were rare. The anametric approach was then adapted and several designers developed TKAs in which articular surfaces were replaced or resurfaced, cruciate ligaments and most of the soft tissue constraints were preserved and the implant surfaces were designed in such a manner that conflict with soft tissue constraints was avoided.

Gunston was the first to experiment on minimally constrained components [4]. His design combined the characteristics of the low friction concept and materials used in the development of the Charnley total hip arthroplasty. The relatively flat tibial component consisted of two separate high density polyethylene surfaces, while the femoral one was narrow, made of steel and had a round shape to replace the posterior portion of femoral condyles (Fig. 3.1). Both components were fixed with bone cement. It was designed to reproduce the polycentric motion of the normal knee so the condition of collateral ligaments and proper ligamentous balance were important. The cruciate ligaments were preserved in order to enhance rotational stability and absorb high stresses on both tibial inserts. Despite the initial encouraging results, this implant failed at a later

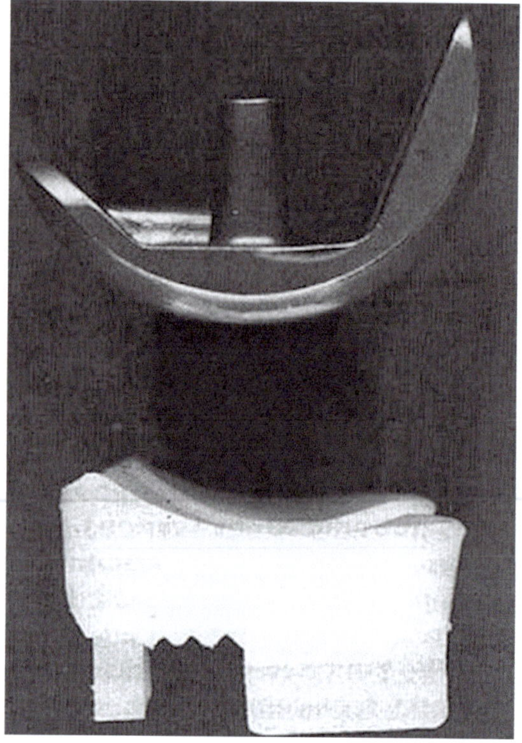

Fig. 3.2 The geometric total knee arthroplasty is shown

stage due to the small contact area, minimal amount of prosthetic material and rotational constraint.

The first metal backed tibial component with modular polyethylene inserts was designed and implanted by Nas Eftekhar at the New York Orthopaedic Hospital in 1969 [5]. It was suggested that metal backing and accurate articular geometry would permit the use of thinner polyethylene inserts. Implants were fixed with cement, but it was the use of long intramedullary stems which would secure fixation. This knee design (Eftekhar Mark I) would evolve into a condylar total knee design (Eftekhar Mark II) (Fig. 3.2). Early in the 1970s, Coventry (Mayo Clinic), Riley (Johns Hopkins), Finerman (UCLA), Turner (Harvard) and Upshaw (Corpus Christi) introduced the first geometric knee arthroplasty (Geomedic or Geometric I Knee) [6]. This design was based on Bob Averill's idea of creating a conforming device which allowed preservation of both cruciate ligaments. The fem-

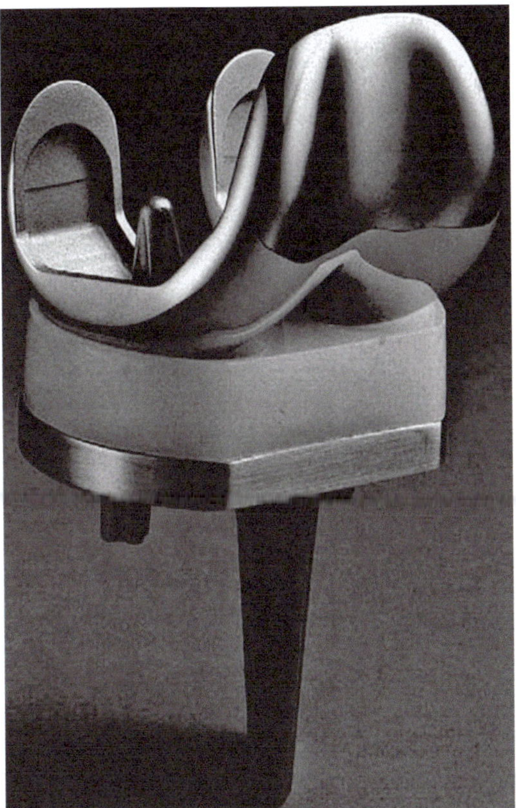

Fig. 3.3 The Eftekhar Mark II total knee arthroplasty is shown

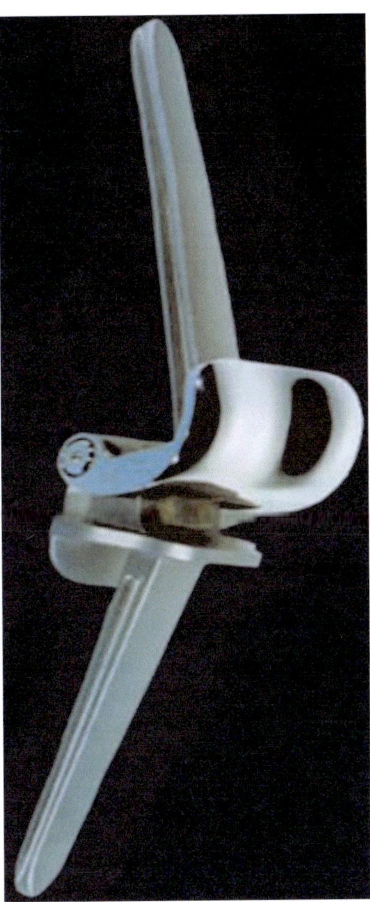

Fig. 3.4 The Guepar hinge total knee arthroplasty is shown

oral components were made of chromium and cobalt and joined together with a narrow metal bar, while the polyethylene tibial insert had three small pegs to improve fixation. The patella was not replaced and both cruciates were preserved (Fig. 3.3). It was designed in order to reduce stresses using a conforming geometry of the femoral and tibial components, but this implant also eventually failed due to rapid and excessive loosening.

The next step in the evolution of this implant was the Geometric II knee. **In** 1975, Zimmer presented two similar geometric knees. In the first, a tibial peg was added in order to improve fixation (Geotibial knee) and in the second, a femoral flange was used in order to improve patellar tracking (Geopatellar knee). Both designs had an increased sagittal radius of curvature of the tibial polyethylene liner in order to increase constraint.

Further designs emerged from these implants – the Multi-Radius, Miller Galante, Miller Galante II, and Nexgen knees. In the same year, Howmedica presented a similar but more anatomical design, the Anametric knee, which would evolve into the porous-coated anatomical knee (PCA) and eventually the Duracon knee.

During the same period, several hinged prostheses were developed, like the Sheehan prosthesis, the Attenborough prosthesis and the most popular Guepar total knee replacement (Fig. 3.4). Despite the initial enthusiasm, however, these prostheses failed because of a high rate of patellofemoral complications, breakage of the implant, early wear and loss of fixation. Nowadays, hinged and rotating hinge arthroplasties are only used in revision and tumour cases.

Outcomes of First Knee Replacements and Evidence-Based Data

The literature is relatively poor regarding the outcomes of first generation knee arthroplasties. An early publication describing a polycentric knee design Scolnick et al. [7] presented satisfactory outcomes of a unicompartmental polycentric knee arthroplasty, but follow-up was only 1 year and it is difficult to draw reliable conclusions. However, the authors supported the use of unicompartmental geometric implants and defined the indications for their use (one compartment osteoarthritis, osteoarthritis unsuitable for valgus upper tibial osteotomy, osteoarthritis after condylar fracture and necrosis and failed prior high tibia osteotomy). Similar results were presented by Jones et al. [8] (a series with unicompartmental polycentric and geometric designs). Follow up was longer (2.6 years), but again too short to be reliable. The main causes of failure in this series were loosening of the tibial implant and unexplained pain. The proposed indications for use were the same as Scolnick et al. and the authors suggest that adequate knee movement and increased levels of independence and activity could be achieved with these implants. Gunston himself presented the results of 89 polycentric knee arthroplasties with 2–7 years follow up [9]. The majority of patients had an improvement in function and mobility, but loosening rates of the prosthetic components were also high (10 %). Bryan and Petersen [10] reported a prognostic assessment of polycentric knees with a 5–7 years follow up. Outcomes were better in the patients with rheumatoid rather than degenerative arthritis and failures occurred due to infection, loosening of the tibial component, dislocation, instability and progression of patellofemoral arthritis. The authors emphasized the need for improving surgical techniques and using more durable and non constrained implants. Probably one of the biggest series with polycentric knee replacements and the longest follow-up was that published by Lewallen et al. [11]. Although the study was retrospective, important conclusions could be made regarding outcomes and complications. The failure rate in this series proved to be high (34 %), with the main causes being instability, loosening, infection and patellofemoral joint pain. According to this study, proper axial alignment was a critical factor in the reduction of complication rates.

Tietjens and Cullen [12] presented the preliminary results of the geometric TKA in 1975. Results were encouraging, but the population sample was small and the follow up short. Three years later, Riley and Hungerford [13] reported the results of 54 geometric knees with a longer follow up (24–64 months). All patients had rheumatoid arthritis and the improvement of pain symptoms and mobility was significant. Patellar pain, flexion contracture and tibial loosening were the causes of the three cases of revision. Finerman et al. [14] reported their early experience with the Geometric II knee. They called it the anametric knee because it was designed to mimic the anatomy of the normal knee. Improvements in pain symptoms and function were attributed to the addition of further sizes and tibial fixation options. An interesting comparative study by Wilson et al. [15] showed no differences in midterm outcomes and revision rates between the Walldius and geometric knee prostheses. Attention to surgical procedures and reduction of technical errors were emphasized by the authors in order to avoid complications. Lowe and McNeur [16] reported a comparative study of Geometric TKA used in two groups of patients with different diagnoses. Patients with rheumatoid and those with degenerative arthritis had similar levels of satisfaction, although more rheumatoid arthritis patients considered their results disappointing. The revision rate was 5 % and the main causes were instability or loosening. In contrast, Hunter et al. [17] supported the use of geometric designs in patients with rheumatoid arthritis demonstrating its benefits in pain relief, good function and low risk of patellofemoral problems. He also recognized that these immunocompromised patients were at risk of developing late infection. Imbert and Caltran [18] analysed the results of 63 first generation Geometric arthroplasties with a follow up of more than 5 years. They reported an increased rate of complications, mainly loosening and infection.

Coventry and Rand [19] also showed similar complication (12 %) and revision rates (20 %) with the use of this implant. All their patients had osteoarthritis and one third of them experienced implant loosening. The 10 year survival of the prosthesis was 69 % with revision or moderate to severe pain as an end point. Eftekhar [5] presented the midterm results of his knee design (4–9 years follow up) in 1983. Although one third of the patients showed evidence of a non progressive radiolucent lines around the tibial component, functional outcome was very satisfactory. Only 2 out of 112 patients had a revision for loosening and deep infection was the major complication.

Concerning the different hinged prostheses, Attenborough [20] reported satisfactory results using the design carrying his name. He classified this implant as a combination of hinged and condylar prostheses and suggested that its characteristics could provide both stability and normal gliding movements during flexion and extension. Short term outcomes showed no loosening and the author suggested the use of this implant in those cases with severe deformities. Cameron and Jung [21] used 27 Guepar II knee replacements in cases with bone loss, non union of tibial or femoral fractures and major instability. The 3 year follow up showed good to excellent results in the majority of patients and a low incidence of loosening. Its use was recommended for these specific indications [21]. Similar indications and results were recorded by Lettin et al. [22] using the Stanmore hinged TKA. The follow up was short (2 years), but again the achievement of stability and deformity correction were emphasized as important benefits of these implants. In contrast, Karpinski and Grimer [23] reported poor results when performing this procedure in revision TKA and proposed its limited use. The Seehan prosthesis produced unsatisfactory results due to design features and faults which were not able to withstand high valgus/varus forces [24]. The publication of unsatisfactory outcomes with the use of hinged prostheses continued with the prospective study of Hui and Fitzgerald [25]. Despite initial encouraging functional results, major complications occurred including sepsis,

loosening and patellar instability. Likewise, other studies reporting outcomes of the Guepar knee showed a high incidence of patellofemoral pain and subluxation, aseptic loosening, flexion contractures and instability [26, 27]. In order to oppose all these recommendations for limited use of the hinged prostheses, Blauth and Hassenpflug [28] presented the long term results of the knee implant having his name. According to the authors, the efficiency of total knee hinged prostheses should not be judged by the results obtained with the pioneer implants, because the designs and techniques were in an immature state. The Blauth prosthesis was found to be very effective with a low incidence of aseptic loosening, instability and patellofemoral problems.

Finally, it is worth mentioning four studies which have reported comparative data across different TKA designs. Insall et al. [29] presented the outcomes of unicondylar, duocondylar, Guepar and geometric implants. The unicondylar implants produced lower rate of complications, but they were used for the less complex cases and the results were not superior to other replacements. The duocondylar implant was recommended for patients with rheumatoid arthritis and mild deformity, while the geometric knee was found to be ideal for osteoarthritis with moderate to severe deformity. The Guepar prosthesis was proposed for complex cases with severe deformities and as a salvage procedure. Despite the short follow up (2–3.5 years), radiologic loosening was high and patellofemoral pain was common [29]. Cracciolo et al. [30] reported the results of a prospective study comparing polycentric and geometric TKAs with a mean follow up of 3.5 years. Pain relief, functional improvement and failure rates were similar in both groups and the authors pointed out the importance of proper choice of design characteristics of the implant. Riley [31] published comparative outcomes between geometric and anametric TKAs. Both designs provided clinically significant improvement in pain and functional activities, but 3 out of 51 geometric components required revision because of loosening. Instead, anametric implants developed radiological loosening only without any clinical manifestation. Another important observation was the development of radiolucent lines, in high rates, around metal backed tibial trays posing questions regarding their safety. The fourth comparative study was published by Thomas et al. in 1991 [32]. The polycentric designs showed higher revision rates than those of total condylar implants and the major causes of revision were loosening, instability and patellofemoral pain. The total condylar prostheses proved to be more durable and the main cause of revision was infection.

Conclusions

The reconstruction of the knee joint is by definition a very difficult and challenging task and its evolution has passed through many stages of experimentation. The results were sometimes encouraging and in some cases disappointing. However, the continuous evaluation of implants, a better understanding of knee anatomy and biomechanics, and improvements in implant design and materials have led to significant overall progress. The preliminary outcomes of the first generation knee replacements were very impressive regarding pain relief, mobility and functional improvement of the patients. Nevertheless, mid and long term evaluations have revealed a high incidence of complications, mainly aseptic loosening, instability and patellofemoral joint problems. As shown above, there is a paucity of strong evidence in the literature, since most studies were retrospective with a short term follow up. However, all the aforementioned studies and publications have enabled us to extract useful information about the design characteristics and function of the primitive implants and comprise a substantial platform for the future growth of TKA.

References

1. Luyckx T, Vanhoorebeeck F, Bellemans J. Should we aim at undercorrection when doing a total knee arthroplasty? Knee Surg Sports Traumatol Arthrosc. 2014; [Epub ahead of print].
2. Laskin RS. New techniques and concepts in total knee replacement. Clin Orthop. 2003;416:151–3.
3. Mayman D. Handheld navigation in total knee arthroplasty. Orthop Clin North Am. 2014;45:185–90.
4. Gunston FH. Polycentric knee arthroplasty. J Bone Joint Surg Br. 1971;53B:272–5.
5. Eftekhar NS. Total knee-replacement arthroplasty. Results with the intramedullary adjustable total knee prosthesis. J Bone Joint Surg Am. 1983;65A:293–309.
6. Coventry MB, Finerman GA, Riley LH, Turner RH, Upshaw JE. A new geometric knee for total knee arthroplasty. Clin Orthop. 1972;83:157–62.
7. Skolnick MD, Bryan RS, Peterson LF. Unicompartmental polycentric knee arthroplasty: description and preliminary results. Clin Orthop. 1975;112:208–14.
8. Jones WT, Bryan RS, Peterson LF, Ilstrup DM. Unicompartmental knee arthroplasty using polycentric and geometric hemicomponents. J Bone Joint Surg Am. 1981;63A:946–54.
9. Gunston FH, MacKenzie RI. Complications of polycentric knee arthroplasty. Clin Orthop. 1976;120:11–7.
10. Bryan RS, Peterson LF. Polycentric total knee arthroplasty: a prognostic assessment. Clin Orthop. 1979;145:23–8.
11. Lewallen DG, Bryan RS, Peterson LF. Polycentric total knee arthroplasty. A ten-year follow-up study. J Bone Joint Surg Am. 1984;66A:1211–8.
12. Tietjens BR, Cullen JC. Early experience with total knee replacement. N Z Med J. 1975;82(544):42–5.
13. Riley Jr LH, Hungerford DS. Geometric total knee replacement for treatment of the rheumatoid knee. J Bone Joint Surg Am. 1978;60A:523–7.
14. Finerman GA, Coventry MB, Riley LH, Turner RH, Upshaw JE. Anametric total knee arthroplasty. Clin Orthop. 1979;145:85–90.
15. Wilson FC, Fajgenbaum DM, Venters GC. Results of knee replacement with the Walldius and geometric prostheses. A comparative study. J Bone Joint Surg Am. 1980;62A:497–503.
16. Lowe GP, McNeur JC. Results of geometric arthroplasty for rheumatoid and osteoarthritis of the knee. Aust N Z J Surg. 1981;51:528–33.
17. Hunter JA, Zoma AA, Scullion JE, Protheroe K, Young AB, Sturrock RD, Capell HA. The geometric knee replacement in polyarthritis. J Bone Joint Surg Br. 1982;64B:95–8.
18. Imbert JC, Caltran M. A follow up study of "geometric" total knee arthroplasty with special reference to the improved "anametric" model. Rev Chir Orthop Reparatrice Appar Mot. 1981;67:499–508.
19. Rand JA, Coventry MB. Ten-year evaluation of geometric total knee arthroplasty. Clin Orthop. 1988;232:168–73.
20. Attenborough CG. The Attenborough total knee replacement. J Bone Joint Surg Br. 1978;60B:320–6.
21. Cameron HU, Jung YB. Hinged total knee replacement: indications and results. Can J Surg. 1990;33:53–7.
22. Lettin AW, Deliss LJ, Blackburne JS, Scales JT. The Stanmore hinged knee arthroplasty. J Bone Joint Surg Br. 1978;60B:327–32.

23. Karpinski MR, Grimer RJ. Hinged knee replacement in revision arthroplasty. Clin Orthop. 1987;220:185–91.
24. Chen SC, Helal B. Preliminary results of the Sheehan total knee prosthesis. Int Orthop. 1980;4:67–71.
25. Hui FC, Fitzgerald Jr RH. Hinged total knee arthroplasty. J Bone Joint Surg Am. 1980;62A:513–9.
26. Bargar WL, Cracchiolo A, Amstutz HC. Results with the constrained total knee prosthesis in treating severely disabled patients and patients with failed total knee replacements. J Bone Joint Surg Am. 1980;62A:504–12.
27. Mascard E, Anract P, Touchene A, Pouillart P, Tomeno B. Complications from the hinged GUEPAR prosthesis after resection of knee tumor. 102 cases. Rev Chir Orthop Reparatrice Appar Mot. 1998;84:628–37.
28. Blauth W, Hassenpflug J. Are unconstrained components essential in total knee arthroplasty? Long-term results of the Blauth knee prosthesis. Clin Orthop. 1990;258:86–94.
29. Insall JN, Ranawat CS, Aglietti P, Shine J. A comparison of four models of total knee-replacement prostheses. J Bone Joint Surg Am. 1976;58A:754–65.
30. Cracchiolo 3rd A, Benson M, Finerman GA, Horacek K, Amstutz HC. A prospective comparative clinical analysis of the first-generation knee replacements: polycentric vs. geometric knee arthroplasty. Clin Orthop. 1979;145:37–46.
31. Riley LH. Total knee arthroplasty. Clin Orthop. 1985;192:34–9.
32. Thomas BJ, Cracchiolo A, Lee YF, Chow GH, Navarro R, Dorey F. Total knee arthroplasty in rheumatoid arthritis. A comparison of the polycentric and total condylar prostheses. Clin Orthop. 1991;265:129–36.

Long Term Survival of Total Knee Arthroplasty. Lessons Learn from the Clinical Outcome of Old Designs. Second Generation of Implants and the Total Condylar TKA

4

Konstantinos Makridis and Theofilos Karachalios

Introduction

Although the knee is classified biomechanically as a hinge joint, its kinematics are more complex, involving motion in variable axes and in three separate planes. Moreover, the stability of the joint is highly dependent on the ligaments and other soft tissues around it (joint capsule, menisci, pes anserinus, iliotibial band, popliteus tendon) [1]. The performance of a satisfactory total knee arthroplasty (TKA) requires a comprehensive knowledge of both anatomy and biomechanics, correct and accurate surgical technique and the use of the appropriate implants. Implant design characteristics should promote normal knee function and minimize the risk of complications [2].

Ideal TKA components must fulfil the following requirements: (a) provide restoration of normal limb alignment; (b) preserve ligaments and soft tissues around the knee as much as possible; (c) provide appropriate ligament balance and knee stability; (d) restore normal knee kinematics, and (e) resist the forces and loads applied to the knee joint. The femoral component must replace the same amount of bone that is resected, while the patellar sulcus should be anatomically shaped with an asymmetric right and left femoral surface. It should also be convex in two planes in order to mimic natural femoral condyles and conform to the concave surfaces of the tibial component. Regarding the tibial component, it has been demonstrated that metal backing decrease polyethylene deformation and influences load transmission to the interface. The use of medullary stems can improve fixation and promote stability in the coronal, sagittal and transverse planes. In contrast, a metal backing design of the patellar component has been shown to rapidly fail because of wear and delamination. Ultra high molecular weight polyethylene is the current material in use as a bearing surface in TKA, and improved manufacturing can critically affect its longevity. Following the initial period of experimentation and clinical trials with primitive TKAs, lessons were learnt and signifi-

K. Makridis, MD
Orthopaedic Department, Center of Biomedical Sciences (CERETETH), University of Thessalia, Larissa, Hellenic Republic

T. Karachalios, MD, DSc (✉)
Orthopaedic Department, Faculty of Medicine, School of Health Sciences, Center of Biomedical Sciences (CERETETH), University of Thessalia, University General Hospital of Larissa, Mezourlo region, Larissa 41110, Hellenic Republic
e-mail: kar@med.uth.gr

© Springer-Verlag London 2015
T. Karachalios (ed.), *Total Knee Arthroplasty: Long Term Outcomes*,
DOI 10.1007/978-1-4471-6660-3_4

cant improvements were performed until the introduction of modern TKAs. The transition from the first generation replacements to the total condylar prostheses was one of the most critical steps in the history of TKA and its evolution will be presented in this chapter.

Total Condylar Knee Prostheses (Second Generation TKAs)

In the 1970s, many new and important innovations were applied to the resurfacing of both the femoral and tibial condyles. The earlier ones which established the use of polyethylene and biological bone cement in total hip replacement and first generation TKAs eventually evolved into Total Condylar TKAs. At that time, there were two well-defined trends in surgical techniques. One was the anatomical approach, in which the articular surfaces were replaced or resurfaced, both cruciate ligaments and most of the soft tissue constraints were preserved and implants were designed in order to avoid conflict with soft tissue constraints. The second was the functional approach, in which knee mechanics were simplified by resection of the condyles and the cruciate ligaments and contact surface areas were maximised in order to decrease polyethylene contact stresses. Restoration of anatomical knee geometry was not the primary purpose of this approach.

In 1970, Kodama and Yamamoto introduced the first anatomical Total Condylar knee [3]. The femoral component had a femoral flange combined with a minimally constrained single piece polyethylene tibial component with a central cut out for preservation of both cruciate ligaments. Press fit fixation was facilitated by the thin femoral capping geometry, the fins on the femoral side and the two anterior staples on the tibial component (Fig. 4.1). This design later evolved as Mark I, II, III and finally the New Yamamoto Micro Fit knee manufactured by Corin. At the same time, Waugh and Smith presented the UCI knee (Fig. 4.2) which consisted of a duplication of femoral condyles and tibial plateaus using casting techniques aiming to achieve unrestricted rotational freedom [4]. The femoral side molds were made in such a way as to attempt to reproduce the multiple radii of curvature.

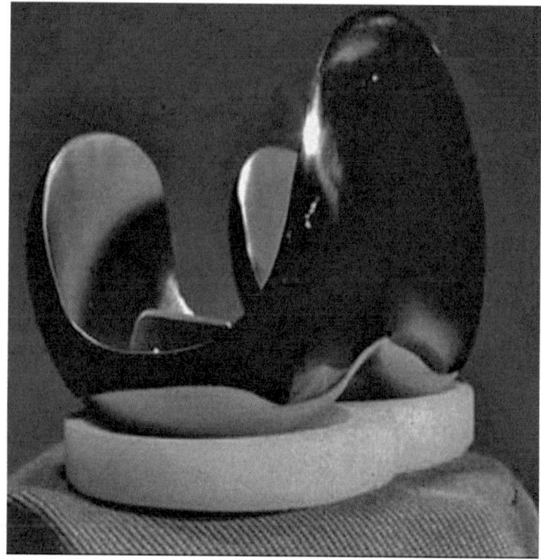

Fig. 4.1 The Kodama-Yamamoto TKA is shown

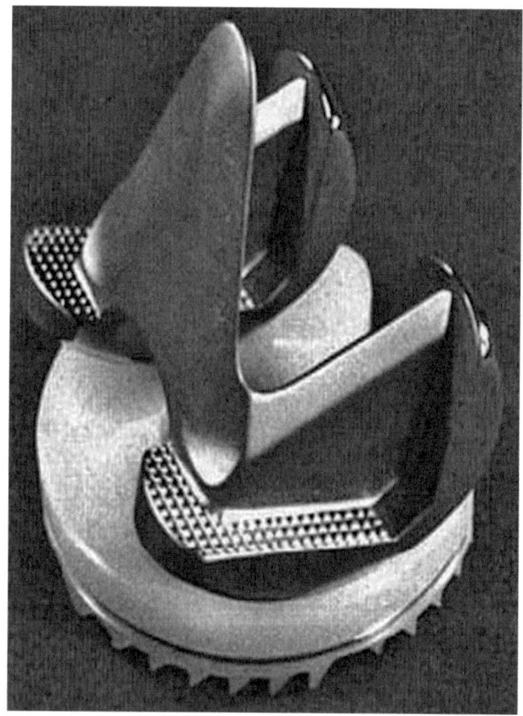

Fig. 4.2 The UCI TKA is shown

The tibial molds were sombrero shaped, which after preparation gave horse shoe shaped tibial components with central and posterior recesses in order to preserve the cruciate ligaments. The patellofemoral compartment was not a priority, so there

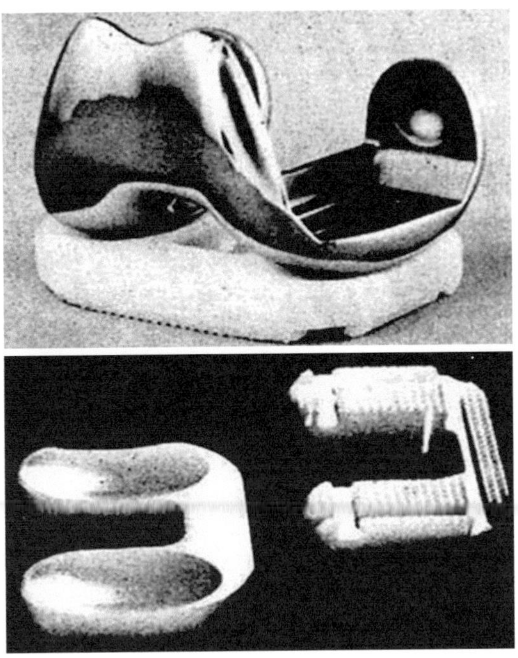

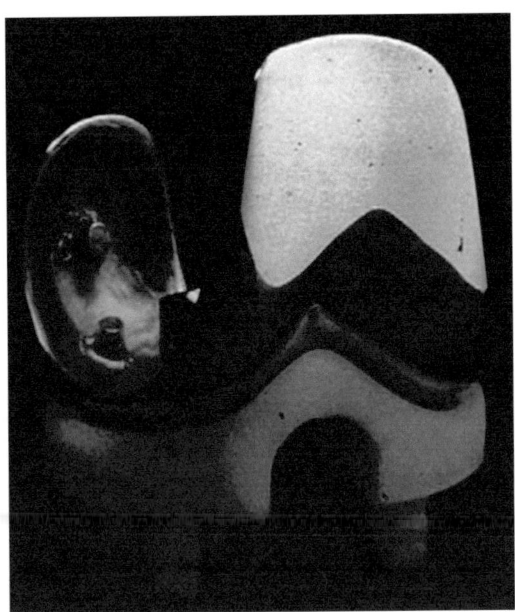

Fig. 4.4 The Leeds TKA is shown

Fig. 4.3 The anatomical TKA is shown

was no femoral flange. This implant later evolved into the Gustillo-Ram and Genesis I and II TKAs.

The Anatomical knee, designed by Townley, was the first TKA with a patellar button (Fig. 4.3). Femoral condyles and patellar flange were asymmetrical, while the largely nonconforming surfaces were designed in order to enhance movement and produce low constraint forces in an effort to decrease loosening [5]. This and the Leeds TKA were the first cemented cruciate retaining tricompartment Total Condylar TKAs. Townley tried to reproduce the normal anatomy of the knee so his design had different radii of curvatures in the frontal and sagittal planes. This design feature was expected to improve range of motion. Moreover, the retention of both cruciate ligaments was thought to promote stability and improve femoral roll back. Generally, Townley recognized and set many of the principles that are still used today in the field of TKA reconstruction. He strongly suggested the restoration of normal mechanical axis and alignment, emphasized proper implant sizing and the use of the thinnest possible polyethylene insert, supported the preservation of both cruciate ligaments to enhance stability and proprioception and noted the importance of patella resurfacing. The Anatomical knee

is now distributed by Biopro as the Total Knee Original, however several other designs have been influenced by its principles including the AGC (Biomet), Axiom (Wright), Natural (Centerpulse), PCA and Duracon (Howmedica).

The Leeds TKA was presented by Bahaa Seedhom at the same time as the Anatomic knee [6]. It had an anterior femoral flange with congruous patellar articulation throughout flexion and there was no need for patellar resurfacing. Femoral condyles were anatomical and asymmetrical and flared posteriorly in order to provide stability in the sagittal plane. Aiming to mimic the normal curvatures of the distal femur, bone surfaces were cut to create curved rather than flat surfaces. The tibial component was a single piece of polyethylene with two oval concaved discs and similar surface geometry to the femoral component allowing substantial anteroposterior and rotational laxity in flexion. An anterior bridge was formed to join the two parts of tibial insert having a recess in the middle to allow for preservation of the cruciate ligaments. There were right and left femoral and tibial components, a trend that would later be adopted by many future manufacturers (Fig. 4.4). Complexities in manufacturing techniques of the femoral and tibial implants and specific marketing

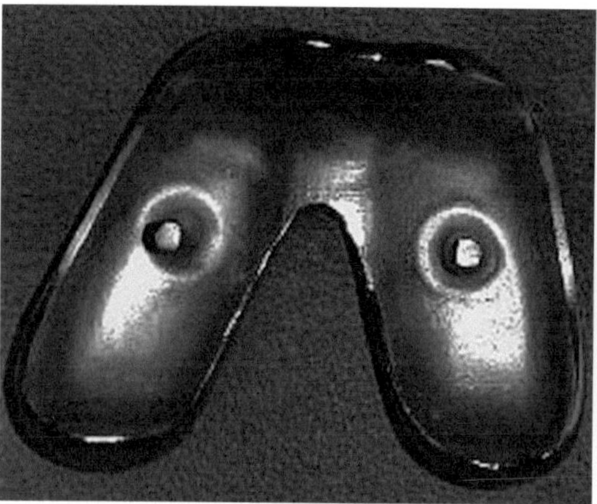
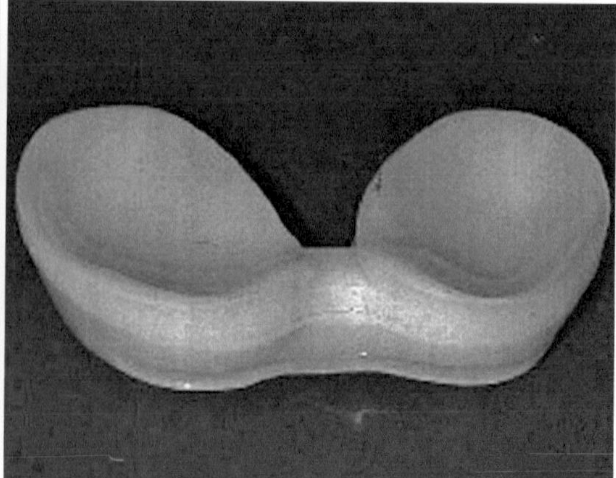

Fig. 4.5 The Ewald TKA is shown

reasons at that time made this knee design less popular among orthopaedic surgeons.

The Ewald TKA consisted of an anatomical cobalt chrome femoral cap articulated with an all polyethylene tibial component (Fig. 4.5). The bearing surfaces were highly conformed in order to increase the contact area; however, the design was highly constrained and was not so popular.

The designs introduced by the Hospital of Special Surgery (HSS) in New York proved to be very influential on the modern TKA. In 1971, Ranawat implanted the Duocondylar knee which was a symmetric, anatomical and cemented implant [7]. The linked femoral component had no anterior flange and both condyles were parallel. There were two separate tibial components providing minimal stability (Fig. 4.6). There was no provision for patellar replacement, but preservation of anterior and posterior cruciate ligaments was predicted. Although this was not a true condylar knee, significant conclusions were drawn from the experience of its use. Mainly, it was considered that resurfacing of the patellofemoral joint should be beneficial, preservation of both cruciate ligaments could probably interfere with the correction of deformities and fixation with cement might be insecure beneath the two separate tibial components. All these features would be taken into account and applied to the design of the next HSS implant, the Duopatella knee. Anatomical design and symmetry were preserved, but an anterior femoral flange was

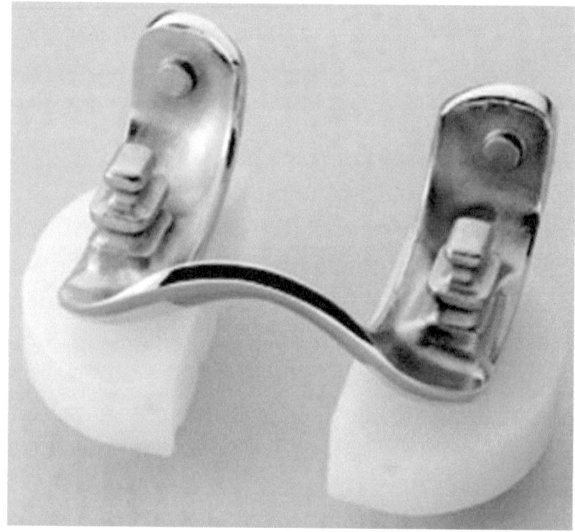

Fig. 4.6 The duocondylar TKA is shown

added in order to solve the problems of the Duocondylar knee. Moreover, a single tibial insert was used with a posterior cut out for preservation of the PCL. The anterior cruciate ligament was planned to be sacrificed. This implant was used in the treatment of patients with polyarticular rheumatoid arthritis with the expectation that the preservation of the PCL would enhance knee flexion. A few years later, the medial tip of the femoral trochlear flange was removed, creating right and left designs based on the asymmetry of the proximal femoral flange in order to reduce the medial overhang in small size knees. The Duopatella implant would evolve into the PFC

Modular and PFC Sigma knee design (Depuy) as well as the Kinematic, Kinematic II, Kinemax and Kinemax Plus systems (Howmedica). At the beginning of 1979, Howmedica presented the PCA knee, which was anatomical with asymmetric medial and lateral femoral condyles similar to the Leeds and the original Townley implants. Its most important feature was the introduction of the porous coating concept. The femoral, tibial and patellar side were metal backed and sintered with 1.5 mm thick cobalt chrome beads.

The first representative of the functional approach concept was introduced during the mid 1960s, the Freeman – Swanson TKA [8]. In order to address the problem of high contact stresses, polyethylene wear and deformities, several suggestions were made. Both cruciate ligaments were resected in order to simplify the kinematics of the knee, reduce femoral rollback and permit a "roller-in-trough" design. Femoral cuts were made to be flat in order to preserve bone and no attempt was made to reproduce knee joint anatomy. A femoral component with a single radius of curvature was designed in order to articulate with a tibial implant of an identical radius, thus enlarging the contact areas considerably. The femoral component had a short stem, placed anteriorly, to fit into the hole left by the intramedullary guide used for alignment, while the tibial part had no stem but a dovetail to promote fixation with the bone (Fig. 4.7). There was only one implant size. Freeman's contribution and innovative ideas were substantial. He emphasized the importance of creating and using specific instruments for proper implant alignment, introduced the use of spacers to check gaps remaining after the bone cuts and he recommended the use of tensor devices for ligament balancing. The first Freeman-Swanson design did not have a real anterior femoral flange and patella tracking was partly based on the femoral component and partly on the native joint. Later on, a long, flat patellar flange was added and the implant was renamed as the Imperial College London Hospital knee (ICLH) (Protek and Howmedica) and later as the Freeman-Samuelson knee.

The first truly satisfactory, widely used and functional cruciate sacrificing implant was the

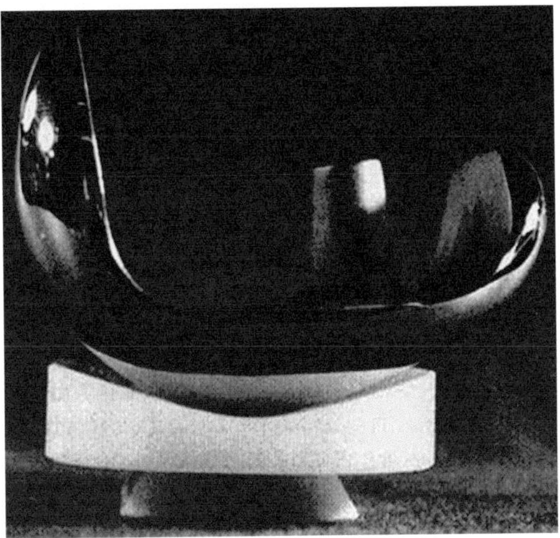

Fig. 4.7 The Freeman-Swanson TKA is shown

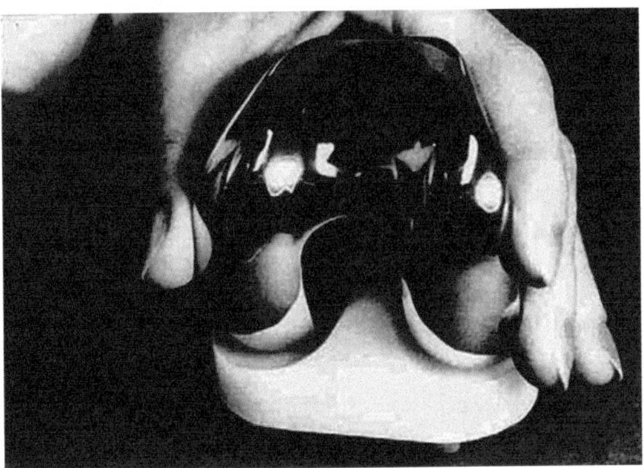

Fig. 4.8 The total condylar TKA is shown

Total Condylar TKA (TC) which was designed and introduced by Insall, Ranawat and Walker (Fig. 4.8). The TC combined the advantages of the anatomical bicondylar and the conforming surface design. The femoral component had a rounded medio-lateral geometry, while the sagittal radius mimicked the natural knee. There was an anterior femoral flange to improve patellar tracking and stability and a patellar button made of polyethylene was also provided. Bearing surfaces were of double dished shapes to provide better stability. The tibial component had a tibial peg to give additional but not primary fixation. Medio-lateral stability was enhanced by a central tibial eminence fitting a femoral intercondylar recess, while over-all knee stability was accomplished by combining joint surface geometry and soft tissue tension. The concept of flat bone cuts, creation of equal and parallel flexion and extension gaps and of careful ligament releasing was substantial. Keeping the principles of Total Condylar knee, Howmedica manufactured two cruciate retaining variants. These were the Cruciate Condylar knee, which preserved both cruciate ligaments, and the Posterior Cruciate Condylar knee, which preserved only the PCL. Some years later, Walker and Insall designed a central tibial post which engaged the femur in flexion in order to promote anteroposterior stability, ensure femoral roll back and avoid complications such as dislocations. This was the Total Condylar II design. The main problems of the Total Condylar knee were increased polyethylene wear, anterior instability and insufficient flexion. Burstein, following biomechanical studies, redesigned the implant shifting the point of contact of the joint more posteriorly and named it the Insall-Burstein Total Condylar knee. Adding a cam mechanism in order to reproduce the progressive rollback function of the PCL, posterior stabilized designs of the Hospital of Special Surgery were produced including the Insall-Burstein Modular posterior stabilized (IBPS II) (Zimmer), the Optetrak posterior stabilized (Exactech) and the Advance posterior stabilized (Wright Mcdical).

Another significant and innovative design based on the functional approach was the mobile bearing knee (bicruciate retaining and rotating platform) introduced by Buechel and Pappas in 1977. The main concept was to achieve lower polyethylene contact stresses, while maintaining knee flexion and to avoid overload of the implant bone interfaces. The femoral component had a small posterior radius of curvature in order to provide normal kinematics during flexion and reduce the risk of polyethylene extrusion. This implant was named the New Jersey Knee System and would later evolve as the Low Contact Stress (LCS) and the LCS Rotating Patellar Replacement knee (DePuy) with the application of bone ingrowth surfaces into the components. Instead of having a dome shaped patella similar to the Total Condylar knee, the design of the patellar button was thick and anatomical in shape in order

to properly fit into the femoral groove. In 1977, Polyzoides and Tsakonas presented another mobile meniscal bearing knee named the Gliding Meniscal knee (Zimmer). Similarly to LCS, articular surfaces in knee flexion were not fully congruent. This implant would later be improved and it evolved into a fully congruent rotational and gliding platform implant called the Rotaglide knee (Corin).

During the decades of 1980 and 1990, only small changes were recorded in existing prostheses. Alterations in the names of the implants did not mean significant modifications or innovations in kinematics, approach or design. Important issues for continuing research were fixation with or without cement, polyethylene wear, use of fixed or mobile bearings and patellofemoral problems.

Long Term Outcomes of Total Condylar Knee Replacements and Evidence Based Data

The evolution of TKA involved not only implant design, fixation techniques, instrumentation and surgical procedure. There was also a significant improvement in the field of research and the performance of quality studies assisting an improved understanding and evaluation of TKA outcomes.

Yamamoto [3] published his initial results in 1979 and these were encouraging. Aseptic loosening appeared not to be a major problem anymore, but interestingly the author suggested that bone cement was harmful to bone and soft tissues and they did not recommend its use [3]. Ten years later, Yamamoto et al. [9] reported the results of the uncemented Mark II TKA. At 2–7 years follow up, the majority of patients showed good to excellent outcomes with a mean flexion of 96.5°. Aseptic loosening was not the major complication, but its incidence was still high (4.4 %).

In 1976, Evanski et al. [10] reported the short term results of the UCI knee. Clinical improvement was satisfactory, but mechanical complications including instability, tibial component loosening or deformation, and patellar problems were common. Nevertheless, the authors recommended the use of this implant. In a similar study several years later, Hamilton [11] emphasized the high incidence of the above complications and discontinued the use of the implant in his practice. The modern evolution of UCI TKA (Genesis TKA) definitely showed better results. In a recent study, with a minimum of 10 years follow up, satisfactory outcome of the cruciate retaining Genesis I TKA regarding range of motion, low risk of clinical loosening and survival rate (96.7 %) was reported [12]. Moreover, a systematic review (level II) performed by Bhandari et al. [13] showed good clinical performance and survival (96.% at 12 years) of the Genesis II knee and further studies with a longer follow up are expected to confirm these results.

In 1985, Townley [14] presented the excellent mid-term results of the Anatomic TKA. Problems related to the patella and loosening of the tibial component were the predominant mechanical complications which required revision. He attributed these complications to implant malalingment, defects in the bone-cement interface and the structural strength of polyethylene.

Duocondylar TKA has generated several problems, in the short term, including knee instability, loosening of the tibial component, and symptoms related to patellofemoral joint [15]. Duopatella TKA addressed all these issues causing failures of the Duocondylar TKA and showed improved outcomes. Outcomes of Kinematic, Kinemax and PFC Sigma were even more promising. Two recent studies [16, 17] have reported outcomes of the PFC Sigma TKA at 10 and 14 years follow up respectively. Functional improvement was significant, aseptic loosening minimal, revision rates low and the 10 year survival rate 97–98 %. Furthermore, a prospective randomised controlled trial showed no statistically significant differences in functional outcome between the PFC Sigma fixed bearing and rotating platform TKA systems in the short term [18]. Concerning Kinematic and Kinemax TKAs, two interesting papers have been published [19, 20] (Fig. 4.9). The first is a biomechanical study evaluating long term PE wear characteristics during movements in the axial, frontal, sagittal and transverse planes. Although wear tracks were slightly different between the two implants, the overall wear rate was similar. The second study

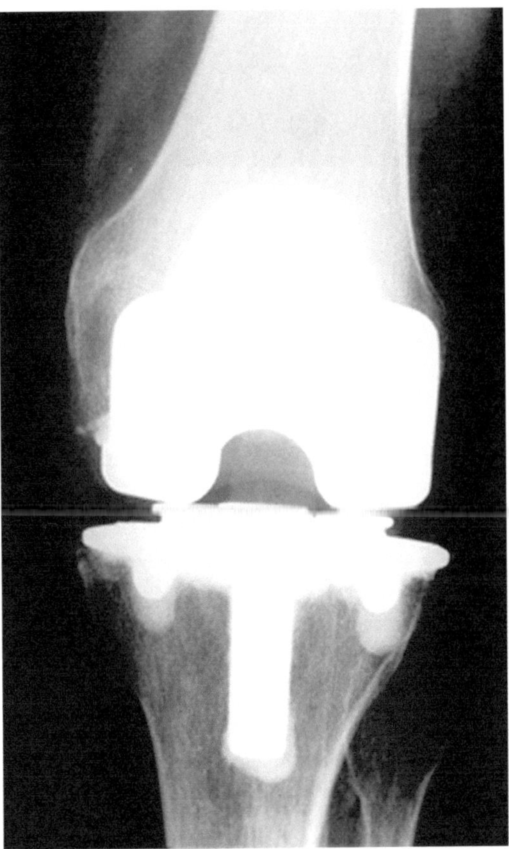

Fig. 4.9 Satisfactory radiological outcome of a Kinemax TKA at 25 years follow up (Courtesy of Th Karachalios)

analysed the 26 year survival of different implant designs. It was found that the Total Condylar, Press Fit Condylar (PFC), Kinematic, Kinemax and Anatomic Modular TKAs had similar satisfactory survival rates with revision as the end point.

Trieb et al. [21] analysed the long term clinical and radiological results of 68 consecutive PCA TKAs performed on patients with rheumatoid arthritis. At a mean follow up of 11 years, clinical results were good, although revision rates were somewhat high. This may be attributed to fatigue type polyethylene wear in this type of prosthesis as shown by Rohrbach et al. [22] in their autopsy and revision retrieval study.

Goldberg and Henderson in 1980 [23] and Herbert and Andersson in 1982 [24] reported their experience with the use of Freeman-Swanson TKA. Correction of deformity, range of motion, and restoration of function appeared to be satisfactory; however, the revision rate was high and major problems were instability, loosening and patellofemoral problems. A few years later, Freeman and Samuelson [25] presented excellent results with the use of their prosthesis. The authors recognized the problems encountered with the use of Freeman-Swanson ICLH implant and described the advantages of the Freeman-Samuelson design.

The literature is relatively rich concerning treatment outcomes of the Total Condylar TKA. Long term follow up studies evaluating the effectiveness of this implant exist. Rodriguez et al. [26] in 2001 published a 20 year follow up study and showed significant durability of the implant. The most common cause for revision was loosening of one or both components. During the same year, Pavone et al. [27] reported their series of 120 arthroplasties and showed that 23 year survival with revision as an end point was 91 %. Huang et al. [28] reported similar findings in their 20 year follow up study. The overall survival rate was 91.9 %, while survival for the all polyethylene tibial component was 96.4 % and for the metal backed tibial component was 88.4 %. Consequently, the authors recommend the use of the more cost effective and durable all polyethylene tibial implant [28].

Long term outcomes were also presented by Buechel et al. [29] concerning rotating implants. Survival rates of patients who underwent primary cementless posterior cruciate retaining meniscal bearing TKAs with an end point revision for any reason was 97.4 % at 10 years and 83 % at 16 years. Survival rates of the primary cemented rotating platform TKAs with the same end point were 97.7 % at 10 and at 20 years. Finally, survival rates of the cementless rotating platform TKA was 98.3 % at 10 years and at 18 years. The outcomes of another rotating platform design were equally good as reported by Polyzoides et al. [30]. Rotaglide TKA showed no mechanical failures, no platform bearing dislocations and satisfactory function.

Conclusions

With the evolution of TKAs, the incidence of complications has been reduced, clinical performance improved and revision rates have decreased. Manufacturing of more durable designs, better understanding of knee kinematics and improvements in surgical techniques have led to significant growth in the field of TKA. The decades of 1970 and 1980 were very productive and many innovative ideas thrived. In the following years of continuous research, many noteworthy studies were reported describing specific design characteristics, their function and their effectiveness. A defining moment in the history of TKA was the development and clinical application of the Total Condylar knee and mobile bearing knee replacements, because they set the standards for modern knee implants.

References

1. Smith PN, Refshauge KM, Scarvell JM. Development of the concepts of knee kinematics. Arch Phys Med Rehabil. 2003;84:1895–902.
2. Dennis DA, Heekin RD, Clark CR, Murphy JA, O'Dell TL, Dwyer KA. Effect of implant design on knee flexion. J Arthroplasty. 2013;28:429–38.
3. Yamamoto S. Total knee replacement with the Kodama-Yamamoto knee prosthesis. Clin Orthop. 1979;145:60–7.
4. Waugh TR, Smith RC, Orofino CF, Anzel SM. Total knee replacement: operative technic and preliminary results. Clin Orthop. 1973;94:196–201.
5. Townley CO. The classic: articular-plate replacement arthroplasty for the knee joint.1964. Clin Orthop. 2005;440:9–12.
6. Seedhom BB, Longton EB, Dowson D, Wright V. Biomechanics background in the design of a total replacement knee prosthesis. Acta Orthop Belg. 1973; 39:164–80.
7. Ranawat CS, Shine JJ. Duo-condylar total knee arthroplasty. Clin Orthop. 1973;94:185–95.
8. Freeman MA, Swanson SA, Todd RC. Total replacement of the knee using the Freeman-Swanson knee prosthesis. 1973. Clin Orthop. 2003;416:4–21.
9. Yamamoto S, Nakata S, Kondoh Y. A follow-up study of an uncemented knee replacement. The results of 312 knees using the Kodama-Yamamoto prosthesis. J Bone Joint Surg Br. 1989;71B:505–8.
10. Evanski PM, Waugh TR, Orofino CF, Anzel SH. UCI knee replacement. Clin Orthop. 1976;120:33–8.
11. Hamilton LR. UCI total knee replacement. A follow-up study. J Bone Joint Surg Am. 1982;64A:740–4.
12. Chalidis BE, Sachinis NP, Papadopoulos P, Petsatodis E, Christodoulou AG, Petsatodis G. Long-term results of posterior-cruciate-retaining Genesis I total knee arthroplasty. J Orthop Sci. 2011;16:726–31.

13. Bhandari M, Pascale W, Sprague S, Pascale V. The Genesis II in primary total knee replacement: a systematic literature review of clinical outcomes. Knee. 2012;19:8–13.
14. Townley CO. The anatomic total knee resurfacing arthroplasty. Clin Orthop. 1985;192:82–96.
15. Ranawat CS, Insall J, Shine J. Duo-condylar knee arthroplasty: hospital for special surgery design. Clin Orthop. 1976;120:76–82.
16. Arthur CH, Wood AM, Keenan AC, Clayton RA, Walmsley P, Brenkel I. Ten-year results of the Press Fit Condylar Sigma total knee replacement. Bone Joint J. 2013;95B:177–80.
17. Patil SS, Branovacki G, Martin MR, Pulido PA, Levy YD, Colwell Jr CW. 14-year median follow-up using the press-fit condylar sigma design for total knee arthroplasty. J Arthroplasty. 2013;28:1286–90.
18. Hanusch B, Lou TN, Warriner G, Hui A, Gregg P. Functional outcome of PFC Sigma fixed and rotating-platform total knee arthroplasty. A prospective randomised controlled trial. Int Orthop. 2010; 34:349–54.
19. Ash HE, Burgess IC, Unsworth A. Long-term results for Kinemax and Kinematic knee bearings on a six-station knee wear simulator. Proc Inst Mech Eng H. 2000;214:437–47.
20. Pradhan NR, Gambhir A, Porter ML. Survivorship analysis of 3234 primary knee arthroplasties implanted over a 26-year period: a study of eight different implant designs. Knee. 2006;13:7–11.
21. Trieb K, Schmid M, Stulnig T, Huber W, Wanivenhaus A. Long-term outcome of total knee replacement in patients with rheumatoid arthritis. Joint Bone Spine. 2008;75:163–6.
22. Rohrbach M, Lüem M, Ochsner PE. Patient and surgery related factors associated with fatigue type polyethylene wear on 49 PCA and DURACON retrievals at autopsy and revision. J Orthop Surg Res. 2008;3:8.
23. Goldberg VM, Henderson BT. The Freeman-Swanson ICLH total knee arthroplasty. Complications and problems. J Bone Joint Surg Am. 1980;62A: 1338–44.
24. Herberts P, Andersson GB. Freeman-Swanson arthroplasty of the knee in rheumatoid arthritis: a 2–7 years experience. Acta Orthop Scand. 1982;53:641–9.
25. Freeman MA, Samuelson KM, Levack B, de Alencar PG. Knee arthroplasty at the London Hospital. 1975–1984. Clin Orthop. 1986;205:12–20.
26. Rodriguez JA, Bhende H, Ranawat CS. Total condylar knee replacement: a 20-year follow-up study. Clin Orthop. 2001;388:10–7.
27. Pavone V, Boettner F, Fickert S, Sculco TP. Total condylar knee arthroplasty: a long-term follow-up. Clin Orthop. 2001;388:18–25.
28. Ma HM, Lu YC, Ho FY, Huang CH. Long-term results of total condylar knee arthroplasty. J Arthroplasty. 2005;20:580–4.
29. Buechel Sr FF, Buechel Jr FF, Pappas MJ, D'Alessio J. Twenty-year evaluation of meniscal bearing and rotating platform knee replacements. Clin Orthop. 2001;388:41–50.
30. Polyzoides AJ, Dendrinos GK, Tsakonas H. The Rotaglide total knee arthroplasty. Prosthesis design and early results. J Arthroplasty. 1996;11:453–9.

Elias Palaiochorlidis and Theofilos Karachalios

Introduction

Total knee arthroplasty (TKA) is one of the most successful surgical procedures excellent 15–20 year survival rates routinely reported by multiple surgeons in large series [1]. It is widely used in the treatment of severe knee osteoarthritis, inflammatory arthritis, posttraumatic arthritis, rheumatoid arthritis, gout and other general arthritic conditions [2]. It is standard procedure in current practice in modern orthopaedics.

Due to its widespread use, orthopaedic surgeons, patients, implant manufacturers, health economic providers and politicians all seek technical data related to long term outcome, complications and cost – benefit issues.

Ideally, in order to estimate TKA outcomes, a globally accepted and validated outcome measure tool, incorporating both objective and subjective recordings, should be used [3]. For decades existing evaluation scales have proved to be insufficient and non-standardized, creating confusion rather than assisting surgeons, patients and authorities to make future decisions [4]. Perhaps a combination of evaluation scales should be used and assessment should be site as well as pathology specific [5].

History

Evaluation of the quality of orthopaedic surgical treatment goes back to the beginning of the specialty. Initially, outcome measures after surgery were based on physical examination and radiological parameters [6]. Progressively, a trend to move from an objective to a subjective evaluation of results has been developed and since the 1980s outcome assessment after orthopedic surgery has focused on the patient's perspective [5]. Behind this trend is the basic observation that nearly all surgeons have treated patients whose objective outcome scores have improved as a result of treatment and who yet have remained unsatisfied [7].

The first published report on total knee arthroplasty is often attributed to Gluck in 1890 [8]. Gluck employed an implant made of ivory for the treatment of knee joints destroyed by tuberculosis. At the time, the only alternatives to this "radical" intervention were amputation, arthrodesis, inter positional arthroplasty, or supervised neglect. Faced with such severe joint disorders, Gluck's surgical interventions were initially

E. Palaiochorlidis, MD, DSc
Orthopaedic Department, Center of Biomedical Sciences (CERETETH), University of Thessalia, Larissa, Hellenic Republic

T. Karachalios, MD, DSc (⊠)
Orthopaedic Department, Faculty of Medicine, School of Health Sciences, Center of Biomedical Sciences (CERETETH), University of Thessalia, University General Hospital of Larissa, Mezourlo region, Larissa 41110, Hellenic Republic
e-mail: kar@med.uth.gr

© Springer-Verlag London 2015
T. Karachalios (ed.), *Total Knee Arthroplasty: Long Term Outcomes*,
DOI 10.1007/978-1-4471-6660-3_5

deemed successful, mostly because the alternatives to the prosthesis were so dismal. Still, Gluck later cautioned about the use of this implant due to unresolved problems with infection. This note of caution underscored the first report on TKA outcomes, and based on the Gluck's warnings inter positional arthroplasty continued as standard treatment for severely diseased knee joints. Inter positional materials included pigs' bladders, fascia lata, patellar bursae, vitallium covers, and cellophane [9]. In 1949, Speed reported on the outcome of 65 inter positional arthroplasties and graded them as good (n=29), fair (17), poor (6) and failures (13) [10]. Miller reported on 37 inter positional arthroplasties in 1952 which demonstrated worse results than Speed [11]. Eleven were reported as good, 8 as fair and 18 as failures. These primitive outcome measures were surgeon derived and did not rely on input from the patients.

In the face of such poor results and with the continued development of manufacturing, of modern anesthesia, aseptic technique and antibiotic prophylaxis, began the modern era of TKA. Shiers reported a case study of two patients using a stainless steel hinged prosthesis [9]. In one patient, heterotopic ossification limited the results, but the other was deemed to be successful. Shiers considered the operation a success because the patient was painfree, could walk with a stick, and could ascend and descend stairs.

Walldius reported encouraging results using a cobalt chromium hinged TKA [12]. Although no formal scoring systems were applied in these studies, the author did consider subjective and objective outcomes in the determination of the success of the operation. The introduction of these implants resulted in a relatively predictable outcome after TKA [13]. The net effect of the success and homogeneity of the second and third generation of implants (survival time with few design modifications) is the emerging emphasis on the quantitative documentation of subtler TKA outcomes [13].

Knee pain is the most common reason for undergoing knee surgery. Disability varies among individuals who undergo knee surgery and depends on pain and loss of function. Disability for an elite athlete may involve inability to perform at a high level of competition, on the other hand, for an elderly individual with knee osteoarthritis, disability may involve difficulties with activities of daily living or walking [14].

A number of individual characteristics are known to affect pain and function after surgery [15]. Individual risk factors which impact on patient outcomes after TKA include age and gender [16–18], antecedent diagnosis [19], body mass index [20, 21], ethnicity [22], psychological distress [23], baseline pain and functional disability [19], comorbidity profile [24], socioeconomic status [25], and severity of radiographic osteoarthritis [26]. Some of these, such as obesity and psychological distress, are potentially modifiable, making accurate and meaningful capture and interpretation of outcome data imperative for both informing those at risk and for developing strategies to mitigate the risk of poor results and dissatisfaction. The objective of treatment must also be taken in account when selecting a tool for assessing TKA. If an inappropriate tool is used to evaluate the outcome of TKA, incorrect treatment decisions can be made for future patients. It is therefore critical to use scales of clinical outcome that are important for the patients who are evaluated, while also being relevant to the surgeon.

A measure of any kind is only useful if it is reproducible (reliable) and accurate (valid). In the assessment of health status, tools must also be able to detect improvement and worsening (responsiveness or sensitivity to change). So when considering selection criteria for a scoring system reliability, validity and responsiveness are essential properties [5].

Reliability equates to the consistency (repeatability) of the system. It is not measured and can only be estimated. In other words, it is the extent to which a measurement gives results that are consistent. It is also known as reproducibility, because repeated administrations of the same questionnaire to stable patients should produce more or less the same result [27]. There are two trends in the estimation of reliability for health status tools. The first is test and retest reliability which involves having patients who are in a stable state respond to a questionnaire at two time interval points. The time period must not be too short, because individuals may remember their prior responses. The time period must also not be too prolonged, which allows for the possibility for clinical change. In general, a time period ranging from 2 days to 2 weeks is used [28].

Validity, in statistics, is the extent to which a concept, conclusion or measurement is well founded and corresponds accurately to the real world. The word "valid" is derived from the Latin validus, meaning strong. The validity of a measurement tool is considered to be the degree to which the tool measures what it claims to measure. Four types of validity are commonly examined and all are relevant to orthopaedic scoring and outcome measurement [28]. *Conclusion* validity asks if there is a relationship between the intervention and the observed outcome. Statistical conclusion validity is the degree to which conclusions about the relationship among variables based on the data are correct or reasonable. This began as questioning whether the statistical conclusion about the relationship between the variables was correct, but now there is a movement towards moving to 'reasonable' conclusions that use: quantitative, statistical, and qualitative data. Statistical conclusion validity involves ensuring the use of adequate sampling procedures, appropriate statistical tests, and reliable measurement procedures. As this type of validity is concerned solely with the relationship that is found among variables, the relationship may be a correlation only. *Internal* validity is similar but examines whether the outcome seen is causal. Internal validity is an inductive estimate of the degree to which conclusions about causal relationships can be made (e.g. cause and effect), based on the measures used, the research setting, and the overall research design. Good experimental techniques, in which the effect of an independent variable on a dependent variable is studied under highly controlled conditions, usually allow for higher degrees of internal validity than, for example, single case designs. Eight kinds of confounding variables can interfere with internal validity (i.e. with the attempt to isolate causal relationships): History, the specific events occurring between the first and second measurements in addition to the experimental variables. Maturation, processes within the participants as a function of the passage of time (not specific to particular events), e.g., growing older, hungrier, more tired, and so on. Testing, the effects of taking a test upon the scores of a second testing. Instrumentation, changes in calibration of a measurement tool or changes in the observers or scorers may produce changes in the obtained measurements. Statistical regression, operating where groups have been selected on the basis of their extreme scores. Selection, biases resulting from differential selection of respondents for the comparison groups. Experimental mortality, or differential loss of respondents from the comparison groups. Selection-maturation interaction, e.g., in multiple-group quasi-experimental designs. *External* validity looks at the ability to generalize the results of one study to other settings, a common practice in orthopaedic discussion. External validity concerns the extent to which the (internally valid) results of a study can be held to be true for other cases, for example to different people, places or times. In other words, it is about whether findings can be validly generalized. If the same research study was conducted on those other cases, would it get the same results? A major factor in this is whether the study sample (e.g. the research participants) is representative of the general population along relevant dimensions. Other factors jeopardizing external validity are: reactive or interaction effect of testing, a pretest might increase the scores on a posttest; interaction effects of selection biases and the experimental variable; reactive effects of experimental arrangements, which would preclude generalization about the effect of the experimental variable upon persons being exposed to it in non- experimental settings; multiple treatment interference, where effects of earlier treatments are not erasable, and finally, *construct* validity. This is the most commonly cited but most demanding concept to understand and refers to an ability to extrapolate study results to different settings. Construct validity refers to the extent to which operationalization of a construct (i.e., practical tests developed from a theory) do actually measure what the theory says they do. Construct validity evidence involves empirical and theoretical support for the interpretation of the construct. Such lines of evidence include statistical analyses of the internal structure of the test including the relationships between responses to different test items. They also include relationships between the test and measures of other constructs. As currently understood, construct validity is not distinct from the support for the substantive theory of the construct that the test is designed to measure. As such, experiments designed to reveal aspects of the causal role of the construct also contribute to construct validity evidence [28].

Responsiveness refers to a scoring system's ability to detect clinically important change over time. Orthopaedic surgeons generally use rating systems to improve in health related quality of life after treatment. An instrument that is not able to measure improvement in a patient who has been treated successfully would not be useful for clinical research or evaluation. Therefore, the characteristic of responsiveness is critical for the practical application of a rating scale. There are many statistical methods that are available to determine responsiveness. The standardized response mean (observed change/standard deviation of change) is most commonly used in orthopaedic research [29]. This statistic incorporates response variance, allowing statistical testing of the response means [30].

Specific and Generic Measures

Specific measures may pertain to a certain pathologic entity (disease-specific), condition (condition-specific), or anatomic location (joint-specific). The focus of these measures does not apply to specific aspects of the condition (or anatomic location), but complaints are usually attributed to the disorder (or anatomic location). For example, a joint specific tool for the knee may ask patients if they have difficulty dressing because of their knee problem. **Generic** measures have a broader perspective including emotional, social, mental, and physical health and do

not restrict attribution to a particular disorder. The advantage of generic health status instruments compared with specific instruments is that they allow comparisons across conditions and treatments. The disadvantage of these tools is that they may not be responsive to clinically important change, because change may be an isolated issue and may not be reflected in the score of this more global measure. The advantage of disease or joint specific measures is that they are generally more responsive to change in the specific phenomenon of interest, and they are more relevant to patients.

The most commonly used generic health status tool is the **Short-form 36** (SF-36). It is a 36-item questionnaire that measures general health and quality of life. It is commonly used in studies of TKA to describe the patient's overall status. A physical component scale and a mental component scale can be derived from the SF-36. It has been validated, it is used widely across medical disciplines, and can be reliably self-administered by the patient. The SF-36 has been used to define disease conditions, to determine the effect of treatment, to differentiate the effect of different treatments, and to compare orthopaedic with other medical disorders. However, a bias of lower over upper extremity function, limitations in assessment of certain physical activities of daily living and the existence of upper and lower limits on the detection of certain changes in quality of life status have been demonstrated with the SF-36. Nevertheless, with an adequate knowledge of its effectiveness and limitations, the SF-36 can be a useful tool in many sectors of orthopaedic surgery [31].

Expectations vary greatly between patients and the mismatch of experience versus expectation after TKA is a potent cause of patient dissatisfaction. Due to earlier surgical intervention, patients now expect not only pain relief, but also correction of any deformity and an early return to physical and recreational activities. Scoring systems have thus evolved to accommodate more active patients at both ends of the age spectrum.

Currently, there is no single best outcome measure for TKA [5]. There are, however, several reliable, responsive and validated systems. The

Western Ontario and McMaster University Osteoarthritis Index (WOMAC) and Oxford-12 disease specific scores are the most frequently used. The WOMAC underwent vigorous psychometric validation before its introduction and requires licensed use from the copyright holders [3]. This may be obtained free online for educational and clinical use (www.womac.org). It is ubiquitous, easy to use and evaluates three domains: pain (5 questions), stiffness (2 questions) and physical function (17 questions), each weighted on a similar computation. The WOMAC Index is sensitive to change and has shown greater efficiency than most other instruments in the assessment of osteoarthritis [32]. A seven-point reduced WOMAC scale has also been developed and retains excellent validity and repeatability in the assessment of total joint replacement [33]. The Oxford-12 knee score (OKS), published in 1998, originally examined 12 items with a possible score of 1–5 for each [34]. It assesses pain, difficulty with washing and drying self, difficulty getting into car/public transport, ability to walk long distances, pain on standing, nocturnal pain, limp, ability to kneel, giving way, ability to shop, descending stairs and interference with work. Scores range from 12 to 60, with 12 being the best outcome. Although simple, it is ranked the highest for a disease specific scale for reliability, content validity and feasibility of use. Many have found the system counter-intuitive [35]. It is now recommended that each question is scored from 0 to 4 with 4 being the best outcome. Thus, the new scoring system ranges from 0 to 48 with 48 representing the most favorable outcome. It is important that any study, which incorporates the OKS, clearly states which method has been used.

In contrast with the patient assessed and equally weighted OKS, the American Knee Society Score (AKSS) is a surgeon assessed weighted score developed through consensus by the Knee Society in 1989 [36]. It comprises two parts, the first addressing pain, stability and range of movement. The second part examines function, with particular reference to walking distance and stair climbing. Maximum scores of 100 are possible in each section. The AKSS has been validated and

is responsive and reproducible. However, it suffers from high inter- and intra-observer variation when the assessments are performed by less experienced doctors and nurses [37]. In an attempt to isolate knee function from other factors, patients are categorized into three types: A, with no contralateral knee disease; B, with substantial arthrosis; and C, with multiple joint involvement. The final knee score is designed to be independent of other factors even in the face of declining function created by comorbidities and polyarthropathy. Unfortunately, the AKSS is not sensitive in revealing problems from the patellofemoral compartment of TKA.

The Hospital for Special Surgery knee rating system was introduced by Insall in 1974. A maximum score of 100 is possible, and it contains six categories scored as follows: pain (30 points), function (22 points), range of motion (18 points), muscle strength (18 points), stability (10 points) and flexion deformity (10 points). Points are subtracted in cases of patients who use walking aids, have lack of extension, or in case of varus or valgus deformity. It has a good inter observer index of relation but poor reproducibility. It emphasizes pain, function and range of motion [38]. The New Jersey Orthopaedic Hospital Score (NJOH) was introduced in 1982. This is a specific outcome measurement scale with a maximum possible score of 100. It contains six categories scored as follows: pain (30 points), function (25 points), range of motion (15 points), muscle strength (8 points), stability (10 points) and flexion deformity (12 points) [39].

The Knee Society Radiological Evaluation System was developed for uniform reporting of radiological results of TKA so comparisons could be made not only between different institutions but also between different implants. The important aspects of satisfactory arthroplasty are featured in the system, such as component position, leg and knee alignment, and the implant-bone interface or fixation. The system is easy to use, quick to use, and covers one page. In addition to the documentation of knee alignment and component position, the system has a numerical score for the implant interface which assesses the quality of fixation. Those features that convert an

Table 5.1 Accuracy and validity of different scoring systems

Scoring system	Validity	Accuracy	Easy of use	Reference
Hospital for special surgery	Yes	Yes/No	Poor	[38]
Oxford knee score	Yes	No	Good	[48]
Sf-36	Yes		Good	[49]
WOMAC	Yes	Yes	Good	[50]
American Knee Society	Yes	No in revision	Fair	[51]
New Jersey orthopaedic hospital score	No		Poor	[39]

image into numbers will enable radiological results to be stored in a data base along with the clinical results. Up to this time, most computerized total joint registries record and store clinical results only. The main disadvantage to this system is the standardization of radiographs for the proper position, rotation, and alignment of the knee. These positioning errors can be reduced if the examiners use multiple sets of knee radiographs, select the most representative films and take measurements [40].

The Bristol Knee Score rating system was published and first used in 1970, and later modified in 1980. It emphasizes knee function, but is not widely accepted [41, 42]. Up to now it seems that WOMAC and Oxford-12 are the most reliable and valid assessments of outcome after TKA.

However, with the increasing use of segmental replacements and osteotomies, scoring systems which examine higher levels of activity are required. The High Activity Arthroplasty Score (HAAS), although not knee specific, can be used to subjectively evaluate a total joint replacement in patients who enjoy an otherwise active lifestyle. This system has been validated in patients receiving either total hip or knee replacements [43].

In the 1990s the Knee Society Clinical Rating System was put forward as a worldwide instrument for assessing the outcome of total or partial knee arthroplasty by evaluating both knee function and patients' functional abilities after TKA [44]. However, it became apparent that not enough details were provided by this scoring system and there were deficiencies and ambiguities, particularly in reporting the contemporary patient functions with TKA. Furthermore, its reliability, responsiveness and validity have been questioned [45]. The KSS was only physician-derived, with inadequate correlation between objective knee scores in physician-assessed scores and subjective, satisfaction scores in patient-derived scores [46]. There was a need to develop a satisfactory Knee Society scoring system, in terms of internal consistency and good validity, in order to meet the needs of contemporary patients who have greater expectations and functional requirements [46]. The New KSS was developed in 2011 with improved responsiveness and reliability. This scoring system integrated an objective physician-derived component with a subjective patient-derived component. Patient perspective is the priority of this system, with patient expectations, satisfaction, and activity levels being well documented via the evaluation of pain relief, functional abilities, satisfaction and expectation fulfillment [47]. In Table 5.1 accuracy and validity of different scoring systems is shown.

Patellofemoral Joint Scoring Systems

It seems that the above scoring systems are not sensitive enough to depict symptoms and problems from the patellofemoral joint of a TKA. This is also a critical disadvantage due to the fact that anterior knee pain and patellofemoral dysfunction are challenging problems after TKA [52]. To the best of our knowledge only few studies present and use specific patellofemoral rating systems [53–55]. The Feller score allocates 30 points for anterior knee pain and 10 points for each of quadriceps strength, ability to rise from a chair and stair climbing [53]. The Kujala score is a scoring questionnaire for anterior knee pain. It allocates points for limping (5), support (5), walking (5), climbing stairs (10), squatting (5), running (10), jumping (10), prolonged sitting with the knees flexed (10), pain(10), swelling (10), abnormal painful patellar movements (subluxations) (10), atrophy of the thigh (5) and flexion deficiency (5), with the maximal sum score being 100 [54]. The patella score presented by the Bristol group allocates points anterior knee pain (2), pain climbing stairs (2), patella tenderness (2), patella crepitus (2) and radiological appearance of patella instability (2) [55]. Recently, a novel outcome measure, the Samsung Medical Center (SMS) patellofemoral scoring system has been published, with emphasis on the evaluation of patellofemoral joint status [52]. It evaluates separately patellofemoral pain and function and then consider them in combination. It lacks items such as limping, swelling, atrophy of the thigh and flexion deficiency that are not specific for patellofemoral problems.

Survival Analysis

Another outcome measure that is widely used in recent literature is survival analysis of TKAs. Survival analysis is defined as a set of methods for analyzing data where the outcome variable is the time until the occurrence of an event of interest e.g. failure of the joint arthroplasty. Survival analysis techniques can be classified into non-parametric (Kaplan Meier product limit method), parametric (exponential methods) and semi-parametric method (Cox-proportional method). The survivorship rate is the percentage of TKAs which have not been revised in any given series of patients for any reason. Generally, it is considered the most often used measure in the literature. It is the most important measure when considering differences between various prosthetic designs. Lastly, it is adjuvant when answering the most difficult patient question, "How long will the knee last". Survival rate depends as well as on patient related factors (body weight, activity) as well as on implant (condylar, unicompartment, posterior cruciate retaining model, posterior stabilized etc.) and surgeon (technique) related factors.

Patient: Reported Outcome Measures (PROMS)

Patients and doctors do not always agree on what constitutes a good postoperative result [56]. For this reason the use of patient reported outcome measures (PROMS) is increasing. PROMS assess the result of TKA from the patient's point of view only [57]. They can be used to evaluate the quality of care delivered by the providers of elective procedures, benchmark their performance and assess the efficacy and cost effectiveness of different approaches and provide a baseline for peer comparison between institutions [57]. Using PROMS, clinicians could achieve best outcomes and improve standards [58]. PROMS are using outcome scores like Oxford Knee Score which has previously been proven to be a reliable, valid outcome score and it is recommended for assessment of large TKA [59]. They also collect information on the effectiveness of care delivered to NHS patients as perceived by the patients themselves. The data adds to the wealth of information available on the care delivered to NHS funded patients to complement existing information on the quality of services [60].

Conclusion

Outcome scoring is vital in the accurate evaluation of TKA. There has been a paradigm shift in the determinants of success over the last two decades, from those based on physical examination and radiographic variables (objective data) to a more patient – centred (subjective data) assessment of outcome [5]. Modern knee surgery has allowed patients' expectations and activity levels to increase but it remains difficult to accurately assess outcome. Evidence in the current literature confirms that few scoring systems have satisfactory levels of reliability and validity [5].

What is clear is that those systems which employ a high degree of patient involvement, such as the Oxford-12 score perform better as a patient-based assessment tool. The generic instruments have a greater potential to measure side-effects or unforeseen effects of treatment, and the WOMAC in particular remains a valid, reliable and responsive measure. However, it is not possible to recommend a single best knee scoring system. Indeed, the ideal of a short, easy to administer, reliable and valid global knee questionnaire does not currently exist.

References

1. Gill GS, Chan KC, Mills DM. 5- to 18-year follow-up study of cemented total knee arthroplasty for patients 55 years old or younger. J Arthroplasty. 1997;12:49–54.
2. Anderson JG, Wixson L, Tsai D, Stulberg SD, Chang RW. Functional outcome and patient satisfaction in total knee patients over the age of 75. J Arthroplasty. 1996;11:831–40.
3. Davies AP. Rating systems for total knee replacement. Knee. 2002;9:261–6.
4. Bellamy N, Goldsmith CH, Buchanan WW, Campbell J, Duku E. Prior scores availability: observations using WOMAC osteoarthritis index. Br J Rheum. 1991;30:150–1.
5. Tilley S, Thomas N. Focus on what knee scoring system. J Bone Joint Surg Br. 2010; Available from: http://www.jbjs.org.uk.
6. Brander VA, Stulberg SD, Adams A, Harden R, Bruehl S, Stanos S, Steven P, Houle T. Ranawat award paper: predicting total knee replacement pain: a prospective. Observational study. Clin Orthop. 2003;416:27–36.
7. Hawker G, Melfi C, Paul J, Green R, Bombardier C. Comparison of a generic SF/36 and a disease specific (WOMAC) instrument in the measurement of outcomes after knee replacement surgery. J Rheumatol. 1995;22:1193–6.
8. Gluck T. Die invaginations methode der Osteo- und Arthroplastik. Ber Klin Wschr. 1890;19:132.
9. Shiers LG. Arthroplasty of the knee. Preliminary report of new method. J Bone Joint Surg (Br). 1954; 36:553–60.
10. Speed JS, Trout PC. Arthroplasty of the knee. A follow-up study. J Bone Joint Surg (Br). 1949;31B:53–60.
11. Miller A, Friedman B. Fascial arthroplasty of the knee. J Bone Joint Surg Am. 1952;34A:55–63.
12. Walldius B. Arthroplasty of the knee using an endo-prosthesis [classical article]. Clin Orthop. 1996;331: 4–10.
13. Dunbar MJ. Subjective outcomes after knee arthroplasty, Thesis. Acta Orthop Scand. 2001;72:Suppl. 301.
14. Marx R. Knee rating scales for clinical outcome. In: Calaghan JJ, Rubash HE, Simonian PT, Wickiewicz TL, Rosenberg AG, editors. The adult knee. Philadelphia: Lippincott Williams & Wilkins; 2002. p. 367–78.
15. Dowsey MM, Choong PFM. Predictors of pain and function following total joint replacement. In: Kinov P, editor. Arthoplasty update. Rijeka: In Tech; 2013.
16. Dowsey MM, Nikpour M, Dieppe P, Choong PF. Associations between pre-operative radiographic changes and outcomes after total knee joint replacement for osteoarthritis. Osteoarthr Cartil. 2012;20:1095–102.
17. Williams DP, Price AJ, Beardetal DJ. The effects of age on patient-reported outcome measures in total knee replacements. Bone Joint J. 2013;95:38–44.
18. Liu SS, Buvanendran A, Rathmell JP, Sawhney M, Bae JJ, Moric M, Perros S, Pope AJ, Poultsides L, Della Valle CJ, Shin NS, McCartney CJ, Ma Y, Shah M, Wood MJ, Manion SC, Sculco TP. A cross-sectional survey on prevalence and risk factors for persistent postsurgical pain 1 year after total hip and knee replacement. Reg Anesth Pain Med. 2012;37:415–22.
19. Judge A, Arden NK, Cooper C, Kassim Javaid M, Carr AJ, Field RE, Dieppe PA. Predictors of outcomes of total knee replacement surgery. Rheumatology. 2012;51:1804–13.
20. Dowsey MM, Liew D, Stoney JD, Choong PF. The impact of pre-operative obesity on weight change and outcome in total knee replacement: a prospective study of 529 consecutive patients. J Bone Joint Surg Br. 2010;92B:513–20.
21. McElroy MJ, Pivec R, Issa K, Harwin SF, Mont MA. The effects of obesity and morbid obesity on outcomes in TKA. J Knee Surg. 2013;26:83–8.
22. Dowsey MM, Broadhead ML, Stoney JD, Choong PF. Outcomes of total knee arthroplasty in English-versus non- English-speaking patients. J Orthop Surg. 2009;17:3059.
23. Paulsen MG, Dowsey MM, Castle D, Choong PF. Preoperative psychological distress and functional outcome after knee replacement. ANZ J Surg. 2011; 81:681–7.
24. Hawker GA, Badley EM, Borkhoff CM, Croxford R, Davies A, Dunn S, Gignac M, Jaglal S, Kreder H, Sale J. Which patients are most likely to benefit from total joint arthroplasty? Arthritis Rheum. 2013;65:1243–52.
25. Clement ND, Jenkins PJ, MacDonald D, Nie Y, Patton J, Breush S, Howie C, Biant L. Socioeconomic status affects the Oxford knee score and short-form 12 score following total knee replacement. Bone Joint J. 2013;95:52–8.
26. Dowsey MM, Dieppe P, Lohmander S, Castle D, Liew D, Choong PFM. The association between radiographic severity and pre-operative function in patients undergoing primary knee replacement for osteoarthritis. Knee. 2012;19:860–5.
27. Streiner DL, Norman GR. Health measurement scales: a practical guide to their development and use. Oxford: Oxford University Press; 1989.
28. Marx R. Knee rating scales. Arthroscopy. 2003;19: 1103–8.
29. Martin DP, Engelberg R, Agel J, Swiontkowski MF. Comparison of the musculoskeletal function assessment questionnaire with the short form-36, the Western Ontario and McMaster Universities Osteoarthritis Index, and the sickness impact profile health-status measures. J Bone Joint Surg Am. 1997; 79A:1323–35.

30. Liang MH, Fossel AH, Larson MG. Comparisons of five health status instruments for orthopaedic evaluation. Med Care. 1990;28:632–42.

31. Patel AA, Donegan D, Todd A. The 36-item short form. J Am Acad Orthop Surg. 2007;15:126–34.

32. Patt JC, Mauerhan DR. Outcomes research in total joint replacement: a critical review and commentary. Am J Orthop (Belle Mead NJ). 2005;34:167–72.

33. Whitehouse SL, Crawford RW, Learmonth ID. Validation for the reduced Western Ontario and McMaster Universities Osteoarthritis Index function scale. J Orthop Surg. 2008;16:50–3.

34. Dawson J, Fitzpatrick R, Murray D, Carr A. Questionnaire on the perceptions of patients about total knee replacement. J Bone Joint Surg (Br). 1998;80B:63–9.

35. Dunbar MJ. Subjective outcomes after knee arthroplasty. Acta Orthop Scand. 2001;S72(301):1–63.

36. Insall JN, Dorr LD, Scott RD, Scott WN. Rationale of the Knee Society clinical rating system. Clin Orthop. 1989;248:13–4.

37. Liow RY, Walker K, Wajid MA, Bedi G, Lennox CM. The reliability of the American Knee Society Score. Acta Orthop Scand. 2000;71:603–8.

38. Insall JN, Ranawat CS, Aglietti P, Shine J. A comparison of four models of total knee-replacement prostheses. J Bone Joint Surg Am. 1976;58A:754–65.

39. Buechel FF. A simplified evaluation system for rating of knee function. Orthop Rev. 1982;11:97–101.

40. Ewald F. The knee society total knee arthroplasty roentgenographic evaluation and scoring system. Clin Orthop. 1989;246:9–12.

41. Mackinnon JG, Young S, Bailey RA. The St Georg sledge in unicompartmental replacement of the knee. J Bone Joint Surg (Br). 1988;70B:217–23.

42. Newman JH, Ackroyd CE, Shah NA. Unicompartmental or total knee replacement: five-year results of a prospective, randomized trial of 102 osteoarthritic knees with unicompartmental arthritis. J Bone Joint Surg (Br). 1998;80B:862–5.

43. Talbot S, Hooper G, Stokes A, Zordan R. Use of a new high-activity arthroplasty score to assess function of young patients with total hip or knee arthroplasty. J Arthroplasty. 2010;25:268–73.

44. Wright JG. Evaluating the outcome of treatment: shouldn't we be asking patients if they are better? J Clin Epidemiol. 2000;53:549–53.

45. Zhang Y. Validation of the new knee society knee scoring system for outcome assessment after total knee arthroplasty. Master of Medical science, The University of Hong Kong; 2013. p. 30.

46. Wright JG, Young NL. The patient\specific index: asking patients what they want. J Bone Joint Surg Am. 1997;79A:974–83.

47. Wylde V, Learmonth I, Potter A, Bettinson K, Lingard E. Patient- reported outcomes after fixed versus mobile-bearing total knee replacement: a multicentre randomized controlled trial using the Kinemax total) knee replacement. J Bone Joint Surg (Br). 2008;90B:1172–9.

48. Judge A, Arden NK, Price A, Glyn-Jones S, Beard D, Carr AJ, Dawson J, Fitzpatrick R. Easing patients for joint replacement: can pre-operative Oxford hip and knee scores be used to predict patient satisfaction following joint replacement surgery and to guide patient selection? J Bone Joint Surg (Br). 2011;93B:1660–4.

49. www.sf-36.com

50. Angst F, Ewert T, Lehmann S, Aeschlimann A, Stucki G. The factor subdimensions of the Western Ontario and McMaster Universities Osteoarthritis Index (WOMAC) help to specify hip and knee osteoarthritis. A prospective evaluation and validation study. J Rheumatol. 2005;32:1324–30.

51. Ghanem E, Pawasarat I, Lindsay A, May L, Azzam K, Joshi A, Parvizi J. Limitations of the Knee Society Score in evaluating outcomes following revision total knee arthroplasty. J Bone Joint Surg Am. 2010;92A:2445–51.

52. Lee CH, Ha CW, Kim S, Kim M, Song YJ. A novel patellofemoral scoring system for patellofemoral joint status. J Bone Joint Surg Am. 2013;95A:620–6.

53. Feller J, Barlett J, Derek L. Patellar resurfacing versus retention in total knee arthroplasty. J Bone Joint Surg (Br). 1996;78B:226–8.

54. Kujala U, Jaakkola L, Koskinen S, Taimela S, Hurme M, Nelimarkka O. Scoring of patellofemoral disorders. Arthroscopy. 1993;9:159–63.

55. Newman JH, Ackroyd CE, Shah NA, Karachalios T. Should the patella be resurfaced during total knee replacement. Knee. 2000;7:17–23.

56. Janse AJ, Gemke RJ, Uiterwaal CS, et al. Quality of life: patients and doctors don't always agree: a meta-analysis. J Clin Epidemiol. 2004;57:653–61.

57. Browne J, Jamieson L, Lewsey J, et al. Patient reported outcome measures (PROMs) in elective surgery: report to the Department of Health, 2007. http://www.lshtm.ac.uk/php/hsrp/research/proms report_12_dec_07.pdf. Date last accessed 5 Apr 2012.

58. Baker P, Dechan D, Lee D, et al. The effect of surgical factors on early patient reported outcome measures following total knee replacement. J Bone Joint Surg (Br). 2012;94B:1058–66.

59. Dunbar MJ, Robertsson O, Ryd L, Lidgren L. Appropriate questionnaires for knee arthroplasty: results of a survey of 3600 patients from The Swedish Knee Arthroplasty Registry. J Bone Joint Surg (Br). 2001;83B:339–44.

60. http://www.hscic.gov.uk/article/3843/Background-information-about-PROMs.

The Long Term Outcome of Total Knee Arthroplasty. The Effect of Age and Diagnosis

Alexander Tsarouhas and Michael E. Hantes

Introduction

Total knee arthroplasty (TKA) is presently considered as one of the most successful and cost effective procedures in orthopaedic surgery from the perspective of patients, surgeons and third party payers. The clinical benefits of the procedure have long been established in terms of objective and self- reported knee scores as well as quality of life measurements. Advances in implant design, instrumentation and surgical technique have gradually increased the long term survival of TKA. A dramatic rise in the incidence of the procedure has also been documented in the developed world running parallel to the global increase in life expectancy.

An increasing recognition of the clinical benefits of the procedure has gradually broadened the indications for TKA both in terms of patient age and preoperative diagnosis. Younger, more active patients as well as elderly individuals, even nonagenarians, are currently considering TKA as an option. In addition, traditional indications of the procedure have expanded in order to include traumatic, degenerative and inflammatory knee pathology (such as rheumatoid-RA and juvenile idiopathic arthritis-JIA). Although TKA has shown predictable improvements of knee pain and function, variable improvement of clinical and functional outcomes and implant survival has been documented. Thus the detection and selection of patients who are more likely to benefit from TKA remains a clinical challenge [1].

Several factors are considered as potential predictors of TKA outcome. Demographic variables (such as age, gender and race), patient related factors (such as pre-operative pain, diagnosis, comorbidities and body mass index), socio-economic status and surgeon related factors (such as technique, experience and surgical volume) have all been implicated in TKA outcomes [2, 3]. The current literature presents abundant comparative data to support the association of each of these factors with TKA. However, defining the predictive value of these factors with accuracy, by means of systematic multivariate analysis, has proven essentially unfeasible. Several methodological issues have largely limited studies of this kind. Because of the large number of confounding factors and their diverse volume, the statistical models used to explain the variability of TKA outcomes have been inadequately powered to adjust for potential predictive factors. In addition, several patient or surgeon related factors may well explain a great part of this variability but are difficult to

A. Tsarouhas, MD, DSc
Private Orthopedic Surgeon, Kalambaka,
Thessaly, Greece

M.E. Hantes, MD, DSc, PhD (✉)
Department of Orthopaedic Surgery,
University Hospital of Larissa, Larissa, Greece

Faculty of Medicine, School of Health
Sciences, University of Thessaly,
Mezourlo 41110 Larissa, Greece
e-mail: hantesmi@otenet.gr

© Springer-Verlag London 2015
T. Karachalios (ed.), *Total Knee Arthroplasty: Long Term Outcomes*,
DOI 10.1007/978-1-4471-6660-3_6

document accurately. For example, patient socio-economic status and variation in surgical technique, surgeon experience and volume are seldom accounted for but are thought to affect overall outcome. Preferential bias may ensue in community based cohorts while response bias may also play a role when self-reported outcomes are measured, because responders tend to be comparably older and have altered mental or psychological status.

Although success rates of TKA in patients of different age and preoperative diagnosis are expected to be variable, their exact effect on TKA outcomes is currently under debate. This chapter aims to review the available literature and present data on specific subgroups of patients regarding the effect of age and diagnosis on TKA outcomes.

The Effect of Age

The mean age at the time of TKA surgery has been estimated at 67.5 years with very few patients aged over 85 years [1]. Recent data from United States registries suggest that the mean age at surgery for patients with non inflammatory arthritis has tended to decrease over recent decades [4]. Although receiving a TKA is considered a function of age, the effect of age on the outcomes of the procedure remains controversial. In their prospective cohort, Jones et al. [5] found that age alone does not affect pain, function or health related quality of life at 6 months after TKA. In contrast, Judge et al. [2] found an association between older age and worse functional outcomes but not pain after TKA. The authors established a smaller effect of age, however, when a multivariate analysis of confounding factors was performed. In line with these findings, Nilsdotter et al. [6] also identified older age as a predictor of postoperative KOOS pain and other symptom scores up to 5 years postoperatively.

Knee Arthroplasty in the Younger Patient

Concerns regarding increased loosening rates and the potential need for multiple revision surgeries have traditionally discouraged younger patients from undergoing TKA. Non operative management as well as other less invasive surgical options, such as arthroscopic debridement and proximal tibial osteotomy, may be considered in patients with specific indications, such as uni-compartmental disease and limb malalignment. However, clinical improvement after knee arthroscopy in the arthritic knee tends to decline over time, whereas patients who undergo TKA after tibial osteotomy may be at higher risk of complications. In addition, delaying TKA surgery is probably not a realistic option when patients continue to experience prolonged pain and increasing disability in performing daily recreational or professional activities, despite routine non operative management. It has been argued that worse outcomes are to be expected when prolonged periods of morbidity have preceded TKA, particularly in achieving a higher level of function.

Over the last decades, satisfactory outcomes have been reported in terms of success rates and implant survival in younger patients undergoing TKA. Gill et al. [7] found a 96.5 % survival rate at 18 years (including patients with osteoarthritis −51.4 %, with rheumatoid arthritis −40.3 % and with other diagnoses −8.3 %). Diduch et al. [8] calculated a survival rate of 87–94 % at 18 years in a mixed population with idiopathic and post-traumatic osteoarthritis. Dalury et al. [9] also found, at an average of 7.2 years follow up, comparable success rates between TKA patients younger than 45 years and those older. However, when patient reported outcomes are considered, findings tend to be more diverse. Self reported outcomes are increasingly thought to better express the success rates of TKA as they incorporate the patient's perspective. In a study of patient reported outcomes after TKA, Williams et al. [10] found comparative Oxford knee and EuroQol scores across different age groups but with a linear trend towards improved outcomes with decreasing age. Interestingly though, a higher dissatisfaction rate was found in patients aged <55 years. The authors suggested that higher activity expectations may differentiate subjective from objective outcomes in younger patient groups. In a recent multi-center study, Parvizi et al. [11] found that approximately one third of young patients who underwent TKA reported residual symptoms and limitations in activity. In line with these findings, Nilsdotter et al. [6] confirmed a decrease in daily living activity scores at 5 years after TKA without however identifying a predictive effect of age on this finding. Interestingly, in a recent survey among young TKA patients (average age 54 years), Barrack et al. [3] found that socioeconomic factors were more strongly associated with satisfaction and functional outcomes than demographic or implant factors. Specifically, low income and minority patients were more likely to be dissatisfied and have functional limitations after TKA.

TKA in the Elderly

Despite an increase in life expectancy and advances in medical treatment the chronological age limit for patients undergoing TKA, among other elective major orthopaedic procedures, remains controversial. Elderly patients have been found to be less likely but equally willing to receive a TKA compared with their younger counterparts [12]. Concerns have been raised regarding the incidence of morbidity and postoperative mortality, with increasing age, in patients undergoing TKA. Elderly patients are considered to suffer from more medical comorbidities pre-operatively and more postoperative complications. A higher likelihood of blood transfusion has also been found in this group of patients [13]. In addition, elderly patients receiving TKA are more likely to be transferred to a rehabilitation facility postoperatively [5]. Most recently, Yoshihara et al. [14] reviewed medical files of US patients aged 80 years and older who underwent TKA between 2000 and 2009. They found an increasing incidence of TKA in this age group as well as an increased number of comorbid conditions suggesting that the indications for surgical treatment have been broadened. The overall in-hospital complication and mortality rates remained stable and decreased over time respectively. However, both parameters were significantly higher compared to patients aged 65–79 years [14]. Similar findings were confirmed by other investigators [15, 16]. These findings indicate that careful patient selection based on surgical indications and aggressive postoperative treatment are essential for achieving optimal outcomes. Patients in these age groups should be informed of the higher risk involved. Whereas higher rates of medical morbidity and post operatively mortality are a concern in the elderly population, clinical outcomes have been encouraging. Berend et al. [17] recorded significant improvements in pain and Knee Society scores in TKA patients older than 89 and a higher survival rate than in age matched controls. In their cohort of nonagenarians receiving TKA, Alfonso et al. [13] found significant pain reduction and slightly higher functional capacity and better survival characteristics compared to age matched controls at a mean follow up of 4.1 years. As expected, most studies of this kind are limited by their short follow up. Overall, these findings suggest that advanced age should not present a contraindication for TKA.

The Effect of Diagnosis

Recent data from large administrative databases in the United States indicate that trends in joint arthroplasty rates in patients suffering from inflammatory and non-inflammatory diseases have significantly changed over the past decades. Total knee arthroplasty rates in non-inflammatory arthritis patients more than doubled from 1991 to 2005, whereas TKA rates for RA and JIA decreased substantially. Interestingly, for both RA and JIA patients, the decrease in arthroplasty rates was most prominent among the younger age groups, resulting in a cumulative decrease of the mean age at the time of TKA for both inflammatory conditions [4].

Rheumatoid Arthritis and TKA

The multisystem disease characteristics of RA have been previously identified as a risk factor for adverse outcomes both in the surgical setting and in the long term. Treatment strategies for RA have undergone significant evolution during the last decades. The advent of potent disease modifying drugs (DMARDs) has obviated surgical treatment for a substantial number of patients and improved the overall quality of life and survival of RA patients. However, despite advances in medical treatment, progressive joint destruction still occurs in a considerable subgroup of patients leading to increasing pain and loss of function. Longer disease duration, erythrocyte sedimentation rate levels at baseline examination and inadequate response to treatment after the first year of follow up all increase the likelihood ratio for TKA during the course of the disease [18]. However, several considerations need to be taken into account in this subgroup of TKA recipients in order to achieve a successful outcome. Poor bone quality, secondary osteonecrosis, cyst formation, soft tissue attenuation, fixed flexion and valgus deformities pose significant technical difficulties in the setting of advanced RA disease.

Overall, satisfactory long term results have been reported for TKA in RA patients in terms of implant survival and knee function. Crowder et al. [19] showed that cemented TKA in the young patient with rheumatoid arthritis is reliable and durable at an average 18 year follow up, with an estimated survivorship of 100 % at 15 years and 93.7 % at 20 years. Similarly, Ito et al. [20] found a 93.7 % survival rate at 15 years and good to excellent HSS knee scores in 77 % of RA patients treated with cemented TKA. However, neither longstanding implant survival nor improved knee function are adequate to predict the functional status of RA patients in the long term. Nishikawa et al. [21] found that at a minimum 10 year follow up, RA patients who received TKA had excellent Knee Society scores but overall poor functional scores and decreased walking ability. The authors suggest that systemic disease progression and multiple joint involvement limited the benefits of successful knee surgery.

The effect of RA diagnosis on the outcomes of TKA has mainly been investigated in comparison to degenerative OA. Because RA is essentially different from OA in terms of pathogenesis, disease progression and prognosis, TKA outcomes would be expected to differ considerably. At baseline, compared to OA patients, RA patients tend to be significantly younger and more frequently female [22]. In addition, due to multi system disease involvement, they carry a higher comorbidity burden, with chronic pulmonary disease being the commonest systemic manifestation of the disorder. To date, available studies have yielded conflicting results. In a multivariate analysis of a large prospective cohort, Judge et al. [2] found that, among other confounding factors, the preoperative diagnosis of RA could predict pain outcomes 6 months after TKA, with RA patients in general experiencing less pain than those with OA. A recent systematic review and meta-analysis of the literature indicated that patients with RA were at higher risk of postoperative infection and early revision following TKA compared to OA patients [23]. In contrast, no differences in late revision, 90 day mortality or venous thromboembolism rates were evident [23]. Infection rates have been reported to be up to three times higher in RA compared to OA patients, which may be attributed to decreased immune system response, due to the disease itself or to immunosuppressive treatment [24].

Juvenile Arthritis and TKA

Juvenile idiopathic arthritis presents certain particularities as it occurs during childhood or adolescence. The knee joint is affected in approximately two thirds of the patients although multiple joint involvement is common. Altered knee anatomy (trumpet shaped deformity with valgus alignment and external tibial rotation), small joint size and compromised bone quality pose considerable challenges for knee replacement surgery. Implantation of knee prostheses in the third and fourth decade of life in patients with a long life expectancy raises higher implant survival expectations as well as concerns about the potential need for revision surgery at a young age. In addition, wound healing problems have been reported with increased frequency as the majority of these patients receive long term immunosuppressive treatment.

Nevertheless, TKA for juvenile idiopathic arthritis has produced encouraging long term outcomes. Quality of life measurements have also been shown to improve significantly after surgery [25]. However, in a retrospective cohort of 349 TKAs, with a 12 year follow up, the mean survivorship of TKA implants in patients with juvenile idiopathic arthritis was found to be inferior compared to younger patients with osteoarthritis or rheumatoid arthritis [26]. This is especially disconcerting because younger patients require better durability of TKA implants.

Conclusion

Total knee arthroplasty is currently considered the optimal treatment for end stage knee arthritis. Although the population which undergoes the procedure currently presents with an expanding range of age and preoperative diagnoses, the effect of these two factors on the long term outcome of the procedure cannot be estimated with accuracy. Hence, a direct interaction between these two variables is evident since younger TKA patients present with different ratios of preoperative diagnosis compared with older ones.

Current literature suggests that joint specific pain relief and functional outcomes achieved are not age dependent. Although in younger patients the continuation of non-operative treatment is advocated for as long as possible and joint preserving surgical alternatives should be considered, TKA is advisable with favorable long term outcomes when function and quality of daily living are severely compromised. Elderly patients may also gain significant clinical improvement from TKA. Provided risk factors are properly assessed and comorbidities are controlled, age should no longer present a barrier to TKA.

The lack of consensus regarding TKA outcomes and their determinants in patients of different knee joint pathology evidently obscures decision making for patient selection, timing of surgery and anticipated clinical outcomes. This is particularly important, given that inflammatory knee arthritis distinctly presents at a younger age and therefore augments the need for long term implant endurance and improved function. Overall, long term outcomes of TKA for inflammatory knee arthritis have been satisfactory when implant survival and knee specific functional scores are considered. Increased perioperative risk of infection and progressive decline of function due to systemic disease progress remain a concern, particularly in RA patients.

References

1. Kane RL, Saleh KJ, Wilt TJ, Bershadsky B. The functional outcomes of total knee arthroplasty. J Bone Joint Surg Am. 2005;87A:1719–24.
2. Judge A, Arden NK, Cooper C, Kassim Javaid M, Carr AJ, Field RE, et al. Predictors of outcomes of total knee replacement surgery. Rheumatology. 2012; 5:1804–13.
3. Barrack RL, Ruh EL, Chen J, Lombardi Jr AV, Berend KR, Parvizi J, et al. Impact of socioeconomic factors on outcome of total knee arthroplasty. Clin Orthop. 2014;472:86–97.
4. Mertelsmann-Voss C, Lyman S, Pan TJ, Goodman SM, Figgie MP, Mandl LA. US trends in rates of arthroplasty for inflammatory arthritis including rheumatoid arthritis, juvenile idiopathic arthritis, and spondyloarthritis. Arthritis Rheum. 2014;66:1432–9.
5. Jones CA, Voaklander DC, Johnston DW, Suarez-Almazor ME. The effect of age on pain, function, and quality of life after total hip and knee arthroplasty. Arch Intern Med. 2001;161:454–60.
6. Nilsdotter AK, Toksvig-Larsen S, Roos EM. A 5 year prospective study of patient-relevant outcomes after total knee replacement. Osteoarthritis Cartilage. 2009;17:601–6.
7. Gill GS, Chan KC, Mills DM. 5- to 18-year follow-up study of cemented total knee arthroplasty for patients 55 years old or younger. J Arthroplasty. 1997;12:49–54.
8. Diduch DR, Insall JN, Scott WN, Scuderi GR, Font-Rodriguez D. Total knee replacement in young, active patients. Long-term follow-up and functional outcome. J Bone Joint Surg Am. 1997;79A:575–82.
9. Dalury DF, Ewald FC, Christie MJ, Scott RD. Total knee arthroplasty in a group of patients less than 45 years of age. J Arthroplasty. 1995;10:598–602.
10. Williams DP, Price AJ, Beard DJ, Hadfield SG, Arden NK, Murray DW, et al. The effects of age on patient-reported outcome measures in total knee replacements. Bone Joint J. 2013;95B:38–44.
11. Parvizi J, Nunley RM, Berend KR, Lombardi AV, Ruh EL, Clohisy JC, et al. High level of residual symptoms in young patients after total knee arthroplasty. Clin Orthop. 2014;472:133–7.
12. Katz BP, Freund DA, Heck DA, Dittus RS, Paul JE, Wright J, et al. Demographic variation in the rate of knee replacement: a multi-year analysis. Health Serv Res. 1996;31:125–40.

13. Alfonso DT, Howell RD, Strauss EJ, Di Cesare PE. Total hip and knee arthroplasty in nonagenarians. J Arthroplasty. 2007;22:807–11.
14. Yoshihara H, Yoneoka D. Trends in the incidence and in-hospital outcomes of elective major orthopaedic surgery in patients eighty years of age and older in the United States from 2000 to 2009. J Bone Joint Surg Am. 2014;96A:1185–91.
15. Memtsoudis SG, Della Valle AG, Besculides MC, Gaber L, Laskin R. Trends in demographics, comorbidity profiles, in-hospital complications and mortality associated with primary knee arthroplasty. J Arthroplasty. 2009;24:518–27.
16. Kreder HJ, Berry GK, McMurtry IA, Halman SI. Arthroplasty in the octogenarian: quantifying the risks. J Arthroplasty. 2005;20:289–93.
17. Berend ME, Thong AE, Faris GW, Newbern G, Pierson JL, Ritter MA. Total joint arthroplasty in the extremely elderly: hip and knee arthroplasty after entering the 89th year of life. J Arthroplasty. 2003;18:817–21.
18. Pantos PG, Tzioufas AG, Panagiotakos DB, Soucacos PN, Moutsopoulos HM. Demographics, clinical characteristics and predictive factors for total knee or hip replacement in patients with rheumatoid arthritis in Greece. Clin Exp Rheumatol. 2013;31:195–200.
19. Crowder AR, Duffy GP, Trousdale RT. Long-term results of total knee arthroplasty in young patients with rheumatoid arthritis. J Arthroplasty. 2005;20(S3):12–6.
20. Ito J, Koshino T, Okamoto R, Saito T. 15-year follow-up study of total knee arthroplasty in patients with rheumatoid arthritis. J Arthroplasty. 2003;18:984–92.
21. Nishikawa M, Owaki H, Takahi K, Fuji T. Disease activity, knee function, and walking ability in patients with rheumatoid arthritis 10 years after primary total knee arthroplasty. J Orthop Surg. 2014;22:84–7.
22. Stundner O, Danninger T, Chiu YL, Sun X, Goodman SM, Russell LA, et al. Rheumatoid arthritis vs osteoarthritis in patients receiving total knee arthroplasty: perioperative outcomes. J Arthroplasty. 2014;29: 308–13.
23. Ravi B, Escott B, Shah PS, Jenkinson R, Chahal J, Bogoch E, et al. A systematic review and meta-analysis comparing complications following total joint arthroplasty for rheumatoid arthritis versus for osteoarthritis. Arthritis Rheum. 2012;64:3839–49.
24. Wilson MG, Kelley K, Thornhill TS. Infection as a complication of total knee-replacement arthroplasty. Risk factors and treatment in sixty-seven cases. J Bone Joint Surg Am. 1990;72A:878–83.
25. Jolles BM, Bogoch ER. Quality of life after TKA for patients with juvenile rheumatoid arthritis. Clin Orthop. 2008;466:167–78.
26. Heyse TJ, Ries MD, Bellemans J, Goodman SB, Scott RD, Wright TM, et al. Total knee arthroplasty in patients with juvenile idiopathic arthritis. Clin Orthop. 2014;472:147–54.

Long Term Outcome of Primary Total Knee Arthroplasty. The Effect of Body Weight and Level of Activity

Polykarpos I. Kiorpelidis, Zoe H. Dailiana, and Sokratis E. Varitimidis

Introduction

Total knee arthroplasty has been a successful treatment in the management of advanced knee osteoarthritis for pain relief, quality of life and function improvement for almost the last 40 years. By the year 2030, it is estimated that in the United States, the demand for total knee replacement will show a 673 % increase from the present day, with the number of operations reaching almost 3.48 million annually [1]. Constant improvement of implant materials and surgical techniques has made this operation one of the most successful procedures in medicine with several studies showing prosthesis survival more than 80–90 % at 15–20 years follow-up [2, 3]. Success rate and revision surgery for aseptic loosening is generally dependent on the degree of wear and osteolysis of the implant. Factors that influence the outcome of total knee arthroplasty are implant design and material, surgical technique and patient related conditions (Fig. 7.1). Body weight and level of activity are also patient specific factors that may affect the durability of total knee arthroplasty (TKA) [4].

P.I. Kiorpelidis, MD
Department of Orthopaedic Surgery and
Musculoskeletal Trauma, Faculty of Medicine,
School of Health Sciences, University of Thessalia,
Larissa, Hellenic Republic

Z.H. Dailiana, MD, DSc
Department of Orthopaedic Surgery, Faculty
of Medicine, School of Health Sciences,
University of Thessalia, 3 Panepistimiou St,
Larissa 41500, Hellenic Republic
e-mail: dailiana@med.uth.gr

S.E. Varitimidis, MD, DSc (⊠)
Department of Orthopaedic Surgery and
Musculoskeletal Trauma, Faculty of Medicine,
School of Health Sciences, University
of Thessalia, Biopolis, 3 Panepistimiou St,
Larissa 41500, Hellenic Republic
e-mail: svaritimidis@ortho-uth.org

Obesity

Association with Osteoarthritis

Obesity nowadays has become a major health issue. The prevalence of obesity nearly doubled from 1980 to 2008 (6.4–12 %) with half of this rise taking place in the last decade. Currently, more than 500 million patients worldwide are considered

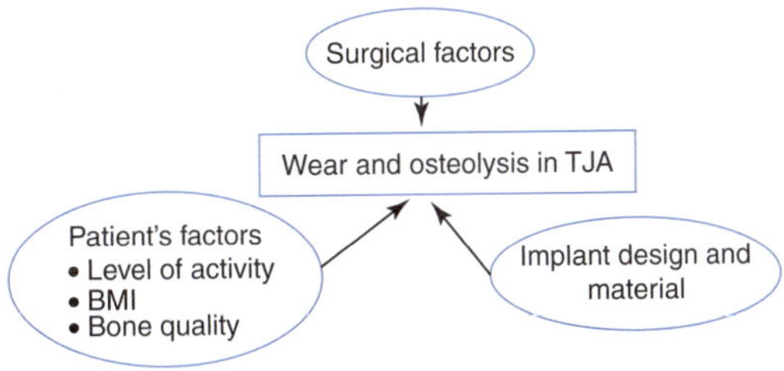

Fig. 7.1 Factors influencing surgical outcome of TJA

© Springer-Verlag London 2015
T. Karachalios (ed.), *Total Knee Arthroplasty: Long Term Outcomes,*
DOI 10.1007/978-1-4471-6660-3_7

to be obese. In 2009–2010, the age adjusted prevalence of obesity was 35.5 % among adult men and 35.8 % among adult women in the U.S. [5, 6]. The development of osteoarthritis has been strongly correlated with obesity by implicating the excessive mechanical load exerted on the knee cartilage as a causative factor. Increased body weight has been found to be more destructive for the knee rather than the hip joint and in relation to the acceptable BMI(<25), there is multiple times increase of possibility for TKA with every increase in the body mass index scale [7–13]. Fehring et al. have suggested that the osteoarthritis risk is fourfold for obese men and fivefold for obese women [14]. It has also been suggested that in patients with a BMI >35, TKA may be required almost 8 years earlier than for those who maintain a normal BMI <25 [15], while another study has shown that morbidly obese patients with gonarthrosis will require TKA 13 years earlier than those with normal BMI [16]. On the other hand, a decrease of 5 kg of body weight (body mass index of 2 units or more) has been shown to decrease the risk of osteoarthritis in women by at least 50 % [17]. Alternatively, 24 % of surgical interventions might be avoided if patients reduce their weight by 5 kg or until their BMI reaches proposed normal levels [13]. During the single leg stance of gait cycle, a force of three to six times of body weight is transmitted across the joint. A study by Messier, revealed a statistically significant direct association between body mass and peak values of compressive forces, resultant forces, abduction moment, and the medial rotation moment of the knee. Each weight loss unit results in a fourfold reduction in the load exerted on the knee per step during daily activities [18]. Biomechanical factors are also considered to be causative factors in the development of knee osteoarthritis. The presence of mechanoreceptors at the surface of chondrocytes, which are activated by increased pressure, induce cartilage degradation by the production of proinflammatory mediators, such as nitric oxide and prostaglandin E2. Proteins produced by the adipose tissue, the adipokines (especially leptin), have also been implicated in the cartilage destruction process. Adipokines along with other cytokines are responsible for the production of nitric

oxide; this interferes with chondrocyte function resulting in the loss of cartilage matrix through induction of apoptosis, activation of metalloproteinases, and inhibition of proteoglycan and type II collagen synthesis [19, 20].

Early Complications

Obesity is defined as an abnormal or excessive accumulation of fat on the human body leading to increased health problems that may reduce life expectancy. Diabetes mellitus, coronary artery disease, hyperlipidemia, hypertension and obstructive sleep apnea are the medical co-morbidities that usually accompany obesity. These comorbidities are theoretically the reason for the higher perioperative complication rates in obese patients. Venous thromboembolism is strongly correlated with obesity and delayed postoperative ambulation, and has been a major concern for the orthopedic community for many years, with several studies being published giving postoperative guidelines for antithrombotic medication prophylaxis. Sixty to 90 % of patients with OSAS (obstructive sleep apnea syndrome) are obese and postoperative respiratory and cardiac complications and length of hospital stay after joint replacement are significantly higher compared to non-obese patients [21]. Anesthesiologists may often be unable to perform spinal anesthesia in obese patients because of excessive body fat, leading to the use of general anesthesia, thus increasing the risk of immediate postoperative respiratory complications (Fig. 7.2). In cases of extreme obesity, the perils of postoperative in-hospital complications are increased 8.44 times, while the odds ratio for length of stay, outpatient complications and readmission rates for every 5 units of BMI >45 are multiplied [22]. These parameters contribute to the increased cost of health care provision.

Classification

Body mass index (BMI) is the calculating tool commonly used to determine and classify categories of severity of obesity in adults (Table 7.1). Obesity is generally defined as a BMI >30 kg/m².

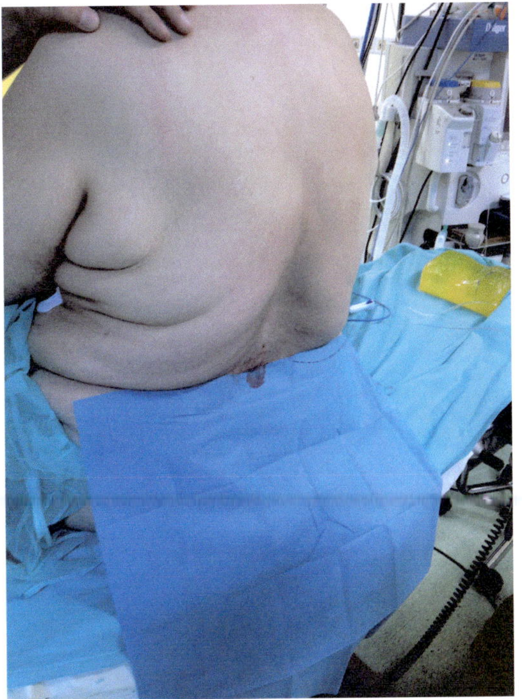

Fig. 7.2 Performing spinal anesthesia on the obese patient

Table 7.1 Categories of severity of obesity are shown

BMI (kg/m²)	Classification	Risk of comorbidities
<18,5	Underweight	Low
18,5–24,99	Normal weight	Average
25–29,99	Overweight – preobese	Increased
30–34,99	Obese (obesity I)	Moderate
35–39,99	Severe obese (obesity II)	Severe
40–49,99	Morbidly-obese	Very severe
>50	Super-obese	Very severe
>60	Super-mega-obese	Very severe

BMI is calculated according to the height and weight of an individual using the formula: $\mathrm{BMI} = \text{weight (kg)/height}^2 \text{ (m}^2)$ or $= [\text{weight (pounds)/height}^2 \text{ (inches}^2)] \times 703$. Even though BMI is the measurement of choice for most health care providers, for many years its validity has been questioned, as if its longevity, having been developed 150 years ago, somehow discredits it. The main concerns are that it does not take into account age or gender and that it cannot distinguish weight associated with muscle mass compared with increased adipose tissue. Newer index screening tools have being developed in order to more accurately assess body fat, such as the body adiposity index (BAI) and the waist-hip ratio (WHR) [23–25]. Nevertheless, BMI still remains an inexpensive tool, which is widely and currently accepted because of its simplicity, for data accumulation.

Long Term Outcomes

Many studies have tried to define the relationship of obesity with TKA regarding postsurgical complications. Wound healing problems, superficial infections, deep infections leading to removal of the prosthesis, fusion or amputation, component malposition and aseptic loosening are all significant related problems that the orthopedic surgeon has to deal with.

Periprosthetic Joint Infection

The association of obesity to periprosthetic joint infection has already been established, with morbidly obese patients showing the highest increase in complication rates. Jamsen et al. [26] revealed an increase in infection rate from 0.37 to 4.66 % in this study group compared with patients with normal BMI in the first postoperative year, while Maliznak et al. [27] found an increased odds ratio of infection of 21.3. Winiarsky et al. [28] reviewing 50 cemented TKA in morbidly obese patients, highlighted the problem of the increased risk of poor wound-healing, infection and avulsion of the medial collateral ligament in this study group. Many other studies with large groups of patients have come to the conclusion that with an increasing BMI, and especially BMI >40 with the presence of diabetes, the probability of periprosthetic joint infection is multiplied [29–34].

Component Malposition

Accurate component alignment plays an important role in the load distribution between knee compartments. Full-length standing hip to ankle

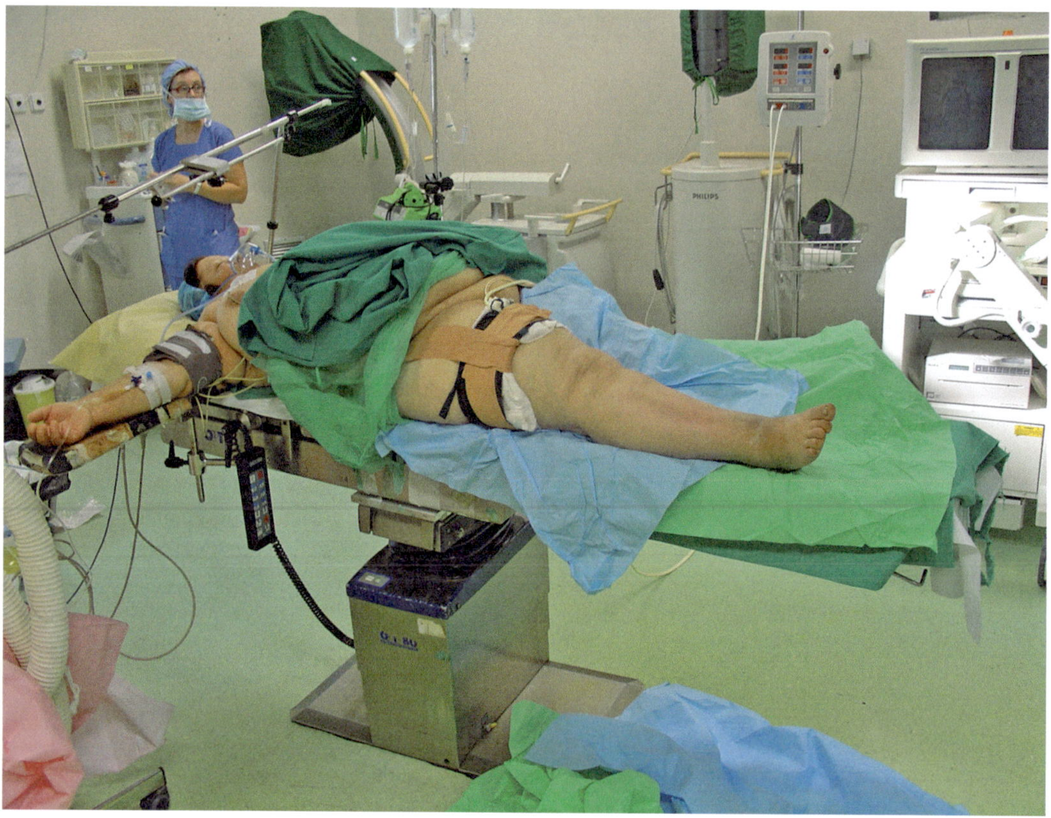

Fig. 7.3 Positioning and proper tourniquet placement is difficult but essential for the success of the operation

X-rays are needed to determine the correct mechanical axis and classify the total knee replacement as aligned or mal-aligned. Precise reconstruction with $0° \pm 3°$ deviation from the mechanical axis, even though other factors may also be important, would result in decreased stresses across the joint line, limiting polyethylene wear and enhancing implant durability [35, 36]. The detrimental effect of obesity in postoperative TKA limb alignment has been identified [37, 38]. Setting up the patient on the operating table and placing the tourniquet is always difficult and time-consuming and should be done with extreme caution, in such a way that surgical operation will not be compromised, especially by tourniquet loosening (Figs. 7.3 and 7.4). In morbidly obese patients especially, thick subcutaneous tissue makes surgical exposure of the joint difficult. Longer mid-lined incisions, eversion of the patella, and increased tourniquet length and width may be required (Figs. 7.5 and 7.6).

Limited vision and the difficulty in accurately positioning the cutting guides may result in a non-successful surgical operation with a poor long-term outcome for the patient [39]. Greater traction of the soft tissue envelope in order to achieve better visualization, longer operating time, poor vascularization of fatty tissue and reduced immune response are all factors that may increase infection rate by 6.7 times in patients with BMI >35 [40]. An anthropometric study in 2008 in severely and morbidly obese patients has attempted to identify those who pose greater surgical difficulties during TKA by proposing new indexes. A suprapatellar index (length of the extremity to be operated on with the circumference of the knee above the upper pole of the patella) below 1.6 is associated with greater surgical difficulty [41]. The femoral and tibial component, when using a femoral intramedullary guide and an extramedullary tibial guide, has the tendency to align in a more varus position in a

Fig. 7.4 Positioning and proper tourniquet placement is difficult but essential for the success of the operation

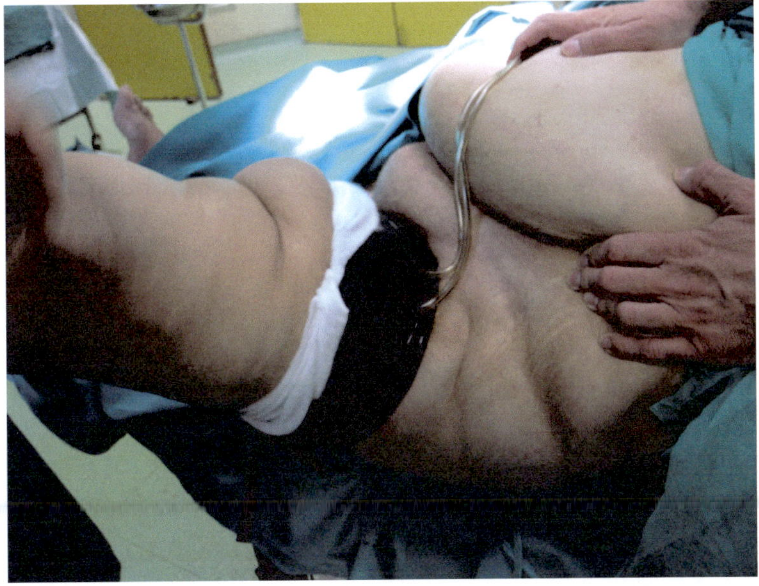

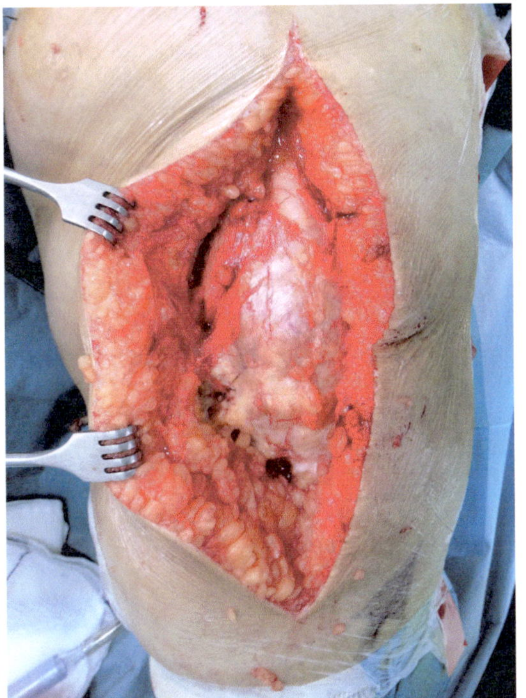

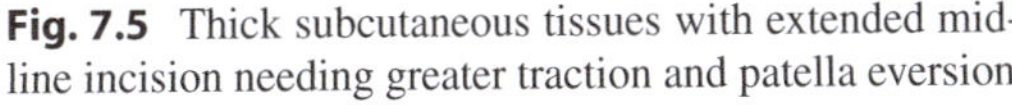

Fig. 7.5 Thick subcutaneous tissues with extended midline incision needing greater traction and patella eversion

Fig. 7.6 Thick subcutaneous tissues with extended midline incision needing greater traction and patella eversion

morbidly obese group [femoral component: 5.0° vs. 6.5° valgus (P<0.05), tibial component: 2.5° vs. 1.0° varus (P<0.05)] [42]. The use of an intramedullary tibial cutting guide makes surgical intervention easier by maintaining the anatomical axis of the tibia as a reference point for correct orientation and reduces operating time [43]. Some authors advocate the use of implant designs with minimal constraint such as posterior stabilized or in cases of severe instability a rotating hinge implant in order to achieve minimal constraint in morbidly obese patients [44]. They also advocate the use of implants with short tibial rods, thus increasing the contact area and reducing the load transferred under the tibial plate and, more recently, the use of trabecular metal tibial components which provide earlier anchoring to the bone [45].

Aseptic Loosening

Obesity has been implicated in aseptic loosening of the TKA components, a phenomenon that can be confirmed by the existence of radiolucent lines in the bone-implant interface. Spicer et al. [46] compared the clinical and radiographic results of 326 TKAs in patients with BMI >30 and 425 TKAs in patients with BMI <30. Although 10 year implant survivorship was similar and linear osteolysis was comparable, focal osteolysis rates were five times increased in the morbidly obese group [46]. Dewan et al. [47] compared 220 cemented tricompartmental TKAs (41 knees in patients with BMI >40) with a mean follow-up of 5.4 years and concluded that morbidly obese patients are 5.4 times more likely to develop patellar radiolucency, have poorer hamstring and quadriceps strength while more patellofemoral problems are encountered. During flexion, the force exerted on the patellofemoral joint is three times the body weight. In increased BMIs, the bigger stresses across the prosthetic joint may reach the threshold for starting patellar radiolucent lines to appear sooner. Studies have shown that the patella attaches to the intercondylar notch of the femoral component at 90–105°, depending on prosthesis design, reaching its highest peak of contact stresses. A decreased deep flexion which is observed in obese patients due to the mechanical stop caused by the greater amount of adipose tissue may enhance stresses responsible for producing patellofemoral symptoms, making ROM even more difficult beyond this point [47]. However, Cavaignac et al. [48] studied 212 unicompartmental knee arthroplasties

and found that 10-year survival rates were almost similar for patients with BMI >30 and BMI <30 (92 % vs 94 %) [48].

Weight Loss After TKA

Obesity and physical activity seem to be strongly correlated after TKA. There is a belief that decreased physical activity because of pain postoperatively will increase body weight. Booth showed in 2002 that only 18 % of obese people lose weight after joint replacement [39]. In 2005 Heisel, investigating weight change in 100 TJA, concluded that neither patients with normal BMI nor obese patients lost weight, while merely overweight patients gained a significant amount. Obesity should thus be treated as an independent disease that is not the result of inactivity due to arthritis [49]. Dowsey et al. in 2010 investigated 529 TKAs at 1 year postoperatively found a clinically significant weight loss of 5 % in 40 (12.6 %) of obese patients, while 107 (21 %) had gained weight [50].

Functional Outcome

Conflicting results emerge from the literature, when comparing functional outcome in obese and non-obese patients (Figs. 7.7 and 7.8). There is a need for better and more organized studies that distinguish the various BMI categories which would generate more comparable data to help reach a general consensus concerning the relationship of obesity and functional outcome. This is especially true for categories of BMI >30 and BMI <40, while data for morbidly obese patients are more conclusive, leading orthopedic surgeons to recommend the loss of excess BMI in these individuals for a better long term outcome. Stickles et al. [51] investigated the outcome of 1,011 TKAs 1 year postoperatively by measuring WOMAC (Western Ontario and McMaster Universities Osteoarthritis Index) and including the SF-36, and concluded that there were no differences between obese and non-obese patients regarding satisfaction and the decision to repeat surgery, but WOMAC scores were

Fig. 7.7 Bilateral TKA in morbidly obese patient with good functional outcome and knee flexion >90° on the right side

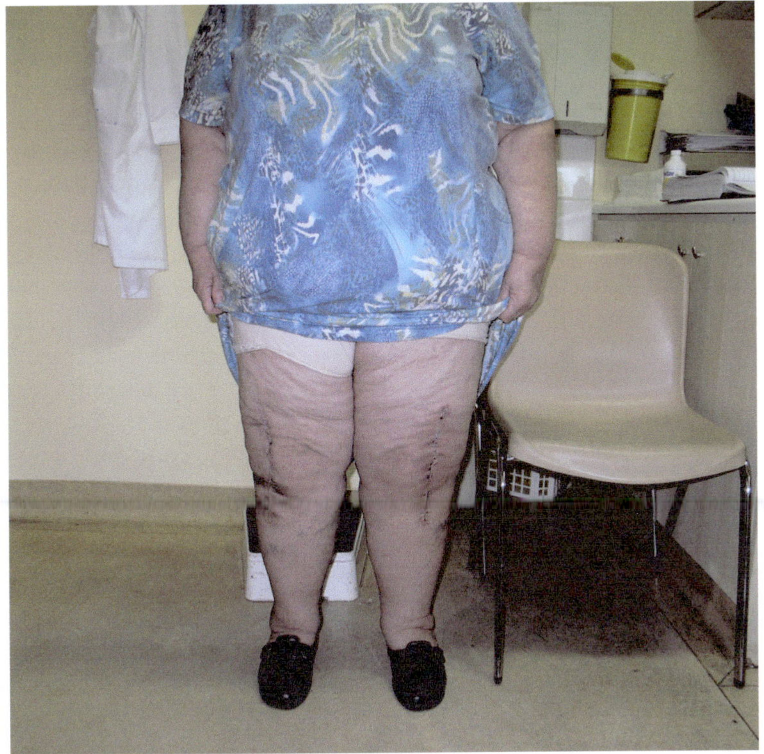

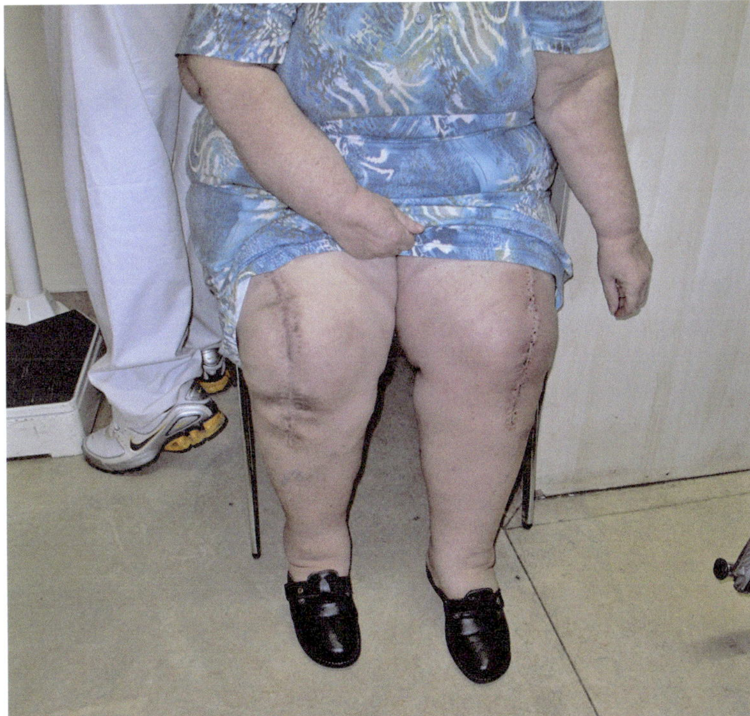

Fig. 7.8 Bilateral TKA in morbidly obese patient with good functional outcome and knee flexion >90° on the right side

lower for those with higher BMI. Also, increased body mass index was associated with more difficulty in ascending or descending stairs at 1 year [51]. In 2012 Colllins et al. [52] published their work on 445 consecutive primary TKAs prospectively followed up to 9 years comparing the clinical outcomes between non-obese and obese (BMI >30) patients. All groups showed great improvements with no significant differences in revision or implant survival rate after 9 years of follow-up. However, lower function scores were seen at all follow-up periods prior to 9 years in the highly obese subset (BMI >35) [52]. In a recent study of 535 cementless TKAs with a mean follow-up of 9 years Jackson et al. [53] found significantly lower HSS scores in obese individuals. In two studies published in 2004 Foran compared TKA outcomes between obese and non-obese patients. In the first study, the author analyzed 78 TKAs performed on obese patients over a 7 year period and found that this group had worse functional outcomes (measured according to the Knee Society Score) than non-obese controls, with the morbidly obese subgroup maintaining the lowest scores [54]. In the second study, the author conducted a 15-year follow-up of 30 non-cemented knee implants in matched case and control groups with no preoperative differences in functional status. At the end of follow-up the non-obese patients had a better Knee Society objective Score (89 vs. 81 in obese patients) [55]. Two studies by Núñez in 2007 [56] and 2009 [57] analysed the factors associated with worse functional outcomes following total knee arthroplasty. Follow-up over 3 and 7 years showed that WOMAC scores, especially on the pain scale, were worse among severely obese patients (BMI >35 kg/m^2) than in non-obese individuals. McElroy et al. [58], in a systematic review, concluded that a BMI >40 at a mean of 5-year follow-up, is associated with lower Knee Society Objective and Function Scores, lower implant survivorship and higher complication rates compared with patients with a BMI within normal range [58]. On the other hand, there are other investigations that do not find significant differences between obese and non-obese patients regarding the outcome of TKA. Singh et al. [59] found that there is no association between BMI and moderate-severe pain in a 5-year primary TKA, implying that obese patients should not be discouraged from total knee replacement. Hamoui et al. [60] compared 30 TKAs in 21 obese patients with 53 TKAs in 41 non-obese patients with a median follow-up of 11.3 years and concluded that KSS scores, osteolysis, radiolucency and revision rates were not statistically significant between these groups. In an even more recent study, 13,673 patients from the British National Joint Registry were assessed according to reported outcome related to TKA using the Oxford Knee Score and general health EuroQol 5D questionnaires. The improvements in patient reported outcome measures were similar, irrespective of BMI, although wound complications were significantly higher at a rate of 17 % in patients with a BMI between 40 and 60 [61]. Issa et al. [62] compared 210 knees in 174 obese patients (BMI >30) with a non-obese control group. There were no differences regarding implant survivorship (98.8 % vs 98.6 %) and the mean postoperative Knee Society Objective and Function scores (90 and 87 points vs 91 and 89 points). However, obese patients had higher complication rates (10.5 % vs 3.8 %) and achieved a significantly lower mean postoperative UCLA activity score [62].

Level of Activity

The level of activity after total knee arthroplasty is associated with patient specific factors such as age, body mass index, gender, presence of other joint replacement and comorbidities. The outcome is usually determined by pain, function and satisfaction and a standardized rating system has been developed for this purpose. The Knee Society (modified) clinical rating system and the University of California at Los Angeles (UCLA) activity rating scale are the ones mainly used.

Biomechanics

Factors influencing polyethylene wear are material properties, thickness of the component, length of stay, load transmitted and contact area. Repeated high loads and cyclic stressing may cause PE fatigue failure leading to earlier wear. The load is highly dependent on body mass index and level of activity. Biomechanical studies have shown that transmitted compressive forces through the tibiofemoral component are: for downhill walking eight times, stair descent six times, and level walking 3.5 times the Body Weight. Slow jogging is eight to nine times and fast jogging more than ten times the Body Weight [63]. The knee is flexed more during the stance phase of jogging (15–45°) than during walking (5–25°) resulting in a fivefold increase in the flexion moment around the knee, making jogging a high-impact force generally not recommended as a post TKA exercise [64].

Age and Activity Level

Implant durability in correlation with patient's age and level of activity has been for many years a matter of discussion, with conflicting data in the literature. Younger patients have been considered to be more active with increased life expectancy, which in turn may lead to high mechanical joint loads and earlier polyethylene wear, component breakage and prosthetic loosening. Implant failure is usually addressed via a revision procedure. There are studies with a small number of subjects younger than 55 years treated with TKA that show an implant survival rate of more than 96 % at 10 years and 87 % at 18 years [65–67]. In a meta-analysis of 13 studies Keeney et al. [68] calculated the initial 6–10 year survival rates as 90.6–99 % and the 15 year survival rates as 85–96.5 % in patients <55 years of age. Heyse et al. [69] reported that the 10 year survivorship of TKA was 95 % and the 20 year survivorship 82 % in patients with juvenile idiopathic arthritis (mean age 30 years). Whether the implant is cemented or cementless does not seem to affect the final result, with femoral component survival rate of 100 % at 17 years, and tibial component survival rate of 100 and 98.7 % respectively at 17 years [70]. UKAs seem to have a better outcome in younger patients with estimated survivorship of 96.5 % at 10 years [71]. Scores of satisfaction, range of motion and ability to kneel in patients under the age of 55 treated with UKA are also higher than those treated with TKA, while the opposite occurs at ages over 65 [72]. Mont compared high and low activity patients at a minimum follow-up of 4 years (mean 7 years) and found no effect of low to moderate impact sports regarding overall satisfaction, rate of revision and clinical and radiographic results [73]. On the contrary, a study by Kim et al. [74] suggested that younger age seems to be the major determinant in polyethylene wear, while infection and aseptic loosening remain secondary causes. Meehan et al. [75] concluded that patients younger than 50 years old had almost 2.5 times (1.36 % vs 3.49) greater risk of mechanical failure rather than periprosthetic infection, and 4.7 times higher revision rates due to aseptic loosening compared with patients older than 65 years of age. Julin et al. [76] evaluated 32,019 TKAs from the Finnish Arthroplasty Register and concluded that after 5 years the implant survival rate was 92 % for patients aged <55 compared to 97 % in patients >65 years of age. Harrysson et al. [77] analyzed revision rates in 21,761 patients older than 60 years and 1,434 patients younger than 60 years and the cumulative revision rates at 8.5 years were almost double in the younger group (13 % vs 6 %). Dy et al. [78] evaluated 310,995 TKAs at 10 years postoperatively and concluded that patients 50–75 years of age had a lower revision rate than patients younger than 50 years (hazard ratio 0.47). Lavernia et al. [79] studied 28 autopsy retrieved polyethylene specimens and suggested that more creep and deformation was strongly associated with increased levels of activity. Kurtz et al. [80] projected the demand for primary and revision TKR in 2030 and concluded that in 340,000 revisions by that time 62 % will be done in the age group less than 65 years. In any case, though, the survivorship of the prosthetic design should be based on patient functional performance rather than age, because younger age does not always correlate with high activity levels [81]. In order to achieve implant durability, constant progress is being made in the improvement of bearing materials and surgical techniques in order to lower polyethylene stresses. For this purpose cross-linking

PE, improved femoral component surface finish, better modular tibial locking mechanisms, and the use of mobile bearing TKA designs have been proposed as materials and designs that will reduce contact stresses and loads transmitted to the fixation interface [82].

Work Activities

Many patients undergoing TKA, especially the younger and more active (less than 60 years old), look forward to starting or returning to presurgery activities. Employment positively affects patient's mental health by increasing individual satisfaction and maintaining the sense of fulfillment and purpose. The time to return to work depends on the physical demands of the patient's job. The recovery time for lighter jobs averages 7 weeks and for heavier, demanding jobs can reach 11 weeks. After 1–3 years with a TKA, the percentage of patients with more demanding jobs still working reaches 91 % [83].

Athletic Activities

Primary and revision total knee replacement have been shown to be extremely effective in pain relief, the key element that enables the elderly to participate in sport and daily living activities, so that they can maintain good health and perhaps prolong life expectancy [84]. Functional outcome is defined as the range of motion, with a minimum of 90° flexion being essential for common daily activities such as climbing and descending stairs and rising from a chair. Variables that affect ROM are preoperative knee flexion, diagnosis, BMI, age, surgical technique, implant design and rehabilitation. Kneeling and squatting seem to be the most difficult activities for osteoarthritic knees and postsurgical improvement in this parameter can boost patient satisfaction [85–87]. The literature shows that unicompartmental knee arthroplasty has better results in terms of kneeling ability when compared with TKA or patellofemoral replacement (PFR) [88]. A study by Ries showed improvement of cardiovascular fitness, with increase in the duration of exercise and maximum workload, in patients undergoing total knee arthroplasty compared with a nonsurgically treated control group [89]. Certainly, there are some rules that patients should follow in order to have a better and longer-lasting outcome. The risk of wear and osteolysis leading to implant failure and aseptic loosening in higher activity levels and high impact sports should be noted. Painless range of motion with good quadriceps and hamstrings muscle function must be restored before participation in sports in order to avoid possible injuries. Table 7.2 shows the recommended sporting activities as described by Swanson et al. [90]. Generally, there is a consensus of more than 95 % among surgeons who recommend (without limitation) walking on even surfaces, climbing stairs, bicycling on even surfaces, swimming and golfing for both THA and TKA. On the contrary, jogging, sprinting and skiing on difficult terrains are strongly discouraged. Nevertheless, there is more flexibility for restrictions in THA concerning walking up stairs, jogging or playing tennis [90]. Even though studies in the literature have shown promising results for participation in athletics after THA, the outcomes after TKA are not so encouraging. Brander et al. [91] showed at a mean follow-up of 25 months in subjects 80 years or older that the ability to walk five blocks increased from 2 to 50 %, while Zahiri et al. [92] showed that walking activity level decreases by 34 % in patients >60 years old. Huch et al. [93] analyzed all sport activities preoperatively and 5 years after TKA in 300 patients with age less than 74 years and found a decrease of 8 %, a percentage that can be explained by increasing age, pain in the operated knee, surgeon's instructions to avoid vigorous activities and patient's rejection of the artificial joint. In the same study, more than 16 % of patients with TKA reported pain at follow-up [93]. Dahm et al. [94] reviewed 1,206 patients who underwent primary TKA with the PFC or Sigma posterior stabilized (DePuy) implant at a mean of 5.7 years (99 % of them with patella resurfacing) and found that 91 % reported satisfaction with their activity level while differences between men and women and age were not statistically significant. Bradbury

Table 7.2 Recommended sport activities for patients with a TKA

Recommended-allowed	Allowed with experience	Not recommended	No conclusion
Low-impact aerobics	Road bicycling	Racquetball	Fencing
Stationary bicycling	Canoeing	Squash	Roller blade/inline skating
Bowling	Hiking	Rock climbing	Downhill skiing
Golf	Rowing	Soccer	Weight lifting
Dancing	Cross-country skiing	Singles tennis	
Horseback riding	Stationary skiing	Volleyball	
Croquet	Speed walking	Football	
Walking	Tennis	Gymnastics	
Swimming	Weight machines	Lacrosse	
Shooting	Ice skating	Hockey	
Shuffleboard		Basketball	
Horseshoes		Handball	
		Jogging	

et al. [95] reviewed 208 TKAs, with 199 of them being uncemented, 5 years after surgery. Patients who participated in sports prior to surgery increased their athletic activities by 65 %. He also found that returning to low impact activities such as bowling was more likely (91 %) than returning to high impact activities such as tennis (20 %). Trying to compare unilateral versus simultaneous bilateral knee arthroplasties, even though the low number of cases (20) may not be sufficient to draw a conclusion, he found that 75 % returned to previous sports activities. Pain relief from both operated knees may be one explanation [95]. Hopper et al. [96] compared 76 total versus 34 unicompartmental knee arthroplasties, according to participation in low-impact athletic activities, preoperatively and 22 months postoperatively. From the 55 and 30 sport participants in the TKA and UKA group accordingly, only 35 (64 %) in the TKA and 29 (97 %) in the UKA group continued their sporting activities. It also seemed that patients with UKA returned earlier to sport and felt that surgery increased their sporting abilities [96]. Another study, reported by Naal et al. [97], on 77 unicompartmental arthroplasties using the Preservation prosthesis (DePuy), found that 73 (95 %) of patients returned to pre-surgery athletic activities, mainly hiking, cycling and swimming, with almost 70 % of them returning less than 6 months from the operation.

References

1. Kurtz SM, Ong K, Lau E, et al. Projections of primary and revision hip and knee arthroplasty in the United States from 2005–2030. J Bone Joint Surg Am. 2007;89A:780.
2. Font-Rodriguez DE, Scuderi GR, Insall JN. Survivorship of cemented total knee arthroplasty. Clin Orthop. 1997;345:79–86.
3. Roberts VI, Esler CN, Harper WM. 15-year follow-up study of 4606 primary total knee replacements. J Bone Joint Surg Br. 2007;89B:1452–6.
4. Tsao AK, Jones LC, Lewallen DG, Implant Wear Symposium 2007 Clinical Work Group. What patient and surgical factors contribute to implant wear and osteolysis in total joint arthroplasty? J Am Acad Orthop Surg. 2008;S1:S7–13.
5. Flegal KM, Carroll MD, Kit BK, et al. Prevalence of obesity and trends in the distribution of body mass index among US adults, 1999–2010. JAMA. 2012;307:491.
6. Finucane MM, Stevens GA, Cowan MJ, et al. National, regional, and global trends in body mass index since 1980: systematic analysis of health examination surveys and epidemiological studies with 960 country-years and 9.1 million participants. Lancet. 2011;377:557–67.
7. Bourne R, Mukhi S, Zhu N, et al. Role of obesity on the risk for total hip or knee arthroplasty. Clin Orthop. 2007;465:185.
8. Mork PJ, Holtermann A, Nilsen TIL. Effect of body mass index and physical exercise on risk of knee and hip osteoarthritis: longitudinal data from the Norwegian HUNT Study. J Epidemiol Community Health. 2012;66:678.
9. Grotle M, Hagen KB, Natvig B, et al. Obesity and osteoarthritis in knee, hip and/or hand: an epidemiological study in the general population with 10 years follow-up. BMC Musculoskelet Dis. 2008;9:132.

10. Lohmander LS, de Verdier MG, Rollof J, et al. Incidence of severe knee and hip osteoarthritis in relation to different measures of body mass: a population-based prospective cohort study. Ann Rheum Dis. 2009;68:490.

11. Wendelboe AM, Hegmann KT, Biggs JJ, et al. Relationships between body mass indices and surgical replacements of knee and hip joints. Am J Prev Med. 2003;25:290.

12. Felson DT, Anderson JJ, Naimark A, et al. Obesity and knee osteoarthritis. Ann Intern Med. 1988;109:18.

13. Coggon D, Reading I, Croft P, McLaren M, Barrett D, Cooper C. Knee osteoarthritis and obesity. Int J Obes Relat Metab Disord. 2001;25:622–7.

14. Odum SM, Springer BD, Dennos AC, Fehring TK. National obesity trends in total knee arthroplasty. J Arthroplasty. 2013;28(8 S):148–51.

15. Gandhi R, Wasserstein D, Razak F, et al. BMI independently predicts younger age at hip and knee replacement. Obes J. 2010;18:2362.

16. Changulani M, Kalairajah Y, Peel T, Field RE. Relationship between obesity and the age at which hip and knee replacement is undertaken. J Bone Joint Surg Br. 2008;90B:360–3.

17. Felson DT, Zhang Y, Anthony JM, Naimark A, Anderson JJ. Weight loss reduces the risk for symptomatic knee osteoarthritis in women. The Framingham Study. Ann Int Med. 1992;116:535–9.

18. Messier SP, Gutekunst DJ, Davis C, DeVita P. Weight loss reduces knee joint loads in overweight and obese older adults with knee osteoarthritis. Arthritis Rheum. 2005;52:2026–32.

19. Guilak F, Fermor B, Keefe FJ, Kraus VB, Olson SA, Pisetsky DS, et al. The role of biomechanics and inflammation in cartilage injury and repair. Clin Orthop. 2004;4:17–26.

20. Pottie P, Presle N, Terlain B, et al. Obesity and osteoarthritis: more complex than predicted! Ann Rheum Dis. 2006;65:17–26.

21. Gupta RM, Parvizi J, Hanssen AD, et al. Postoperative complications in patients with obstructive sleep apnea syndrome undergoing hip or knee replacement: a case – control study. Mayo Clin Proc. 2001;76:897.

22. Schwarzkopf R, Thompson SL, Adwar SJ, et al. Postoperative complication rates in the "super-obese" hip and knee arthroplasty population. J Arthroplasty. 2012;27:397.

23. Gupta S, Kapoor S. Body adiposity index: its relevance and validity in assessing body fatness of adults. ISRN Obes. 2014;22:243–94.

24. Freedman DS, Thornton JC, Pi-Sunyer FX, Heymsfield SB, Wang J, Pierson Jr RN, Blanck HM, Gallagher D. The body adiposity index (hip circumference/height(1.5)) is not a more accurate measure of adiposity than is BMI, waist circumference, or hip circumference. Obesity. 2012;20:2438–44.

25. Suchanek P, Kralova Lesna I, Mengerova O, Mrazkova J, Lanska V, Stavek P. Which index best correlates with body fat mass: BAI, BMI, waist or WHR? Neuro Endocrinol Lett. 2012;33:78.

26. Jämsen E, Nevalainen P, Eskelinen A, et al. Obesity, diabetes, and preoperative hyperglycemia as predictors of periprosthetic joint infection: a single-center analysis of 7181 primary hip and knee replacements for osteoarthritis. J Bone Joint Surg Am. 2012;94A: e101.

27. Malinzak RA, Ritter MA, Berend ME, et al. Morbidly obese, diabetic, younger, and unilateral joint arthroplasty patients have elevated total joint arthroplasty infection rates. J Arthroplasty. 2009;24(6 S):78–82.

28. Winiarsky R, Barth P, Lotke P. Total knee arthroplasty in morbidly obese patients. J Bone Joint Surg Am. 1998;80A:1770–4.

29. Dowsey MM, Choong PF. Obese diabetic patients are at substantial risk for deep infection after primary TKA. Clin Orthop. 2009;467:1577–81.

30. Patel AD, Albrizio M. Relationship of body mass index to early complications in knee replacement surgery. Arch Orthop Trauma Surg. 2008;128:5–9.

31. Chesney D, Sales J, Elton R, Brenkel IJ. Infection after knee arthroplasty a prospective study of 1509 cases. J Arthroplasty. 2008;23:355–9.

32. Pulido L, Ghanem E, Joshi A, Purtill JJ, Parvizi J. Periprosthetic joint infection: the incidence, timing, and predisposing factors. Clin Orthop. 2008;466:1710–5.

33. Bordini B, Stea S, Cremonini S, Viceconti M, De Palma R, Toni A. Relationship between obesity and early failure of total knee prostheses. BMC Musculoskelet Disord. 2009;10:29.

34. Gino MMJ, Kerkhoffs MD, Servien E, Dunn W, Dahm D, Jos A, Bramer M, Haverkamp D. The influence of obesity on the complication rate and outcome of total knee arthroplasty a meta-analysis and systematic literature review. J Bone Joint Surg Am. 2012; 94A:1839–44.

35. Parratte S, Pagnano MW, Trousdale RT, et al. Effect of postoperative mechanical axis alignment on the fifteen-year survival of modern, cemented total knee replacements. J Bone Joint Surg Am. 2010;92A:2143.

36. Werner FW, Ayers DC, Maletsky LP, et al. The effect of valgus/varus malalignment on load distribution in total knee replacements. J Biomech. 2005;38:349.

37. Ritter MA, Davis KE, Meding JB, et al. The effect of alignment and BMI on failure of total knee replacement. J Bone Joint Surg Am. 2011;93A:1588.

38. Estes CS, Schmidt KJ, McLemore R, Spangehl MJ, Clarke HD. Effect of body mass index on limb alignment after total knee arthroplasty. J Arthroplasty. 2013;28(8 S):101–5.

39. Booth RE. Total knee arthroplasty in the obese patient: tips and quips. J Arthroplasty. 2002;17(4 S):69.

40. Namba RS, Paxton L, Fithian DC, Stone ML. Obesity and perioperative morbidity in total hip and total knee arthroplasty patients. J Arthroplasty. 2005;20(3S): 46–50.

41. Lozano L, Núñez M, Segur JM, et al. Relationship between knee anthropometry and surgical time in total knee arthroplasty in severely morbidly obese patients. A new prognostic index of surgical difficulty. Obes Surg. 2008;18:1149–53.

42. Krushell RJ, Fingeroth RJ. Primary total knee arthroplasty in morbidly obese patients: a 5- to 14-year follow-up study. J Arthroplasty. 2007;22(2S):77.

43. Lozano L, Segur JM, Maculé F, et al. Intramedullary versus extramedullary tibial cutting guide in severely obese patients undergoing total knee replacement. Randomized study of 70 patients with Body Mass Index >35 kg/m². Obes Surg. 2008;18:1599–604.

44. Lozano LM, López V, Ríos J, Popescu D, Torner P, Castillo F, Maculé F. Better outcomes in severe and morbid obese patients (BMI >35 kg/m²) in primary Endo-Model rotating-hinge total knee arthroplasty. Sci World J. 2012;2012:249391.

45. Lozano LM, Núñez M, Sastre S, Popescu D. Total knee arthroplasty in the context of severe and morbid obesity in adults. Open Obes J. 2012;4:1–10.

46. Spicer DD, Pomeroy DL, Badenhausen WE, et al. Body mass index as a predictor of outcome in total knee replacement. Int Orthop. 2001;25:246.

47. Dewan A, Bertolusso R, Karastinos A, et al. Implant durability and knee function after total knee arthroplasty in the morbidly obese patient. J Arthroplasty. 2009;24(1 S):89.

48. Cavaignac E, Lafontan V, Reina N, Pailhé R, Wargny M, Laffosse JM, Chiron P. Obesity has no adverse effect on the outcome of unicompartmental knee replacement at a minimum follow-up of seven years. Bone Joint J. 2013;95B:1064–8.

49. Heisel C, Silva M, dela Rosa MA, Schmalzried TP. The effects of lower-extremity total joint replacement for arthritis on obesity. Orthopedics. 2005;28:157–9.

50. Dowsey MM, Liew D, Stoney JD, Choong PF. The impact of preoperative obesity on weight change and outcome in total knee replacement. A prospective study of 529 consecutive patients. J Bone Joint Surg Br. 2010;92B:513–20.

51. Stickles B, Phillips L, Brox WT, et al. Defining the relationship between obesity and total joint arthroplasty. Obes Res. 2001;9:219.

52. Collins RA, Walmsley PJ, Amin AK, Brenkel IJ, Clayton RA. Does obesity influence clinical outcome at nine years following total knee replacement? J Bone Joint Surg Br. 2012;94B:1351–5.

53. Jackson M, Sexton S, Walter W, et al. The impact of obesity on the mid-term outcome of cementless total knee replacement. J Bone Joint Surg Br. 2009;91B:1044.

54. Foran JRH, Mont MA, Rajadhyaksha AD, et al. Total knee arthroplasty in obese patients: a comparison with a matched control group. J Arthroplasty. 2004;19:817.

55. Foran JRH, Michael AM, Etienne G, Jones LC, Hungerford S. The outcome of total knee arthroplasty in obese patients. J Bone Joint Surg Am. 2004;86A:1609–15.

56. Núñez M, Núñez E, del Val JL. Health-related quality of life and costs in patients with osteoarthritis on waiting list for total knee replacement. Osteoarthritis Cartilage. 2007;15:1001–7.

57. Núñez M, Lozano L, Núñez E, et al. Total knee replacement and health-related quality of life: factors influencing long-term outcomes. Arthritis Rheum. 2009;61:1062–9.

58. McElroy MJ, Pivec R, Issa K, Harwin SF, Mont MA. The effects of obesity and morbid obesity on outcomes in TKA. J Knee Surg. 2013;26:83–8.

59. Singh JA, Gabriel SE, Lewallen DG. Higher body mass index is not associated with worse pain outcomes after primary or revision total knee arthroplasty. J Arthroplasty. 2011;26:366.

60. Hamoui N, Kantor S, Vince K. Crookes PF long-term outcome of total knee replacement: does obesity matter? Obes Surg. 2006;16:35–8.

61. Baker P, Petheram T, Jameson S, et al. The association between body mass index and the outcome of total knee arthroplasty. J Bone Joint Surg Am. 2012;94:1501–8.

62. Issa K, Pivec R, Kapadia BH, Shah T, Harwin SF, Delanois RE, Mont MA. Does obesity affect the outcomes of primary total knee arthroplasty? J Knee Surg. 2013;26:89–94.

63. Kuster MS, Wood GA, Stachowiak GW, Gatchter A. Joint load considerations in total knee replacement. J Bone Joint Surg Br. 1997;79B:109–13.

64. D'Lima DD, Steklov N, Patil S, Colwell Jr CW. The Mark Coventry award: in vivo knee forces during recreation and exercise after knee arthroplasty. Clin Orthop. 2008;466:2605–11.

65. Diduch D, Insall J, Scott W, Scuderi GR, Font-Rodrigues D. Total knee replacement in young, active patients: long-term follow-up and functional outcome. J Bone Joint Surg Am. 1997;79A:575–82.

66. Duffy G, Trousdale R, Stuart M. Total knee arthroplasty in patients 55 years old or younger: 10- to 17-year results. Clin Orthop. 1998;356:22–7.

67. Ranawat C, Padgett D, Ohashi Y. Total knee arthroplasty for patients younger than 55 years. Clin Orthop. 1989;248:27–33.

68. Keeney JA, Eunice S, Pashos G, Wright RW, Clohisy JC. What is the evidence for total knee arthroplasty in young patients?: a systematic review of the literature. Clin Orthop. 2011;469:574–83.

69. Heyse TJ, Ries MD, Bellemans J, Goodman SB, Scott RD, Wright TM, Lipman JD, Schwarzkopf R, Figgie MP. Total knee arthroplasty in patients with juvenile idiopathic arthritis. Clin Orthop. 2014;472:147–54.

70. Kim YH, Park JW, Lim HM, Park ES. Cementless and cemented total knee arthroplasty in patients younger than fifty five years. Which is better? Int Orthop. 2014;38:297–303.

71. Biswas D, Van Thiel GS, Wetters NG, Pack BJ, Berger RA, Della Valle CJ. Medial unicompartmental knee arthroplasty in patients less than 55 years old: minimum of two years of follow-up. J Arthroplasty. 2014;29:101–5.

72. Von Keudell A, Sodha S, Collins J, Minas T, Fitz W, Gomoll AH. Patient satisfaction after primary total and unicompartmental knee arthroplasty: an age-dependent analysis. Knee. 2014;21:180–4.

73. Mont MA, Marker DR, Seyler TM, Gordon N, Hungerford DS, Jones LC. Knee arthroplasties have similar results in high- and low-activity patients. Clin Orthop. 2007;460:165–73.

74. Kim KT, Lee S, Ko DO, Seo BS, Jung WS, Chang BK. Causes of failure after total knee arthroplasty in osteoarthritis patients 55 years of age or younger. Knee Surg Relat Res. 2014;26:13–9.

75. Meehan JP, Danielsen B, Kim SH, Jamali AA, White RH. Younger age is associated with a higher risk of early periprosthetic joint infection and aseptic mechanical failure after total knee arthroplasty. J Bone Joint Surg Am. 2014;96A:529–35.

76. Jaakko J, Jämsen E, Puolakka T, Konttinen YT, Moilanen T. Younger age increases the risk of early prosthesis failure following primary total knee replacement for osteoarthritis. A follow-up study of 32,019 total knee replacements in the Finnish Arthroplasty Register. Acta Orthop Scand. 2010;81:413–9.

77. Harrysson OL, Robertsson O, Nayfeh JF. Higher cumulative revision rate of knee arthroplasties in younger patients with osteoarthritis. Clin Orthop. 2004;421:162–8.

78. Dy CJ, Marx RG, Bozic KJ, Pan TJ, Padgett DE, Lyman S. Risk factors for revision within 10 years of total knee arthroplasty. Clin Orthop. 2014;472:1198–207.

79. Lavernia CJ, Sierra RJ, Hungerford DS, Krackow KLavernia CJ, Sierra RJ, Hungerford DS, Krackow K. Activity level and wear in total knee arthroplasty: a study of autopsy retrieved specimens. J Arthroplasty. 2001;16:446–53.

80. Kurtz SM, Lau E, Ong K, Zhao K, Kelly M, Bozic KJ. Future young patient demand for primary and revision joint replacement: national projections from 2010 to 2030. Clin Orthop. 2009;467:2606–12.

81. Keeney JA, Nunley RM, Wright RW, Barrack RL, Clohisy JC. Are younger patients undergoing TKAs appropriately characterized as active? Clin Orthop. 2014;472:1210–6.

82. Dennis DA. Trends in total knee arthroplasty. Orthopedics. 2006;29(9S):13–6.

83. Lombardi AV, Nunley RM, Berend KR, Ruh EL, Clohisy JC, Hamilton WG, Della Valle CJ, Parvizi J, Barrack RL. Do patients return to work after total knee arthroplasty? Clin Orthop. 2014;472:138–46.

84. Singh JA, Lewallen DG. Patient-level improvements in pain and activities of daily living after total knee arthroplasty. Rheumatology. 2014;53:313–20.

85. Weiss JM, Noble PC, Conditt MA, Kohl HW, Roberts S, Cook KF, Gordon MJ, Mathis KB. What functional activities are important to patients with knee replacements? Clin Orthop. 2002;404:172–88.

86. Hassaballa MA, Porteous AJ, Newman JH, Rogers CA. Can knees kneel? Kneeling ability after total, unicompartmental and patellofemoral knee arthroplasty. Knee. 2003;10:155–60.

87. Kim TK, Kwon SK, Kang YG, Chang CB, Seong SC. Functional disabilities and satisfaction after total knee arthroplasty in female Asian patients. J Arthroplasty. 2010;25:458–64.

88. Hassaballa MA, Porteous AJ, Learmonth ID. Functional outcomes after different types of knee arthroplasty: kneeling ability versus descending stairs. Med Sci Monit. 2007;13:77–81.

89. Ries MD, Philbin EF, Groff GD, Sheesley KA, Richman JA, Lynch F. Improvement in cardiovascular fitness after total knee arthroplasty. J Bone Joint Surg Am. 1996;78A:1696–701.

90. Swanson EA, Schmalzried TP, Dorey FJ. Activity recommendations after total hip and knee arthroplasty: a survey of the American Association for Hip and Knee Surgeons. J Arthroplasty. 2009;24:120–6.

91. Brander VA, Malhotra S, Jet J, Heinemann AW, Stulberg SD. Outcome of hip and knee arthroplasty in persons aged 80 years and older. Clin Orthop. 1997;345:67–78.

92. Zahiri CA, Schmalzried TP, Szuszczewicz ES, Amstutz HC. Assessing activity in joint replacement patients. J Arthroplasty. 1998;13:890–5.

93. Huch K, Muller KAC, Sturmer T, Brenner H, Puhl W, Gunther KP. Sports activities 5 years after total knee or hip arthroplasty: the Ulm Osteoarthritis Study. Ann Rheum Dis. 2005;64:1715–20.

94. Dahm DL, Barnes SA, Harrington JR, Sayeed SA, Berry DJ. Patient-reported activity level after total knee arthroplasty. J Arthroplasty. 2008;23:401.

95. Bradbury N, Borton D, Spoo G, Cross MJ. Participation in sports after total knee replacement. Am J Sports Med. 1998;26:530–5.

96. Hopper GP, Leach WJ. Participation in sporting activities following knee replacement: total versus unicompartmental. Knee Surg Sports Trauma Arhosc. 2008;16:973–9.

97. Naal FD, Fischer M, Preuss A, Goldhahn J, von Knoch F, Preiss S, Munzinger U, Drobny T. Return to sports and recreational activity after unicompartmental knee arthroplasty. Am J Sports Med. 2007;35:1688.

Long Term Clinical Outcome of Total Knee Arthroplasty. The Effect of the Severity of Deformity

Panagiotis Megas, Anna Konstantopoulou, and Antonios Kouzelis

Introduction

Total knee arthroplasty (TKA) is the gold standard for treatment of knee osteoarthritis demonstrating excellent long term results in terms of functional outcome and revision rates [1–3]. Joint deformity is due to a combination of factors such as extra or intra articular deformity, bone destruction and defects, soft tissue contractures and ligamentous imbalance. When bone deformity is located in the femoral and/or tibial metaphysis it can usually be addressed in a one stage TKA procedure (Fig. 8.1), while diaphyseal deformities are often reconstructed with staged procedures (Fig. 8.2). Soft tissue imbalance combined with severe deformity renders TKA a rather challenging procedure, demanding clear knowledge of the structures which stabilize the knee joint and surgical experience in reconstructing difficult cases. Proper joint alignment and ligament balance enhance implant longevity and are associated with rewarding functional outcomes [4, 5].

In this review, the effect of the severity of the arthritic knee deformity on the long term performance of TKA is evaluated.

P. Megas, MD, DSc (✉) • A. Konstantopoulou, MD
A. Kouzelis, MD, DSc
Department of Orthopaedics and Traumatology,
University Hospital of Patras,
Rion GR-26504, Greece
e-mail: panmegas@gmail.com

Knee Joint Deformity

Malalignment in the frontal plane is a common manifestation of knee arthritis, and it remains uncertain whether it is a cause or a consequence of the degenerative pathway [6]. Knee joint alignment, as determined by the mechanical axis, can be measured on long full limb radiographs as the angle formed by the intersection of the line connecting the centers of the femoral head and intercondylar notch (femoral mechanical axis) with the line connecting the centers of tibial spines and the ankle talus (tibial mechanical axis) [7, 8]. In the neutral knee, the two axes should be collinear, forming the load bearing axis, where the knee center should be located [9]. A knee can be described as being varus when alignment is >0° in the varus direction, and valgus when alignment is >0° in the valgus direction [7]. An alternative way of indicating varus and valgus malalignment on radiographic imaging is using angle values <180° and >180° respectively [6]. Although the use of the mechanical axis is considered the gold standard, alignment on the frontal plane can be safely determined by the anatomical axis using a pre-existing plain radiograph of the knee, or by certain clinical measures, avoiding unnecessary radiation exposure and facilitating assessment for researchers and clinicians [6]. Increased valgus deformity poses the risk of patellofemoral osteoarthritis progression [10]. Fixed flexion deformity is another common angular deformity seen

© Springer-Verlag London 2015
T. Karachalios (ed.), *Total Knee Arthroplasty: Long Term Outcomes*,
DOI 10.1007/978-1-4471-6660-3_8

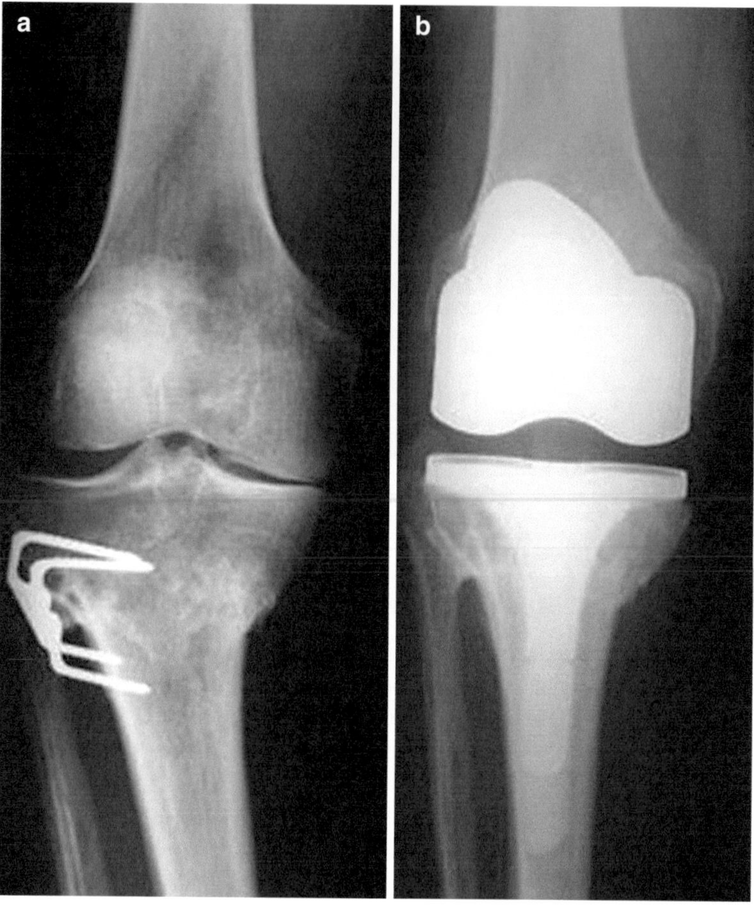

Fig. 8.1 Varus osteoarthritic knee with tibial metaphyseal deformity, (**a**) preoperative radiograph, (**b**) postoperative radiograph following single stage TKA

in knees with indications for TKA. The lack of full knee extension results in greater quadriceps contraction, altered gait kinematics and overloading of the contralateral limb [11].

Varus Deformity

Varus deformity is the most common angular contraction of the knee joint indicated for primary TKA [6, 12] (Fig. 8.3). Arthritic knees with varus deformity are characterized by cartilage and/or bone loss (mainly tibia) in the medial compartment. As a result of the angulation, soft tissues and ligaments of the medial side undergo contracture and must be released in order to achieve neutral limb alignment in TKA [12]. Concerning the definition of severe varus deformity, there is a lack of consistency within the available literature.

Some authors define severely varus deformed arthritic knees as bearing a femoral mechanical axis/tibial mechanical axis angle of 8° or at least 10–12° in varus [8, 13, 14]. Other studies use angles of >15° or 20° [15–18]. These variations possibly reflect the authors' decision to divide the available patient population into subgroups, in order to make assumptions related to the preoperative joint deformity. Angulations of more than 20° around the joint metaphysis usually require a procedure additional to TKA to efficiently restore limb alignment [4]. According to Engh [5], the choice of ligament release technique depends on the severity of varus deformity. Almost all surgeons are familiar with soft tissue release of the medial side of the proximal tibia. Joint line release with sub periosteal fractional detachment of the superficial and deep medial collateral ligaments has proven successful for mild to moderate varus

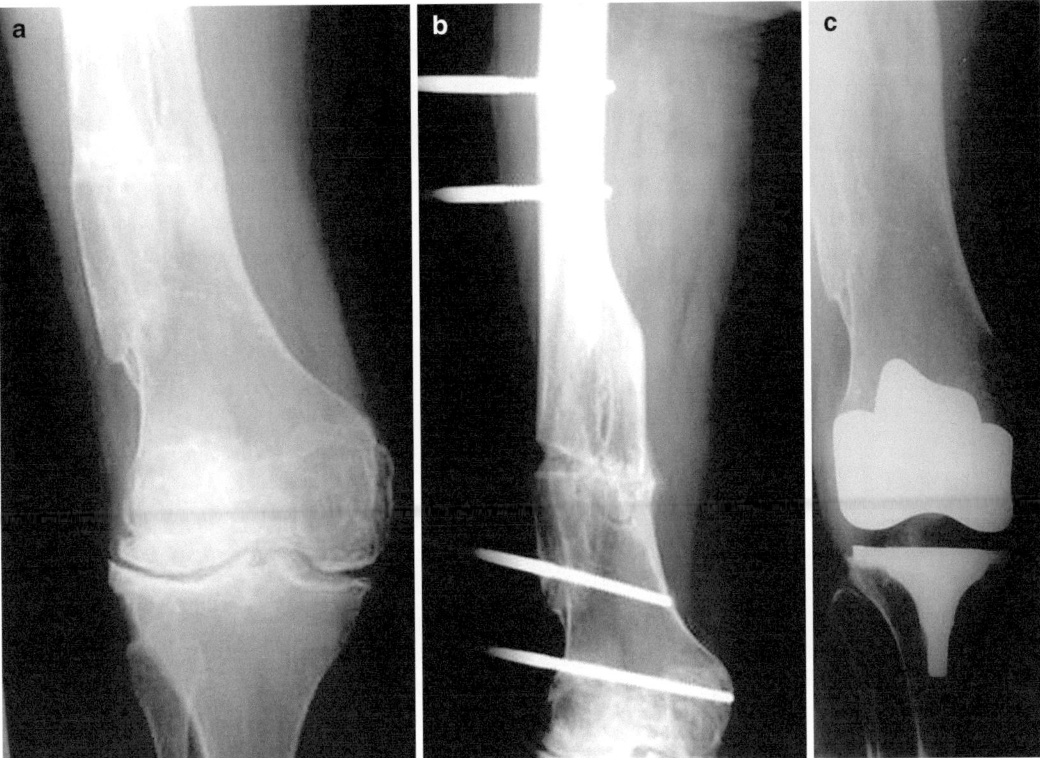

Fig. 8.2 Valgus osteoarthtitic knee with femoral diaphyseal deformity, (**a**) preoperative radiograph, (**b**) radiograph showing extraarticular corrective osteotomy, (**c**) postoperative radiograph following staged TKA

deformity. When it comes to severe varus deformity with fixed flexion contraction, an epicondylar osteotomy to release the collateral ligaments from the femur is useful. Thus, not only is balancing of the varus deformity achieved, but also better access to the posterior contracted structures of the knee. Posterior cruciate ligament and sometimes the popliteus tendon are the causes of these combined contractures. In such cases, balancing of the posterior cruciate ligament or sacrificing it and the use of a more constrained implant are commonly used options [5]. Extensive medial release can inevitably result in increased medial flexion gap and the mandatory use of a thicker polyethylene insert or a more constraint prosthesis [12].

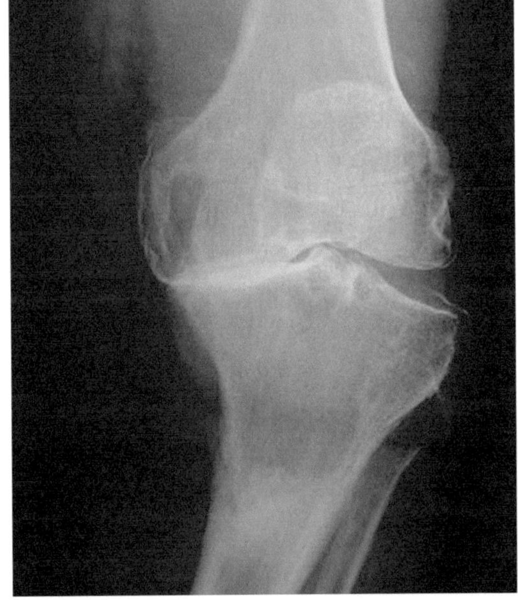

Fig. 8.3 Radiograph showing severe varus deformity of a left osteoarthritic knee

Surgical Technique

Various surgical techniques have been used in order to successfully reconstruct severe deformities during TKA. Mullaji et al. [19] used medial extra articular tibial osteotomy combined with selective posteromedial release. In all cases posterior cruciate substituting implants were used with tibial stem extenders and bone grafting, when necessary, based on the size of tibial bone defects. These authors report very good mid- term results regarding stability and deformity correction [19]. Meftah et al. [20] proposed a posteromedial capsulotomy, piecrust incising of the superficial medial collateral ligament and manipulations under valgus stress, in an attempt to minimize complications derived from extensive medial release. Satisfactory mid-term results for severe varus and fixed flexion were reported in terms of deformity correction, reduced incidence of over release and instability, hematoma formation, and the need for constrained prosthesis [20]. Dixon et al. [18], in a small series of patients, proposed a technique of downsizing, lateralizing of the tibial component and removing the excess proximal medial tibial bone in order to achieve loosening of the medial side and correction of severe varus deformity. In the most cases, non-constraining implants were used. The authors claim excellent clinical and radiologic results and stable correction in mid-terms [18]. According to their opinion, longer term data is necessary in order to identify possible increased polyethylene wear due to tibial prosthesis lateralization. Mullaji et al. [21] described a sliding medial condylar osteotomy performed under navigation guidance. Correct repositioning of the condylar fragment and knee ligament balancing was optimized by computer assisted navigation and the authors reported satisfactory mid-term results [21].

Few long term clinical outcome studies are available. Ritter et al. [22] suggested that patients with severe deformity should not be excluded from surgical treatment having as sole criterion the deformity itself. They report mid to long term results with no significant difference in terms of function, alignment or implant failure rates compared to a control group without severe deformity [22]. In all cases, different types of posterior cruciate ligament retaining prostheses were used. In their opinion constrained implants can be used in extreme cases. Kharbanda et al. [15] evaluated the use of grafting techniques for the reconstruction of bone defects in primary TKA for severe varus knees and identified the indications for structural or impaction grafting, depending on the extent of bone defect. Long term outcome was excellent, justifying the use of such cost effective, biological agents. Implants with stem extenders were used in almost all cases [15]. Karachalios et al. [23] studied the clinical outcome of severe varus and valgus arthritic knees reconstructed with the use of posterior cruciate retaining prosthesis. Outcomes of the varus subgroup were comparable to those of arthritic knees without severe deformity.

The hypothesis that computer assisted surgery (CAS) can efficiently contribute to the satisfactory reconstruction of severe knee deformities in TKA has been recently tested (Fig. 8.4). Several authors have attempted to correlate navigation guided TKA to better early postoperative results but failed to provide longer term superiority. Hsu

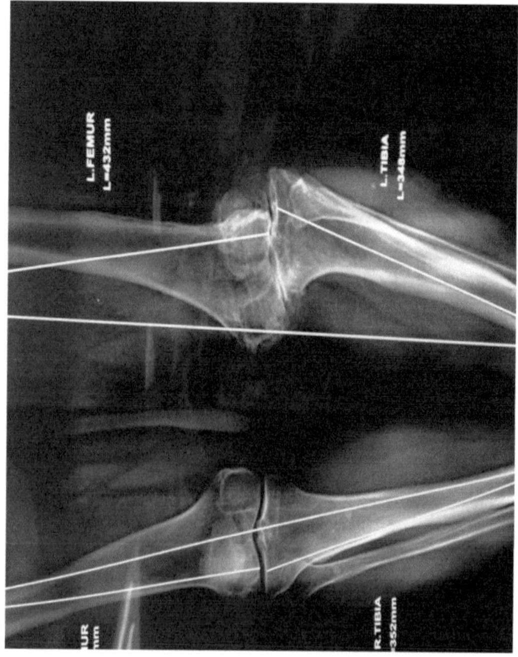

Fig. 8.4 Complex combined femoral and tibial deformity. Indications for computer assisted surgery

et al. [14] supported the accuracy of CAS reconstruction despite the fact that severe deformity negatively affected the postoperative axis. Bae et al. [17] positively correlated the severity of varus deformity with postoperative alignment, while Maniwa et al. [16] found no such correlation or higher rate of complications. Moon et al. [12] suggested that the preoperative degree of varus deformity and proximal tibia vara, among other clinical and radiological parameters, were the only determinants of the accuracy of varus deformity reconstruction. In a meta-analysis of twenty nine studies, results favored the use of computer navigated compared to conventional TKA, without taking into consideration the severity of deformity [24].

Valgus Deformity

Arthroplasty in the valgus knee is a challenging procedure not only for the surgeon, but also in terms of instrumentation [25] (Fig. 8.5). It should not be considered the reverse of varus deformity, as it is different and far more demanding [5, 26] (Fig. 8.6). Distal femoral anatomy is often distorted with the lateral femoral condyle abnormally small, almost dysplastic. Lateral ligaments are contracted and medial soft tissue structures stretched. Required asymmetric resections of the femoral condyles for limb alignment can cause further ligamentous imbalance [5]. Thus soft tissue balanced release becomes a crucial element for satisfactory TKA outcome [25, 27, 28]. Appropriate limb alignment should be obtained intraoperatively by symmetrical flexion and extension gaps and a centralized patella position [25, 29]. Deformities of the adjacent joints may be also present and should be addressed. Valgus flat foot is often associated with valgus knee deformity. The surgeon can consider correction of these deformities prior to TKA in order to ensure proper alignment and function [26].

Valgus deformity greater than or equal to $20°$ is considered severe by some authors [22, 30], while others accept smaller angles ($10–15°$) as the lower limit to severe deformity [28, 29, 31]. Ligament structure parameters such as medial

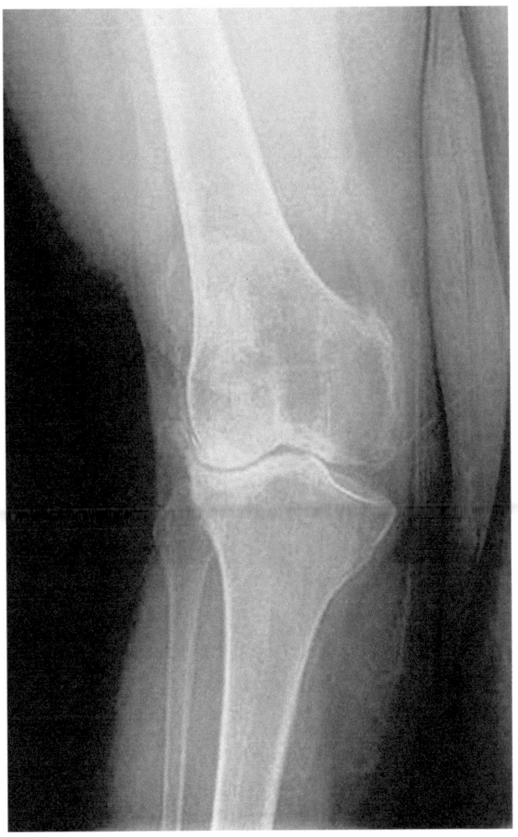

Fig. 8.5 Radiograph showing severe valgus deformity of a right osteoarthritic knee

collateral ligament insufficiency and the potential of posterior cruciate ligament sacrifice, favoring the use of a constrained prosthesis, should be taken into consideration [30]. Several authors claim higher failure rates and difficulties in revision of constrained prostheses and they suggest the use of these implants in the elderly and less demanding patients [32]. Peroneal nerve palsy can occur when treating knees with severe valgus deformity. When knee alignment is restored, the nerve is stretched. Spinal or epidural anesthesia may induce this complication and hide its symptoms [26]. Rajgopal et al. [30] have suggested that the operated knees should be placed in $10°$ of flexion during the early postoperative period in order to avoid peroneal nerve elongation [30].

All authors highlight the importance of proper lateral soft tissue release. Ritter et al. [22] noted that surgeons tend to slightly undercorrect severe deformities. Koskinen et al. [33] suggested that

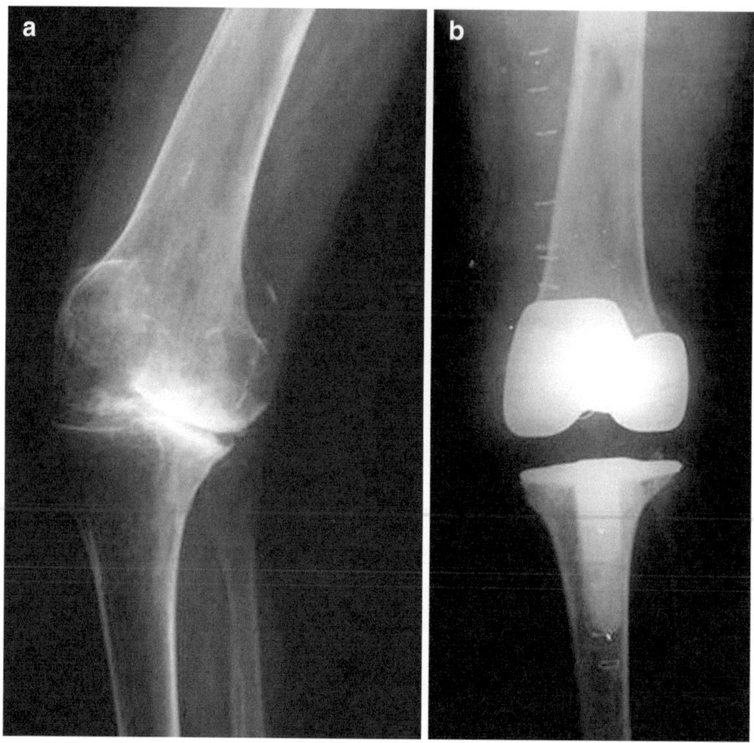

Fig. 8.6 Severe valgus deformity of a right osteoarthritic knee, (**a**) preoperative radiograph, (**b**) postoperative radiograph showing satisfactory limp alignment

residual valgus deformity increases the risk of revision and all patients with preoperatively severe valgus deformity should be followed up regularly, especially for implant wear and late onset instability. Various authors report satisfactory long term outcomes using cruciate retaining implants, in terms of alignment, revision and delayed instability [22, 27, 30]. Politi et al. [29] used a lateral cruciform retinacular release in combination with posterior cruciate retaining implants and demonstrated satisfactory mid to long term results. Nikolopoulos et al. [31] used a lateral parapatellar approach and tibial tubercle osteotomy instead of the standard medial parapatellar approach and reported satisfactory functional long term results. Radulescu et al. [26] do not favor the lateral approach due to soft tissue complications and inappropriate wound coverage after deformity correction. Zhou et al. [34] favor the lateral approach but also suggest that medial collateral ligament reconstruction and tibial

tubercle osteotomy have a high complication rate and increased surgery time. Augmentation of the deficient lateral condyle is an option but the indications and results of this technique are inconsistent in the literature [33, 34]. Ranawat et al. [28] have described a combination of inside-out release technique which involves the capsule, the iliotibial band, appropriate bone cuts and the use of posterior stabilized implants, and reported satisfactory long term outcomes. Marked valgus deformity which requires extensive posterolateral release in combination with medial collateral ligament insufficiency undermines the stability of the arthroplasty in the long term. Knees with such an intraoperative ligamentous imbalance should be replaced with a more constrained implant in order to ensure satisfactory long term results [22, 30, 33]. Zhou et al. [34] treated a series of severe valgus knees with marked osseous deficiency using different techniques and implants (cruciate-retaining, posterior stabilized or hinged knees), individualizing the decision based on the degree of soft tissue contraction, bone loss and intraoperative stability. They reported excellent long term results, supporting the use of the less possible constrained prostheses, especially in cases of younger patients. In their opinion, having in mind a future revision, preservation of bone stock offers satisfactory long term outcome. Finally, Karachalios et al. [23] studied the clinical outcome of severe varus and valgus arthritic knees reconstructed with the use of posterior cruciate retaining prostheses. Outcomes of the valgus subgroup were also comparable to those of arthritic knees without severe deformity. However, in valgus deformities, when exceeding 30°, a high incidence of extensor mechanism complications were observed (Fig. 8.7).

Fixed Flexion Deformity and Range of Motion

Flexion contracture is commonly encountered in knees undergoing TKA (61 %) and it is often associated with varus deformity [35, 36]. Mild deformities can be passively corrected intraoperatively [11]. Severe deformities require surgical techniques such as posterior osteophyte removal, posterior capsule and posterior cruciate ligament release, and appropriate femoral bone resections [11, 37]. Residual flexion affects gait kinematics, posing a contraction overload to the quadriceps and subsequent pressure on the patellofemoral joint. Patients are dissatisfied due to residual functional disability [35, 37]. Even though mild flexion contractions may resolve gradually after surgery, most become permanent, highlighting

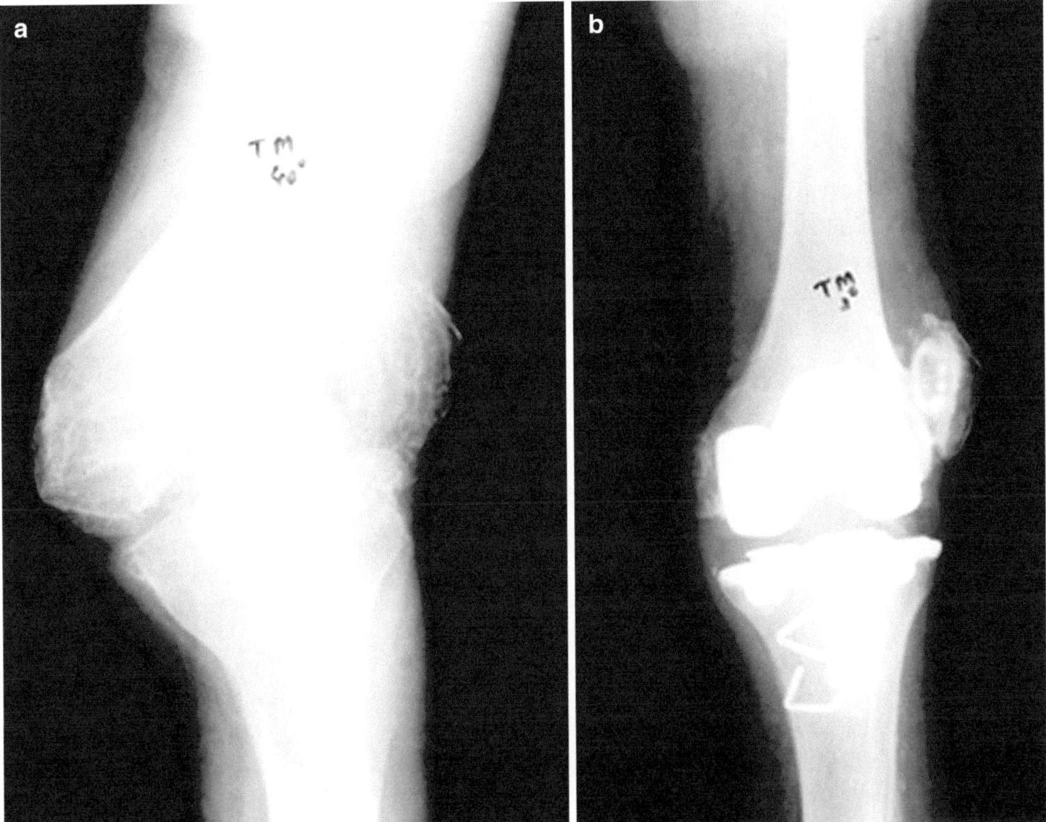

Fig. 8.7 Severe valgus deformity (40°) of a left osteoarthritic knee, (**a**) preoperative radiograph, (**b**) postoperative radiograph showing dislocation of the patella

the importance of intraoperative correction and postoperative maintenance with focused physiotherapy [11].

In full knee extension the angle of flexion contracture is 0°. The more limited the extension the greater is the angle. A range of 5° towards flexion or hyperextension is considered normal [36]. An angle greater than or equal to 20° of fixed flexion contracture can be considered as a severe deformity [38]. Rheumatoid knees suffer from flexion contractures more severely and more often than osteoarthritic knees [36]. Another term often met in literature is "stiff knee", which refers to knees with a range of motion of less than 50° [39].

Satisfactory postoperative range of motion is an important predictor of TKA outcome and a dominant parameter of most knee scoring systems. Ninety degrees of flexion is the minimum required for usual everyday living [40, 41]. In particular, 67° of knee flexion is required for the gait's swing phase, 83 and 90° for climbing or descending stairs respectively, and 93° for rising from a chair [40]. In western societies, the current lifestyle of seniors does not require more than 110–115°, while cultural and religious behaviors of other populations have higher demands [42].

Acute postoperative range of motion is a limited predictor of TKA clinical outcome [43]. Many authors have attempted to correlate various clinical factors, as far as range of motion is concerned, with short and mid-term TKA outcome. However, preoperative diagnosis and preoperative range of motion seem to affect the postoperative result more [44]. Rheumatoid knees undergoing arthroplasty have more satisfactory results concerning correction of flexion contractures [36]. Other studies suggest that limited preoperative range of motion is the only important variable, having a negative influence on postoperative range of motion in mid-terms [45, 46]. Other authors take also into account preoperative malalignment in the frontal plane [47] and intraoperative procedures such as removal of posterior osteophytes and soft tissue release, demonstrating that the achievement of good intraoperative range of motion can be correlated with a good postoperative result [48]. Computer assisted surgery appears to be more accurate in assessing flexion deformities and provides surgeons with the necessary data in order to restore knee extension and have a good intraoperative range of motion [35].

Long term data is contradictory. Stair ascending and descending is significantly improved 7 years after TKA when compared to mid-term values [49]. Long term outcomes in patients with a preoperative fixed flexion deformity are similar to those without preexisting deformity. Ten years after surgery, these patients present with continuous improvements [50]. Patients with rheumatoid knees also have equally good long term outcomes compared to those with osteoarthritis [51, 52]. Concerning stiff, osteoarthritic knees, authors report good long term outcomes and functional improvements which overcome the intraoperative difficulties and early high complication rates [53, 54].

A relatively new development in knee arthroplasty is high flexion TKA implants specifically designed to achieve higher postoperative knee flexion. However, no long term data related to the survival or to the functional performance of these implants are yet available [55]. Present studies do not support any advantages over the conventional implants and further longer term research is necessary [55, 56]. On the other hand, there is growing evidence that increased range of motion is not the patient's primary concern – he/she is mainly looking for relief from osteoarthritic pain [55].

References

1. Lützner J, Hübel U, Kirschner S, Günther KP, Krummenauer F. Long-term results in total knee arthroplasty. A meta-analysis of revision rates and functional outcome. Chirurg. 2011;82:618–24.
2. Feng B, Weng X, Lin J, Jin J, Wang W, Qiu G. Long-term follow-up of cemented fixed-bearing total knee arthroplasty in a Chinese population: a survival analysis of more than 10 years. J Arthroplasty. 2013;28:1701–6.
3. Mont MA, Pivec R, Issa K, Kapadia BH, Maheshwari A, Harwin SF. Long-term implant survivorship of cementless total knee arthroplasty: a systematic review of the literature and meta-analysis. J Knee Surg. 2014;27(5):369–76.
4. Tria Jr AJ. Management of fixed deformities in total knee arthroplasty. J Long Term Eff Med Implants. 2004;14(1):33–50.

5. Engh GA. The difficult knee: severe varus and valgus. Clin Orthop. 2003;416:58–63.

6. Hinman RS, May RL, Crossley KM. Is there an alternative to the full-leg radiograph for determining knee joint alignment in osteoarthritis? Arthritis Rheum. 2006;55:306–13.

7. Cahue S, Dunlop D, Hayes K, Song J, Torres L, Sharma L. Varus-valgus alignment in the progression of patellofemoral osteoarthritis. Arthritis Rheum. 2004;50:2184–90.

8. Saragaglia D, Blaysat M, Mercier N, Grimaldi M. Results of forty two computer-assisted double level osteotomies for severe genu varum deformity. Int Orthop. 2012;36:999–1003.

9. Cooke TD, Sled EA, Scudamore RA. Frontal plane knee alignment: a call for standardized measurement. J Rheumatol. 2007;34:1796–801.

10. Teichtahl AJ, Wluka AE, Cicuttini FM. Frontal plane knee alignment is associated with a longitudinal reduction in patella cartilage volume in people with knee osteoarthritis. Osteoarthritis Cartilage. 2008;16:851–4.

11. Su EP. Fixed flexion deformity and total knee arthroplasty. J Bone Joint Surg Br. 2012;94B(S11):112–5.

12. Moon YW, Kim JG, Han JH, Do KH, Seo JG, Lim HC. Factors correlated with the reducibility of varus deformity in knee osteoarthritis: an analysis using navigation guided TKA. Clin Orthop Surg. 2013;5:36–43.

13. Ahn JH, Back YW. Comparative study of two techniques for ligament balancing in total knee arthroplasty for severe varus knee: medial soft tissue release vs. Bony resection of proximal medial tibia. Knee Surg Relat Res. 2013;25:13–8.

14. Hsu WH, Hsu RW, Weng YJ. Effect of preoperative deformity on postoperative leg axis in total knee arthroplasty: a prospective randomized study. Knee Surg Sports Traumatol Arthrosc. 2010;18:1323–7.

15. Kharbanda Y, Sharma M. Autograft reconstructions for bone defects in primary total knee replacement in severe varus knees. Indian J Orthop. 2014;48:313–8.

16. Maniwa K, Ishibashi Y, Tsuda E, Yamamoto Y, Inoue R, Otsuka H. Accuracy of image-free computer navigated total knee arthroplasty is not compromised in severely deformed varus knees. J Arthroplasty. 2013;28:802–6.

17. Bae DK, Song SJ, Heo DB, Tak DH. Does the severity of preoperative varus deformity influence postoperative alignment in both conventional and computer-assisted total knee arthroplasty? Knee Surg Sports Traumatol Arthrosc. 2013;21:2248–54.

18. Dixon MC, Parsch D, Brown RR, Scott RD. The correction of severe varus deformity in total knee arthroplasty by tibial component downsizing and resection of uncapped proximal medial bone. J Arthroplasty. 2004;19:19–22.

19. Mullaji AB, Padmanabhan V, Jindal G. Total knee arthroplasty for profound varus deformity: technique and radiological results in 173 knees with varus of more than 20 degrees. J Arthroplasty. 2005;20:550–61.

20. Meftah M, Blum YC, Raja D, Ranawat AS, Ranawat CS. Correcting fixed varus deformity with flexion contracture during total knee arthroplasty: the "inside-out" technique: AAOS exhibit selection. J Bone Joint Surg Am. 2012;94A:e66.

21. Mullaji AB, Shetty GM. Surgical technique: computer-assisted sliding medial condylar osteotomy to achieve gap balance in varus knees during TKA. Clin Orthop. 2013;471:1484–91.

22. Ritter MA, Faris GW, Faris PM, Davis KE. Total knee arthroplasty in patients with angular varus or valgus deformities of > or = 20 degrees. J Arthroplasty. 2004;19:862–6.

23. Karachalios T, Sarangi PP, Newman JH. Severe varus and valgus deformities treated by total knee arthroplasty. J Bone Joint Surg Br. 1994;76:938–42.

24. Mason JB, Fehring TK, Estok R, Banel D, Fahrbach K. Meta-analysis of alignment outcomes in computer-assisted total knee arthroplasty surgery. J Arthroplasty. 2007;22:1097–106.

25. Pape D, Kohn D. Soft tissue balancing in valgus gonarthrosis. Orthopade. 2007;36:657–8.

26. Radulescu R, Badila A, Japie I, Ciobanu T, Manolescu R. Primary total knee arthroplasty in severe valgus knee. J Med Life. 2013;6:395–8.

27. Elkus M, Ranawat CS, Rasquinha VJ, Babhulkar S, Rossi R, Ranawat AS. Total knee arthroplasty for severe valgus deformity. Five-to-fourteen-year follow-up. J Bone Joint Surg Am. 2004;86A:2671–6.

28. Ranawat AS, Ranawat CS, Elkus M, Rasquinha VJ, Rossi R, Babhulkar S. Total knee arthroplasty for severe valgus deformity. J Bone Joint Surg Am. 2005;87A(S1):271–84.

29. Politi J, Scott R. Balancing severe valgus deformity in total knee arthroplasty using a lateral cruciform retinacular release. J Arthroplasty. 2004;19:553–7.

30. Rajgopal A, Dahiya V, Vasdev A, Kochhar H, Tyagi V. Long-term results of total knee arthroplasty for valgus knees: soft-tissue release technique and implant selection. J Orthop Surg (Hong Kong). 2011;19:60–3.

31. Nikolopoulos DD, Polyzois I, Apostolopoulos AP, Rossas C, Moutsios-Rentzos A, Michos IV. Total knee arthroplasty in severe valgus knee deformity: comparison of a standard medial parapatellar approach combined with tibial tubercle osteotomy. Knee Surg Sports Traumatol Arthrosc. 2011;19:1834–42.

32. Pour AE, Parvizi J, Slenker N, Purtill JJ, Sharkey PF. Rotating hinged total knee replacement: use with caution. J Bone Joint Surg Am. 2007;89A:1735–41.

33. Koskinen E, Remes V, Paavolainen P, Harilainen A, Sandelin J, Tallroth K, Kettunen J, Ylinen P. Results of total knee replacement with a cruciate-retaining model for severe valgus deformity–a study of 48 patients followed for an average of 9 years. Knee. 2011;18:145–50.

34. Zhou X, Wang M, Liu C, Zhang L, Zhou Y. Total knee arthroplasty for severe valgus knee deformity. Chin Med J (Engl). 2014;127(6):1062–6.

35. Gallie PA, Davis ET, Macgroarty K, Waddell JP, Schemitsch EH. Computer-assisted navigation for the assessment of fixed flexion in knee arthroplasty. Can J Surg. 2010;53:42–6.

36. Tew M, Forster IW. Effect of knee replacement on flexion deformity. J Bone Joint Surg Br. 1987;69B:395–9.
37. Scuderi GR, Kochhar T. Management of flexion contracture in total knee arthroplasty. J Arthroplasty. 2007;22:20–4.
38. Berend KR, Lombardi Jr AV, Adams JB. Total knee arthroplasty in patients with greater than 20 degrees flexion contracture. Clin Orthop. 2006;452:83–7.
39. Aglietti P, Windsor RE, Buzzi R, Insall JN. Arthroplasty for the stiff or ankylosed knee. J Arthroplasty. 1989;4:1–5.
40. Kettelkamp DB, Johnson RJ, Smidt GL, Chao EY, Walker M. An electrogoniometric study of knee motion in normal gait. J Bone Joint Surg Am. 1970;52(4):775–90. Available from http://jbjs.org/content/52/4/775.long
41. Chiu KY, Ng TP, Tang WM, Yau WP. Review article: knee flexion after total knee arthroplasty. J Orthop Surg (Hong Kong). 2002;10:194–202.
42. Li PH, Wong YC, Wai YL. Knee flexion after total knee arthroplasty. J Orthop Surg (Hong Kong). 2007;15:149–53.
43. Bade MJ, Kittelson JM, Kohrt WM, Stevens-Lapsley JE. Predicting functional performance and range of motion outcomes after total knee arthroplasty. Am J Phys Med Rehabil. 2014;93:579–85.
44. Kotani A, Yonekura A, Bourne RB. Factors influencing range of motion after contemporary total knee arthroplasty. J Arthroplasty. 2005;20:850–6.
45. Gatha NM, Clarke HD, Fuchs R, Scuderi GR, Insall JN. Factors affecting postoperative range of motion after total knee arthroplasty. J Knee Surg. 2004;17:196–202.
46. Sancheti KH, Sancheti PK, Shyam AK, Joshi R, Patil K, Jain A. Factors affecting range of motion in total knee arthroplasty using high flexion prosthesis: a prospective study. Indian J Orthop. 2013;47:50–6.
47. Kawamura H, Bourne RB. Factors affecting range of flexion after total knee arthroplasty. J Orthop Sci. 2001;6:248–52.
48. Ritter MA, Harty LD, Davis KE, Meding JB, Berend ME. Predicting range of motion after total knee arthroplasty. Clustering, log-linear regression, and regression tree analysis. J Bone Joint Surg Am. 2003;85A:1278–85.
49. Van der Linden ML, Rowe PJ, Myles CM, Burnett R, Nutton RW. Knee kinematics in functional activities seven years after total knee arthroplasty. Clin Biomech (Bristol, Avon). 2007;22:537–42.
50. Cheng K, Ridley D, Bird J, McLeod G. Patients with fixed flexion deformity after total knee arthroplasty do just as well as those without: ten-year prospective data. Int Orthop. 2010;34:663–7.
51. Ito J, Koshino T, Okamoto R, Saito T. 15-year follow-up study of total knee arthroplasty in patients with rheumatoid arthritis. J Arthroplasty. 2003;18:984–92.
52. Van Loon CJ, Wisse MA, de Waal Malefijt MC, Jansen RH, Veth RP. The kinematic total knee arthroplasty. A 10- to 15-year follow-up and survival analysis. Arch Orthop Trauma Surg. 2000;120:48–52.
53. Kim Y-H, Kim J-S. Does TKA improve functional outcome and range of motion in patients with stiff knees? Clin Orthop. 2009;467:1348–54.
54. Rajgopal A, Ahuja N, Dolai B. Total knee arthroplasty in stiff and ankylosed knees. J Arthroplasty. 2005;20:585–90.
55. Murphy M, Journeaux S, Russell T. High-flexion total knee arthroplasty: a systematic review. Int Orthop. 2009;33:887–93.
56. Endres S. High-flexion versus conventional total knee arthroplasty: a 5-year study. J Orthop Surg (Hong Kong). 2011;19:226–9.

Long Term Clinical Outcome of Total Knee Arthroplasty. The Effect of Surgeon Training and Experience

Nikolaos Roidis, Gregory Avramidis, and Petros Kalampounias

Introduction

Total Knee Arthroplasty (TKA) is one of the most common elective procedures performed worldwide, as it is considered an effective intervention for patients suffering from advanced knee osteoarthritis. It is a relatively easy, safe and cost-effective solution that provides relief from pain and disability and offers increased function and thus, improvement in quality of life. The success rate and beneficial outcomes have led to a vastly increasing number of operations performed annually, with an expected 3.5 million procedures in the U.S. alone over the next 20 years, a sixfold increase over current estimates [1, 2].

Despite the satisfactory outcomes of TKA, patients continue to experience complications and adverse effects, and to report poor subjective outcomes following TKA at an estimated level of 20 % [3–5]. A number of factors have been identified as influencing TKA outcome, including patient-related factors such as gender and medical comorbidity, technical factors such as surgical exposure and alignment of the prosthesis, and provider factors such as hospital and surgeon procedure volumes and experience.

In the field of Surgery and Orthopaedics there is an ongoing debate as to the influence of surgeon and center volume on surgical outcome. Many authors contend that complex surgeries such as TKA should be performed in specialist centers by experienced surgeons performing a high volume of operations annually. These claims are based on studies focusing on outcomes of patients with cardiovascular disease (i.e., acute myocardial infarction) who were admitted to Specialist Hospitals and Centers and who were clearly found to show significantly better outcomes compared to those treated in non-specialist facilities. Furthermore, rehabilitation and other important ancillary services may be more accessible to higher-volume providers. Based on these observations, it is expected that specific orthopaedic surgery (such as TKA) performed in specialist centers by high volume surgeons will produce better patient outcomes and will minimize complications, morbidity and cost at the same time improving long term outcomes [6].

Definitions and Eligibility Criteria

Patient outcomes include mortality, morbidity (pulmonary embolus, deep venous thrombosis, sepsis, myocardial infarction, or pneumonia), surgical complications (surgical site infection, bleeding and subsequent need for blood transfusion, urinary tract infection, GI bleeding etc.),

N. Roidis, MD, DSc (✉) • G. Avramidis, MD
P. Kalampounias, MD
3rd Orthopaedic Department, KAT Hospital,
Nikis 2, Kifisia, Athens 14561, Hellenic Republic
e-mail: roidisnt@hotmail.com

© Springer-Verlag London 2015
T. Karachalios (ed.), *Total Knee Arthroplasty: Long Term Outcomes*,
DOI 10.1007/978-1-4471-6660-3_9

length of hospital stay (LOS), discharge disposition, readmissions, and reoperations within the first 30 days after discharge as well as long-term follow up of the implant and patient satisfaction.

Throughout the literature, patients included in relevant studies and surveys met the following criteria [7]: (a) age >65 years; (b) absence of certain risk factors (pathologic fracture, conversion of previous TKA, infection of knee or thigh during admission) which tend to cause substantially higher rates of post-operative adverse outcome compared with primary TKA patients; and (c) availability of detailed demographic data including race and sex. Surgeons are divided according to the total number of operations performed annually, although there is much controversy regarding exact classification parameters (low / medium/high volume). Low volume (LV) ranges from <3 to <52 TKAs per year, whereas high volume (HV) expands from >5 to >70 TKAs per year, depending on each study's criteria and thresholds [7–10]. Similarly, hospitals are divided into low volume (<25 TKA per year) or high volume (>200 TKA per year) and they also classified as (a) Training Centers, (b) Teaching Hospitals or at least affiliated with a Medical School, (c) Acute care facilities and (d) Highly Specialized Centers [11]. Depending on surgeon experience, training and availability of specific facilities, variations of the TKA procedure have been identified which may influence the final outcome. These variations include surgical approach and exposure (parapatellar or subvastus – standard or MIS), computer/robotic assisted placement of the components etc.

Surgical Volume and Outcome

There are a large number of papers examining surgical volume and outcome in a wide spectrum of surgical procedures and specialties. In a recent systematic review, Chowdhury et al. examined 163 articles covering 13 surgical specialties [12]. Of the papers reviewed 74.2 % and 74 % showed a significantly better outcome in hospitals with higher volumes and higher surgeon volume respectively. Specialization resulted in

significantly better outcomes with 91 % of studies showing a significant improvement in positive outcome; however, this benefit varied amongst specialties [12].

Effect of Volume on Mortality

Surgical mortality is a rare occurrence in elective orthopaedic practice [7, 13, 14]. However, there are a number of papers which indicate such an association in elective total knee replacement. It is suggested that the higher the volume the lower the risk of mortality [7, 8, 15–17]. Interestingly, there is no difference between highly specialized centers and non-specialized hospitals. In one study, it has been shown that there is no relation between surgeon volume and surgical mortality [18].

Effect of Volume on Morbidity

The lowest complications rates (and consequently the lowest morbidity rates) occur amongst surgeons in the highest volume groups. Low volume surgeons (<52 patients/year) had higher transfusion rates due to postoperative anemia and higher occurrence of postoperative infection [19, 20]. When surgeon volume increased above 200 TKR a year, it was also associated with a decreased risk of myocardial infarction (MI), pulmonary embolus (PE), deep surgical site infection and in some cases, mortality [21–27]. A 5 year meta-analysis study reviewing over 200,000 TKRs concluded that lower volume hospitals were associated with an increased rate of PE [18]. It was reported that there is a decreased risk of respiratory complications when a surgeon performs a minimum of 50 TKRs a year [7, 8]. The incidence of hemorrhage (upper G.I. or other) was significantly higher in high volume and specialized centers, probably due to more intensive use of pharmacologic thromboembolism prophylaxis [13, 14, 28]. A statistically significant decrease in transfusion rate following TKA performed by HV surgeons compared to LV surgeons (4 % vs 13 %) was also reported [19]. A statistically significant association between low surgeon volume and infection rates either in hospital (almost twice as high) [26], or 1 year postoperatively (almost 2.5 times higher rate) [22], has been suggested. Neither study specified whether this was deep or superficial site infection. A statistically significant decrease in pneumonia rates following TKA performed by HV surgeons (1.02 % HV vs 1.68 % LV) is reported by some authors [7, 8]. Finally, a significant increase in TKA operation time for LV surgeons (165 min vs 135 min) should be considered as an aggravating factor due the increase of intraoperative risks [24]. Regarding hospitalization, significantly higher lengths of stay (LOS) were observed in low volume units and surgeons (mean of 5 days in HV as opposed to 7 days in LV centers and surgeons), with no influence on outcome, however [10, 20, 21, 29, 30].

It must be stated that modern, less invasive operating techniques (MIS/Mini-Sub/Midvastus exposure) as well as computerized/robotic assisted placement of the components (that usually require advanced surgeon training and skill) mainly affect the immediate postoperative co-morbidity factors (less soft tissue damage and blood loss, reduced need for analgesia, earlier patient mobilization etc.) and "technical" details (improved radiographic component alignment leading to correct mechanical axis and prosthesis function) [31–33]. Recent literature suggests that the long-term clinical outcome remains uninfluenced by such procedures.

Effect of Volume on Clinical Outcome

For TKR, crude analysis shows no relationship between surgeon and hospital volume and readmission rate to hospital within a year. However, there is good evidence that the rate of readmission was reduced in Training Centers [18]. There is evidence of a higher risk of revision surgery within 6 months in HV Hospitals, although this finding is possibly due to the fact that highly specialized centers tend to take up more complex patient cases which often require reoperation. Patients operated on by low-volume surgeons in low-volume hospitals presented lower WOMAC functional status scores at 2 year follow up (<60 on a scale of 0–100) when compared to patients operated on by higher volume surgeons or/and in higher volume hospitals [7, 8]. Other studies have also demonstrated that higher surgical and hospital volumes result in more favorable patient outcomes [7, 34, 35]. Patients operated on by LV surgeons were more likely to report an inability to flex the knee to 90°, and more likely to report an inability to achieve full extension at 2 year follow up [8]. It is suggested that surgeon volume is a greater predictor of favorable outcome than hospital volume, but there is also evidence that both surgeon and hospital volume influence outcome. It seems that TKA mid-term survival does not depend on surgeon volume [26]. Moreover, no association between surgeon volume and 3 year and 1 year revision rate, respectively, has been observed [21, 30].

Findings with regard to TKA costs warrant a brief mention. In particular, TKA costs were markedly higher in low volume non-specialized hospitals than in high volume Units and Centers of Excellence, probably due to the difference in LOS and a higher incidence of adverse effect at the former. It was also found that academic medical centers typically have higher costs when compared with other hospitals [16, 17, 36]. However, at least some of the higher costs that have been observed in teaching hospitals seem to be related to the greater complexity of patient populations served by these hospitals [37].

Literature Against the Association of Surgical Volume and Outcome

Sharkey et al. have questioned the concept of a linear relationship between increasing volume and reducing complication rates [38]. They report a plateau with respect to complication rates at higher volumes. Complication and mortality rates in their unit, which performed 1,000 hip arthroplasties annually, did not differ markedly from units performing >100 arthroplasties [38]. The most crucial predictor of outcome was found to be patient characteristics rather than volume [27, 30]. Kreder et al. [21] do not support the regionalization of services based on patient outcomes. Additionally, Hamilton and Ho [39], found that there was no significant outcome advantage in high volume hospitals. Feinglass et al. [40] found no hospital volume effect on complication rates, which they attribute to the fact that most procedures in their study were performed in relatively high volume hospitals, with less than 2 % of TKA performed by institutions performing less than ten TKRs annually. Additionally, they found that complication rates declined over the 7-year study period, which they attribute to improved safety and decreased length of stay.

Surgical Threshold

Should there be a minimum volume threshold for certain orthopaedic procedures? Schulz and Smektala [41] and Schräder and Ewerbeck [42] were unable to deduce a minimum threshold value, whereas Norton et al. [11] have suggested a minimum of 50 TKAs per surgeon annually in order to diminish adverse outcomes, while indicating more than 100 TKAs would be preferable. Katz et al. [7] support the recommendation of a minimum of 50 TKAs a year, reporting a decreased risk of respiratory complications when the operating surgeon performed a minimum of 50 TKR a year. When this number was increased to a minimum of 200 TKAs a year it was also associated with a decreased risk of myocardial infarction (MI), pulmonary embolus (PE), deep infection and mortality [7]. Hervey et al. [15] report that even a minimum volume of 15 TKAs a year decreased mortality rate. In their paper Luft et al. [43] found that hospitals performing 50–100 THAs a year had mortality rates almost as low as hospitals performing more than 200 THAs a year.

Conclusions

It has been demonstrated (data mined from registries of major Healthcare, either Public or Private, Organizations) that higher volume Units/Surgeons are usually associated with improved outcomes. Factors explaining these findings are widely available in the current literature. Highly skilled surgeons achieve good outcomes and as they gain experience are better able to select patients suitable for surgery.

Training and education regarding the specific condition they are treating should therefore lead to improved outcomes [43].

Whilst low volume units and lack of standardization may cause few problems within the standard National Health Systems (NHS) provision of total joint arthroplasties, findings from several studies raise concerns about the standards of care within private practice and independent sector run treatment centers (ISTCs) whose data are not included in hospital episode statistics (HES) or in national registries. Often, there is no source of valid data on volumes within private hospitals. If there is, data is relatively poor, and made up of large numbers of different surgeons performing a few cases each, and taking varying approaches to the procedures. Similar concerns have recently been raised by the President of the Royal College of Surgeons (UK) concerning the standards and quality of operations performed by surgeons arising from various educational programs run by the UK's ISTCs. Both private hospitals and ISTCs should be obliged to make their data available to HES and to the hip replacement registry, in order allow their activities to be examined and compared with NHS hospitals [44].

Understanding the relationship between provider volume and outcomes for TKA is critical in order to understand discussions concerning 'centralization' or 'regionalization' and overall efforts to improve quality and outcomes of care in TKA. The principle behind centralization or regionalization is that improved patient outcomes can be achieved by concentrating complex surgical procedures in regional centers, or "centers of excellence". Better equipped units employing highly qualified and skilled nursing staff, well versed and experienced surgeons can easily achieve a high level of organizational standards and clinical practice and apply standardization of procedures in order to minimize adverse or unpredictable incidents that tend to cause the majority of undesirable outcomes.

Many volume outcome studies, which have been utilized in order to prove the efficacy of centralization, rarely examine the same variable. Marlow et al., in a recent review, report that there is a trend towards increased hospital volume significantly affecting patient morbidity and length of stay. However, for each of the remaining parameters of hospital/surgeon volume and patient morbidity, mortality and length of stay, this report does not definitively demonstrate a statistically significant association. It has been demonstrated that there is a more commonly reported association between increased hospital volume and reductions in patient morbidity and length of stay. The authors believe that research into the differences in hospital clinical guidelines for the treatment of patients after either primary or revision knee arthroplasty may identify beneficial practices used in high-volume hospitals, which can be applicable to low-volume hospitals. The centralization evidence base is growing; however, this research needs to include examinations of the impact of hospital clinical guidelines as well as hospital/patient variables. Despite these conclusions regarding volume and outcome, little can be said either to promote or renounce the idea of the centralization of knee arthroplasty procedures based on the existing data. It is apparent, however, that before services are reallocated or centralized, a prospective contemporary study should be conducted which will address the aforementioned limitations of the published literature.

References

1. Kurtz S, Ong K, Lau E, Mowat F, Halpern M. Projections of primary and revision hip and knee arthroplasty in the United States from 2005 to 2030. J Bone Joint Surg Am. 2007;89A:780–5.
2. Hawker G, Wright J, Coyte P, Paul J, Dittus R, Croxford R, et al. Health-related quality of life after knee replacement. J Bone Joint Surg Am. 1998;80A:163–73.
3. Callahan CM, Drake BG, Heck DA, Dittus RS. Patient outcomes following tricompartmental total knee replacement. A meta-analysis. JAMA. 1994;271:1349–57.
4. Fortin PR, Clarke AE, Joseph L, Liang MH, Tanzer M, Ferland D, et al. Outcomes of total hip and knee replacement: preoperative functional status predicts outcomes at six months after surgery. Arthritis Rheum. 1999;42:1722–8.
5. Fortin PR, Penrod JR, Clarke AE, St-Pierre Y, Joseph L, Belisle P, et al. Timing of total joint replacement affects clinical outcomes among patients with osteoarthritis of the hip or knee. Arthritis Rheum. 2002;46:3327–30.
6. Williams SC, Koss RG, Morton DJ, Loeb JM. Performance of top-ranked heart care hospitals on evidence-based process measures. Circulation. 2006;114:558–64.
7. Katz JN, Barrett J, Mahomed NN, Baron JA, Wright RJ, Losina E. Association between hospital and surgeon procedure volume and the outcomes of total knee replacement. J Bone Joint Surg Am. 2004;86A:1909–16.
8. Katz JN, Mahomed NN, Baron JA, Barrett JA, Fossel AH, Creel AH, et al. Association of hospital and surgeon procedure volume with patient-centered outcomes of total knee replacement in a population-based cohort of patients age 65 years and older. Arthritis Rheum. 2007;56:568–74.
9. Manley M, Ong K, Lau E, Kurtz SM. Total knee arthroplasty survivorship in the United States Medicare population: effect of hospital and surgeon procedure volume. J Arthroplasty. 2009;24:1061–7.
10. Styron JF, Koroukian SM, Klika AK, Barsoum WK. Patient vs provider characteristics impacting hospital lengths of stay after total knee or hip arthroplasty. J Arthroplasty. 2011;26:1418–26.
11. Norton EC, Garfinkel SA, McQuay LJ, Heck DA, Wright JG, Dittus R, et al. The effect of hospital volume on the in-hospital complication rate in knee replacement patients. Health Serv Res. 1998;33:1191–210.
12. Chowdhury MM, Dagash H, Pierro A. A systematic review of the impact of volume of surgery and specialization on patient outcome. Br J Surg. 2007;94:145–61.
13. Cram P, Lu X, Kates SL, Singh JA, Li Y, Wolf BR. Total knee arthroplasty volume, utilization, and outcomes among Medicare beneficiaries, 1991–2010. JAMA. 2012;308:1227–36.
14. Cram P, Vaughan-Sarrazin MS, Wolf B, Katz JN, Rosenthal GE. A comparison of total hip and knee replacement in specialty and general hospitals. J Bone Joint Surg Am. 2007;89A:1675–84.
15. Hervey SL, Purves HR, Guller U, Toth AP, Vail TP, Pietrobon R. Provider volume of total knee arthroplasties and patient outcomes in the HCUP-nationwide inpatient sample. J Bone Joint Surg Am. 2003;85A:1775–83.
16. Taylor Jr DH, Whellan DJ, Sloan FA. Effects of admission to a teaching hospital on the cost and quality of care for Medicare beneficiaries. N Engl J Med. 1999;340:293–9.
17. Taylor HD, Dennis DA, Crane HS. Relationship between mortality rates and hospital patient volume for medicare patients undergoing major orthopaedic surgery of the hip, knee, spine, and femur. J Arthroplasty. 1997;12:235–42.
18. Judge A, Chard J, Learmonth I, Dieppe P. The effects of surgical volumes and training centre status on outcomes following total joint replacement: analysis of the Hospital Episode Statistics for England. J Pub Health. 2006;28:116–24.

19. Baker P, Dowen D, McMurtry I. The effect of surgeon volume on the need for transfusion following primary unilateral hip and knee arthroplasty. Surgeon. 2011;9:13–7.

20. Bozic KJ, Maselli J, Pekow PS, Lindenauer PK, Vail TP, Auerbach AD. The influence of procedure volumes and standardization of care on quality and efficiency in total joint replacement surgery. J Bone Joint Surg Am. 2010;92A:2643–52.

21. Kreder HJ, Grosso P, Williams JI, Jaglal S, Axcell T, Wal EK, et al. Provider volume and other predictors of outcome after total knee arthroplasty: a population study in Ontario. Can J Surg. 2003;46:15–22.

22. Muilwijk J, van den Hof S, Wille JC. Associations between surgical site infection risk and hospital operation volume and surgeon operation volume among hospitals in the Dutch nosocomial infection surveillance network. Infect Control Hosp Epidemiol. 2007;28:557–63.

23. Nunley RM, Lachiewicz PF. Mortality after total hip and knee arthroplasty in a medium-volume university practice. J Arthroplasty. 2003;18:278–85.

24. Ong K, Lau E, Manley M, Kurtz SM. Patient, hospital, and procedure characteristics influencing total hip and knee arthroplasty procedure duration. J Arthroplasty. 2009;24:925–31.

25. Schroer WC, Calvert GT, Diesfeld PJ, Reedy ME, LeMarr AR. Effects of increased surgical volume on total knee arthroplasty complications. J Arthroplasty. 2008;23:61–7.

26. Wei MH, Lin YL, Shi HY, Chiu HC. Effects of provider patient volume and comorbidity on clinical and economic outcomes for total knee arthroplasty: a population-based study. J Arthroplasty. 2010;25:906–12.

27. Yasunaga H, Tsuchiya K, Matsuyama Y, Ohe K. Analysis of factors affecting operating time, postoperative complications, and length of stay for total knee arthroplasty: nationwide web-based survey. J Orthop Sci. 2009;14:10–6.

28. Cram P, Cai X, Lu X, Vaughan-Sarrazin MS, Miller BJ. Total knee arthroplasty outcomes in top-ranked and non-top-ranked orthopedic hospitals: an analysis of Medicare administrative data. Mayo Clin Proc. 2012;87:341–8.

29. Husted H, Hansen HC, Holm G, Bach-Dal C, Rud K, Andersen KL, et al. What determines length of stay after total hip and knee arthroplasty? A nationwide study in Denmark. Arch Orthop Trauma Surg. 2010;130:263–8.

30. Paterson JM, Williams JI, Kreder HJ, Mahomed NN, Gunraj N, Wang X, et al. Provider volumes and early outcomes of primary total joint replacement in Ontario. Can J Surg. 2010;53:175–83.

31. Alcelik I, Sukeik M, Pollock R, Misra A, Shah P, Armstrong P, et al. Comparison of the minimally invasive and standard medial parapatellar approaches for primary total knee arthroplasty. Knee Surg Sports Traumatol Arthrosc. 2012;20:2502–12.

32. Bathis H, Perlick L, Tingart M, Luring C, Zurakowski D, Grifka J. Alignment in total knee arthroplasty. A comparison of computer-assisted surgery with the conventional technique. J Bone Joint Surg (Br). 2004;86:682–7.

33. Hetaimish BM, Khan MM, Simunovic N, Al-Harbi HH, Bhandari M, Zalzal PK. Meta-analysis of navigation vs conventional total knee arthroplasty. J Arthroplasty. 2012;27:1177–82.

34. Lavernia CJ, Guzman JF. Relationship of surgical volume to short-term mortality, morbidity, and hospital charges in arthroplasty. J Arthroplasty. 1995;10:133–40.

35. Soohoo NF, Zingmond DS, Lieberman JR, Ko CY. Primary total knee arthroplasty in California 1991 to 2001: does hospital volume affect outcomes? J Arthroplasty. 2006;21:199–205.

36. Yuan Z, Cooper GS, Einstadter D, Cebul RD, Rimm AA. The association between hospital type and mortality and length of stay: a study of 16.9 million hospitalized Medicare beneficiaries. Med Care. 2000;38:231–45.

37. Khuri SF, Najjar SF, Daley J, Krasnicka B, Hossain M, Henderson WG, et al. Comparison of surgical outcomes between teaching and nonteaching hospitals in the Department of Veterans Affairs. Ann Surg. 2001;234:370–82; discussion 82–3.

38. Sharkey PF, Shastri S, Teloken MA, Parvizi J, Hozack WJ, Rothman RH. Relationship between surgical volume and early outcomes of total hip arthroplasty: do results continue to get better? J Arthroplasty. 2004;19:694–9.

39. Hamilton BH, Ho V. Does practice make perfect? Examining the relationship between hospital surgical volume and outcomes for hip fracture patients in Quebec. Med Care. 1998;36:892–903.

40. Feinglass J, Amir H, Taylor P, Lurie I, Manheim LM, Chang RW. How safe is primary knee replacement surgery? Perioperative complication rates in Northern Illinois, 1993–1999. Arthritis Rheum. 2004;51:110–6.

41. Schulze Raestrup U, Smektala R. Are there relevant minimum procedure volumes in trauma and orthopedic surgery? Zentralbl Chir. 2006;131:483–92.

42. Schrader P, Ewerbeck V. Experience in orthopaedic surgery with minimum provider volumes. Der Chirurg; Zeitschrift fur alle Gebiete der operativen Medizin. 2007;78:999–1011.

43. Luft HS, Hunt SS, Maerki SC. The volume-outcome relationship: practice-makes-perfect or selective-referral patterns? Health Serv Res. 1987;22:157–82.

44. Marlow NE, Barraclough B, Collier NA, Dickinson IC, Fawcett J, Graham JC, et al. Centralization and the relationship between volume and outcome in knee arthroplasty procedures. ANZ J Surg. 2010;80:234–41.

Long Term Clinical Outcome of Total Knee Arthroplasty. The Effect of Limp Alignment, Implant Placement and Stability as Controlled by Surgical Technique

John Michos and Theofilos Karachalios

Introduction

The numbers of total knee arthroplasties (TKAs) performed per year is increasing rapidly. In the year 2005, 533,000 procedures were performed in the US and it is estimated that by the year 2030, the numbers of procedures will reach the level of three million per year [1]. Outcomes of TKA are satisfactory with a reported survival of 95.9 % at 15 years with revision for any reason, of 97 % with revision for mechanical failure and of 98.8 % with revision for aseptic loosening as an end point [2]. Other studies have also reported excellent results with a survival rate ranging from 90 to 98 % at the level of 10–15 years follow up [3–7]. Ritter et al. [8] and Lachiewicz et al. [9] have also reported survival rates of 95 % and 96.8 %, with revision for aseptic loosening as an end point at a minimum 15 years follow up. Common reasons for TKA failure have been identified (e.g., polyethylene wear, aseptic loosening, instability, infection, arthrofibrosis, malalignment or malposition, deficient extensor mechanism, avascular necrosis of the patella, periprosthetic fracture and isolated patellar implant failures) [10], while the most common reasons for reoperation are extensor mechanism problems, infection and instability [11, 12]. Sharkey et al. [10] have shown that the most prevalent cause of early failure in their series was infection (17.5 %), and for late failure polyethylene wear (25 %). Moreover, infection and surgical technique errors were the main reasons for early reoperations (within 5 years of the primary procedure) in an evaluation of 440 revision TKAs [13].

Normal knee alignment and stability are three of the main targets of TKA and can be achieved taking into consideration the following three inter-related elements; (a) the normal or prosthetic knee joint should be centered on the mechanical axis of the lower extremity, (b) appropriate level of joint line should be restored and (c) stability should be achieved by fractional release of contracted ligaments. Ligament release does not cause instability. Failure to align the knee in three planes and release the tight ligaments does cause instability, unreliable function and excessive wear. Several authors argue that the above elements are very important for the long term survival and functional performance of TKA [13–21].

In this review, the effect of limp alignment, appropriate implant placement and stability, as

J. Michos, MD, DSc
Senior Consultant Orthopaedic Surgeon,
D' Orthopaedic Department,
Asklepieion General Hospital, Boula, Athens

T. Karachalios, MD, DSc (⊠)
Orthopaedic Department, Faculty of Medicine,
School of Health Sciences, Center of Biomedical
Sciences (CERETETH), University General Hospital
of Larissa, University of Thessalia,
Mezourlo region, Larissa 41110, Hellenic Republic
e-mail: kar@med.uth.gr

© Springer-Verlag London 2015
T. Karachalios (ed.), *Total Knee Arthroplasty: Long Term Outcomes*,
DOI 10.1007/978-1-4471-6660-3_10

controlled by surgical technique, on the long term outcome of TKA will be presented following an analysis papers on surgical technique and long term quality studies.

The Effect of Restoration of the Mechanical Axis

Satisfactory TKA depends on many factors, including restoration of the mechanical axis of the limb, ligament balancing, component orientation and size. Correct alignment is one of the most important factors for implant long time survival [14, 15] (Fig. 10.1). It is well accepted that the tibial component should implanted at 90° to the tibial anatomical axis in the coronal plane and at 3–7° of posterior inclination (posterior slope) to the anatomical axis in the sagittal plane depending on the implant design. The orientation of the femoral component in the coronal plane should be at approximately 6° of valgus (usually 5–7°), which is the difference between the anatomical and mechanical axis of the femur. In the sagittal plane the femoral component should be implanted in a neutral position (no flexion or extension) in order to prevent overstuffing of the anterior part of the joint, or notching of the femoral cortex. The longevity of TKA is strongly related to the restoration of the mechanical axis of the limb and to the appropriate orientation of the components in all planes. Malpositioning of both components (especially of the tibial tray) is important in the long term survival of TKA (Fig. 10.2). Postoperative varus limb alignment is associated with a higher incidence of implant failure when compared to anatomical limb alignment [10–21]. It seems that valgus limb alignment is better tolerated than varus. Bargen et al. [22] has reported a higher incidence of failure in varus compared to valgus tibiofemoral alignment (91 % vs 11 %) (Fig. 10.3). Aglietti et al. [23] found that any tibial component with a varus angle of more than 2° in relation to the anatomical axis of the tibia was related to a considerably greater occurrence of radiolucent line. Green et al. [24] also showed that the alignment of the tibial tray has a considerable effect on loads

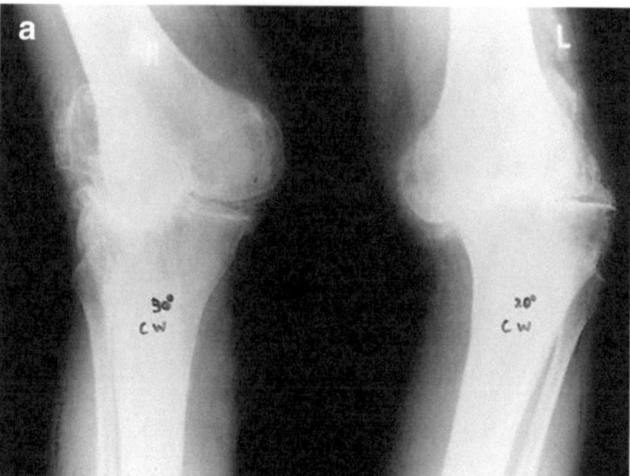
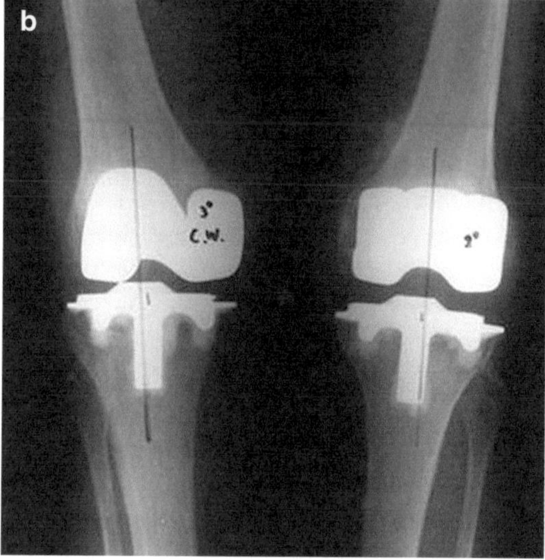

Fig. 10.1 Bilateral severe valgus and varus knee deformity, (**a**) preoperative radiographs, (**b**) postoperative radiographs showing satisfactory correction

applied to the tibial condyles. Tibial tray implanted in varus more of than 3° is a factor associated with loosening and failure, especially if it is combined with BMI of more than 33.7 [14]. The mode of failure associated with varus tibial trays is that of medial tibial condyle bone collapse [14].

The Effect of Preoperative Deformity and Soft Tissue Contractures

In varus knee deformity (Fig. 10.4), which is the most common of the osteoarthritic knee deformities, the medial structures are contracted. These structures include the deep and superficial medial collateral ligament, posterior and posteromedial capsule and posterior cruciate ligament, depending on the severity of the deformity. Whiteside has shown [25] that, when the knee is tight in flexion only, the superficial medial

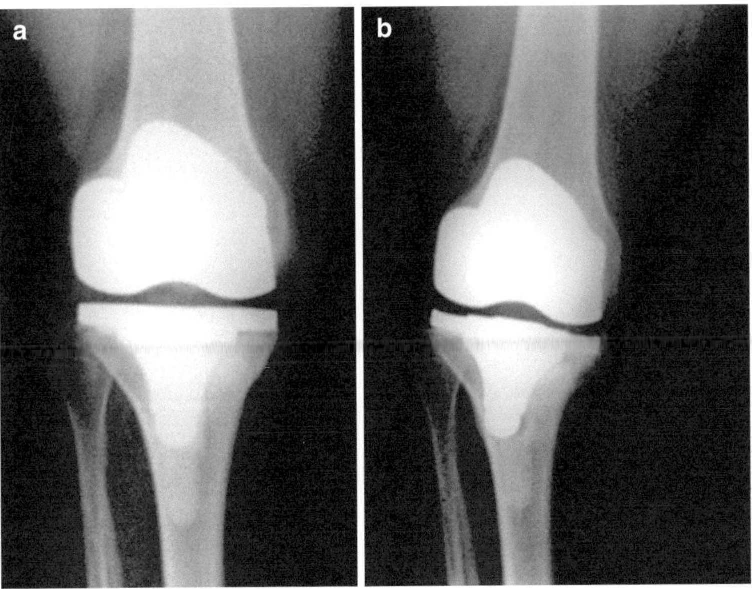

Fig. 10.2 The effect of varus placement of the tibial component, (**a**) immediate postoperative radiograph, (**b**) early aseptic loosening and varus drift of the component at 5 years follow up

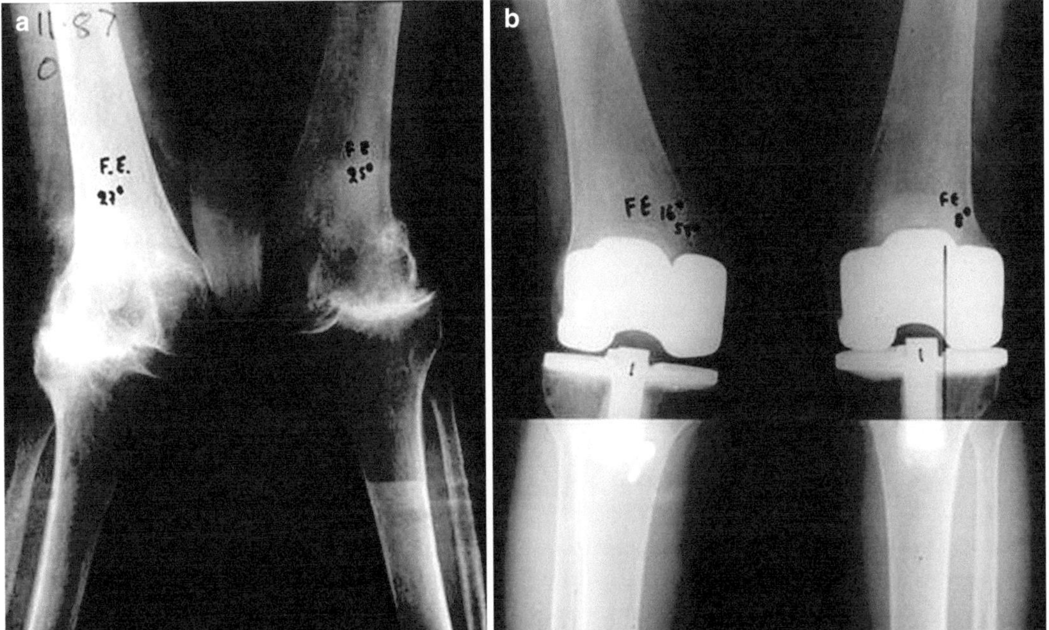

Fig. 10.3 Bilateral valgus knee deformities, (**a**) preoperative radiographs, (**b**) postoperative radiographs of well functioning TKA with valgus under correction of the right knee

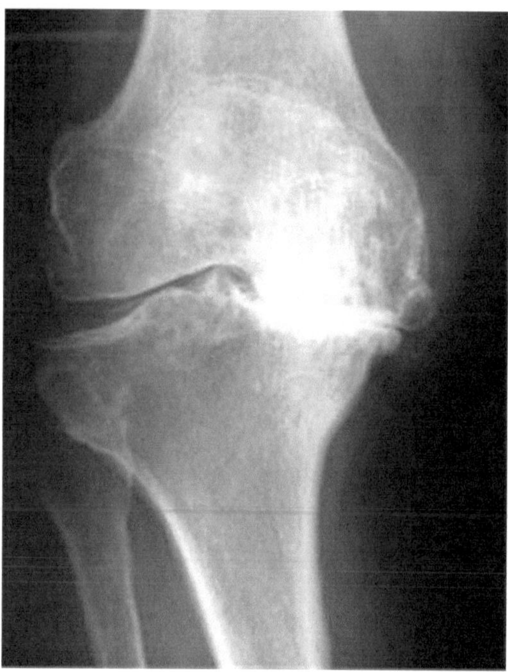

Fig. 10.4 Radiographs of a varus osteoarthritic knee joint

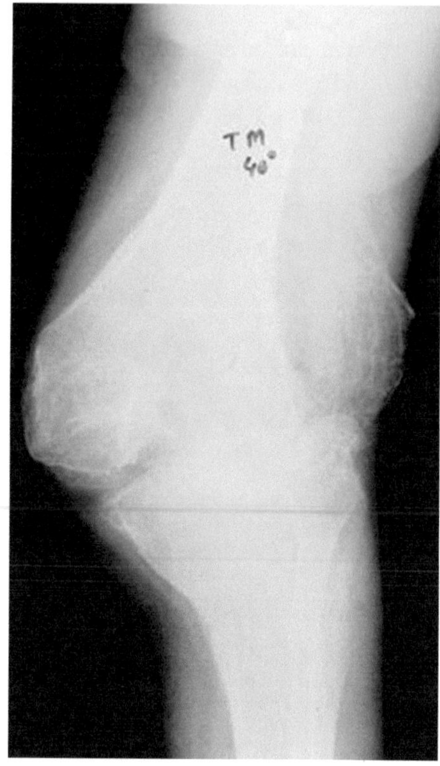

Fig. 10.5 Radiographs of a valgue osteoartheitic knee joint

collateral ligament is mainly responsible for the contracture, while when it is tight in extension, the deep medial collateral ligament is the cause of contracture. When the knee is tight in both flexion and extension, all the above structures contribute to medial tightness and need balanced release [26]. In order to restore the tibiofemoral axis it is necessary to remove the osteophytes from the upper lip of the medial tibial condyle and the medial femoral condyle in combination with a balanced release of the medial structures. The deep medial collateral ligament is sub periosteally elevated from the upper medial tibial condyle and its detachment can be extended to the posteromedial part of the condyle (if needed). The superficial medial collateral ligament is next sub periosteally elevated with the use of an elevator or a curved osteotome and, finally, even hamstring insertion may be necessary to elevate it. In severe varus deformities the correction is facilitated by the removal of the posterior cruciate, or by detachment of its inscrtion from the posterior tibia, as it has been shown that a contracted posterior cruciate contributes to the deformity on the

coronal plane [27]. The procedure is performed stage by stage and the alignment and stability is tested after each surgical step. The goal is to achieve a normal laxity of 2 mm as estimated by a symmetrical joint opening of both the medial and lateral sides. Fixed flexion deformity is corrected by careful removal of the posterior osteophytes using a curved osteotome, and further release of the posterior capsule from its insertion in the posterior part of the condyles.

Valgus knee deformity (Fig. 10.5) is less common than varus. It accounts for 10–15 % of all knee deformities, and is more difficult to correct. It has been reported that TKA in knees with severe varus deformity results in superior outcome when compared to those of knees with severe valgus deformity. This superiority has been attributed to incomplete tibiomemoral axis correction in the valgus knees [28]. Bone deformities and soft tissues contractures are also encountered and are responsible for surgical technical difficulties during balanced restoration of the axis. In contrast to the varus knee, where the medial compartment is distorted, in valgus knees the lateral femoral condyle is usually mainly affected, being hypoplastic posteriorly and distally.

The lateral stabilizing structures are contracted and require balanced release. These elements include capsule-ligament units (lateral collateral ligament, posterolateral and posterior capsule, and posterior cruciate ligament) and musculo-tendinous structures (iliotibial band, the popliteal tendon, lateral gastrocnemius and biceps tendon). Several techniques for release of the contracted elements have been suggested, but no standardized method has been established [25, 26, 29]. It has been shown that the iliotibial band and the posterolateral capsule are mainly responsible for tightness of the knee in extension, while the popliteal tendon and the lateral collateral ligament are mainly responsible for tightness in flexion [30]. During correction of the deformity and balanced release of the structures, the iliotibial band is first detached from Gerdy's tubercle, if the knee is tight in extension, then the popliteal tendon and the lateral collateral ligament are subperiosteally elevated from the lateral femoral condyle in order to overcome tightness in flexion. The posterolateral capsule can be released using the "pie crust technique" or with a horizontal cautery cut at the level of the joint line, if further correction is necessary, in order to achieve balanced correction of the deformity [31]. The Posterior cruciate ligament can be released at its tibial insertion, or even resected, if further correction is required. Release of the posterior cruciate ligament further contributes to appropriate alignment in the coronal plane [31]. In order to restore the mechanical axis in severely deformed valgus knees, other techniques have also been proposed such as approaching the knee through the lateral side with or without tibial tubercle osteotomy. It is claimed that this procedure facilitates the balanced release of the contracted elements [32–34]. In severely deformed knees, the extensive release of the structures, which is required for correction of the deformity, may lead to instability. In such cases a constrained implant design should be used. In cases with an incompetent medial collateral ligament a constrained implant design should also be used. Sliding lateral femoral condyle osteotomy is another proposed technique for valgus correction, as the osteotomised fragment moves distally with the lateral contracted elements attached on it. Distal transposition releases tension and fixation with screws is then performed [35]. A thorough search of the literature has revealed that papers related to balanced release of the contracted structure describe the technique in only a relatively small number of patients and little data is given regarding the effect on the long term outcome of the TKA.

The Effect of Restoring the Joint Line and Balancing the Extension and Flexion Gap

Joint line height should be corrected with appropriate restoration of both femoral and tibial bone defects and balanced release of contracted structures in both the coronal and sagittal plane. In order to achieve this excessive removal of bone during femoral and tibial osteotomies should be avoided. The attempt to balance large extension and flexion gaps with the use of thick polyethylene only is the usual cause of joint line elevation (Fig. 10.6). Mid and long term studies have shown inferior outcomes and a high incidence of complications in TKAs in which there is a deviation from the anatomic line of more than 5 mm [36]. Posterior offset of the femoral implant should ideally be equal to the preoperative posterior offset of the femoral condyles (sagittal plane), in order to restore the joint line in flexion (Fig. 10.7). In order to avoid residual instability it is very important to have symmetric balancing of the collateral ligaments and equal flexion and extension gaps (Fig. 10.8). Minimal mediolateral laxity of 1–2 mm in extension, and equal flexion and extension gaps (tested in extension and with the knee at 90° of flexion when lifting up the femur and rotating the tibia) are considered the ideal result which enhances long term outcome [37]. If flexion is tighter than the extension gap

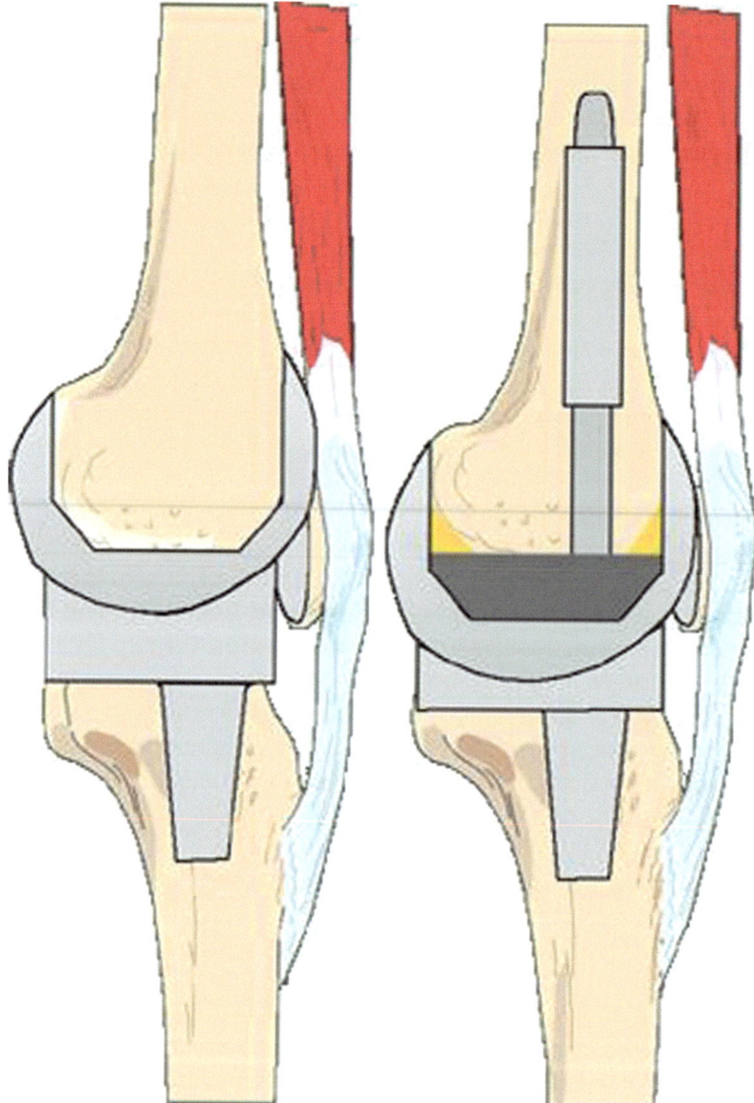

Fig. 10.6 Elevation of the joint line using a thick polyethylene liner (*left*). In order to avoid this effect, bone defect should be reconstructed (*right*)

and a posterior cruciate retaining implant is used, an attempt to increase the posterior tibial slope may solve the problem. If a tight flexion gap is due to a tight posterior cruciate ligament only and not to tight collaterals, partial release of the posterior cruciate ligament insertion from the tibia could be an helpful intervention.

Ligamentous imbalance or excessive posterior tibial slope has been shown to cause increased translational and rotational moments leading to a higher concentration of stresses on the joint surfaces and further subluxation [38]. Residual instability related to surgical technique may lead to high stress concentration and excessive polyethylene wear compromising clinical outcome and longevity of the TKA. Thus when dealing with severe knee deformities, surgeons should be prepared to use implants with higher degrees of constraint. In cases of inflammatory arthritis, such as rheumatoid arthritis, posterior cruciate

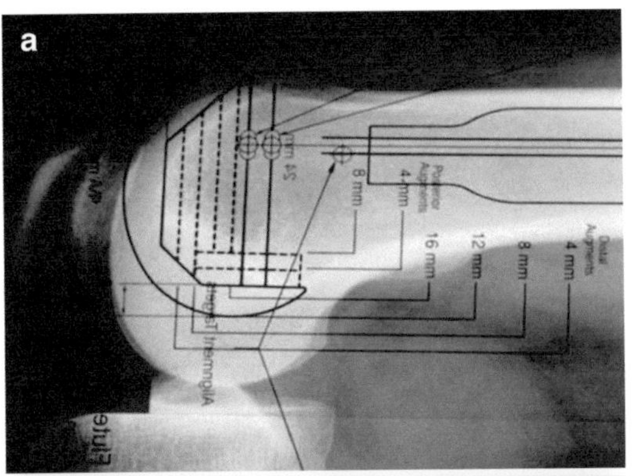

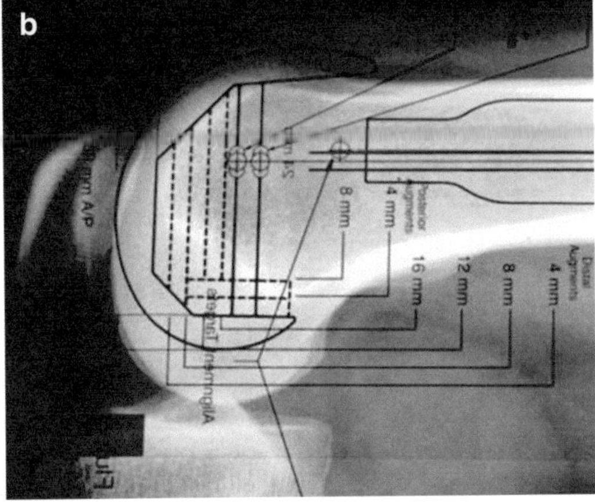

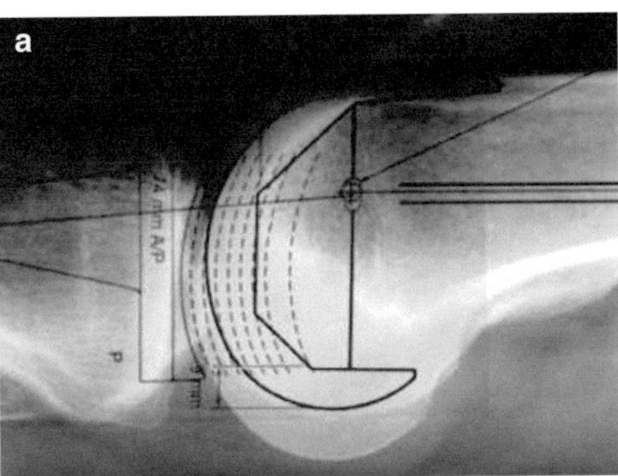

Fig. 10.7 The effect of anterior offset (**a**) and posterior offset (**b**) on the flexion gap and anterior patellofemoral overstuffing is shown

retaining TKA implants should be used with caution, anticipating the possibility of later rupture of the posterior cruciate ligament due to disease activity resulting in pain, effusion and anteroposterior instability [39].

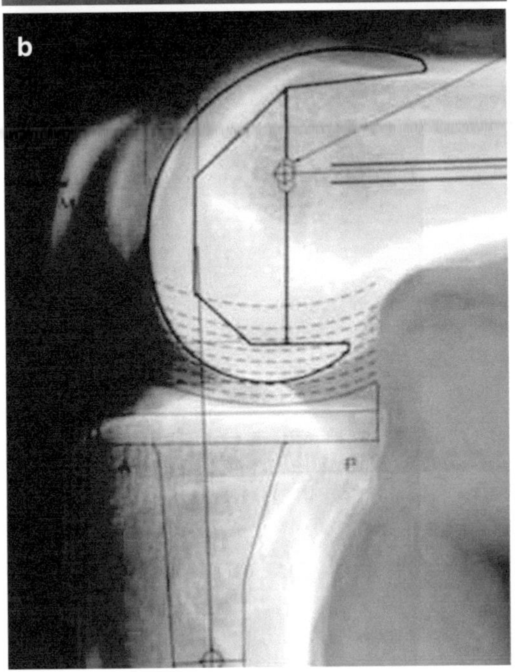

Fig. 10.8 The same component – polyethylene composite thickness in extension (**a**) and flexion (**b**) ensures equal soft tissue balancing and stability

The Effect of Appropriate Anteroposterior and Rotational Placement of the Components

Bone resection from the distal and posterior femur and proximal tibia creates a flexion and an extension gap. Equalization and balance of these gaps is very important for the outcome of the procedure. Instrumentation systems used for femoral bone cuts are either anterior referencing, posterior referencing or both (Fig. 10.9). With posterior referencing systems, if implant size is to be changed, the anterior cut of the femur is altered while the posterior femoral condyle cut remains unchanged. Thus downsizing the component may cause anterior notching, while upsizing may lead to overstuffing of the patellofemoral space.

With anterior referencing systems, the selected anterior femoral cut is not affected by up or downsizing the guide, while the thickness of the bone to be resected from the posterior condyles is changed thus affecting the flexion gap.

Equally important is also the appropriate rotational placement of both components. Malrotation

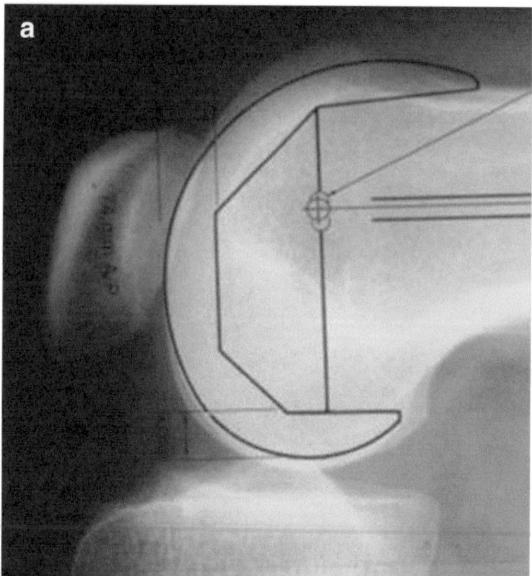

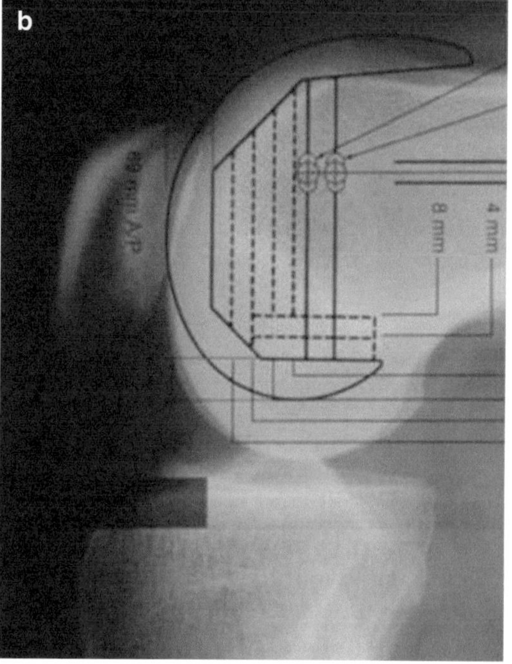

Fig. 10.9 The effect of up (**a**) and down (**b**) sizing of the femoral component on the flexion gap is shown

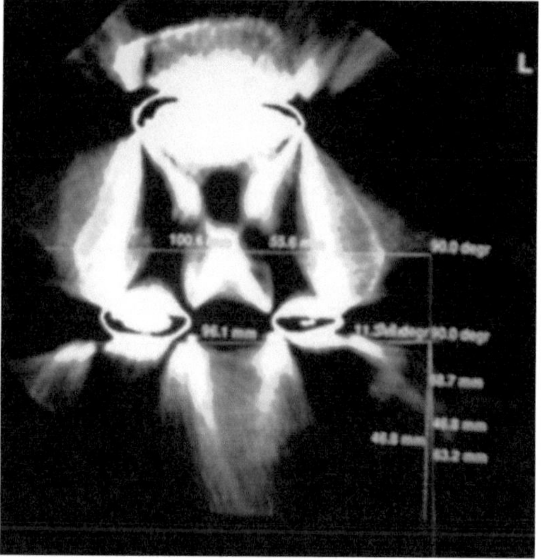

Fig. 10.10 Transverse CT-scan section showing that femoral component is rotationally aligned parallel to the transepicondylar axis

of either the tibial or femoral component will cause abnormal patellofemoral tracking and asymmetrical gaps, with undesired consequences. Correct rotation of the femoral component will allow the patella to slide in the groove without high strain, from full extension to full flexion. The transepicondylar axis is suggested and commonly used as a guide for this purpose, as it has been shown that it is 3–5° externally rotated in relation to the posterior condylar line (Fig. 10.10). However, the centers of the epicondyles are often difficult to define, because of the bulk of soft tissues and their broad bases [40–42]. More accurate positioning can be achieved by using the anteroposterior axis, which is the line joining the deepest point of the trochlear groove and the most lateral edge of the posterior cruciate ligament femoral insertion, as described by Hanada and Whiteside and called "Whiteside line" [43, 44] (Fig. 10.11). Insall and Scott have proposed the flexion gap technique, consisting of cutting the posterior condyles in a fashion parallel to the tibial cut, with the knee flexed at 90°, after balancing the collateral ligaments [45]. With this technique, the femoral component is routinely implanted in slight external rotation of the femur [46]. Another drawback is that ligament release is performed in extension and bony cuts in flexion. If the posterior condylar line is used as a guide for rotational positioning of the femoral implant, asymmetric wear of the posterior parts of the condyles often seen in valgus deformed knees should be taken into consideration in order to avoid undesirable internal rotation of the component and subsequent patellar

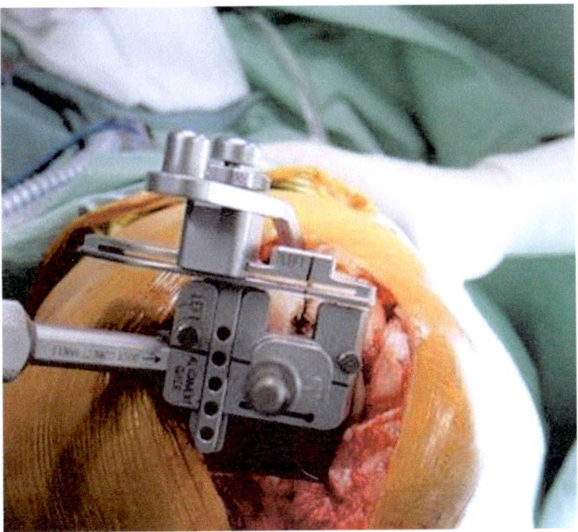

Fig. 10.11 Femoral cutting jig aligned parallel to the (Whiteside) line

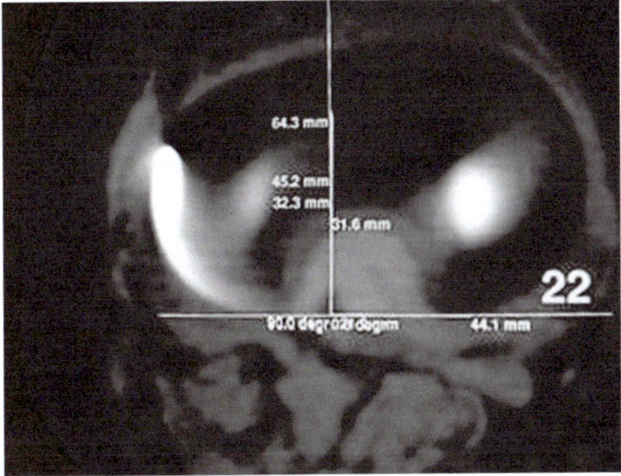

Fig. 10.12 Transverse CT-scan section showing the appropriate rotational placement of the tibial tray

instability [47]. Tibial tray rotation also affects patellofemoral alignment and thus excessive internal rotation should be avoided (Fig. 10.12). The central point of the tray must be in line with the junction of the inner and medial third of the tibial tuberosity [48].

The Effect of Instrumentation for Femoral and Tibial Cuts

For appropriate femoral alignment and component placement intramedullary systems have been shown to offer superior accuracy and are always used [49]. Concerning tibial alignment, there is considerable debate as to whether intramedullary or extramedullary systems provide more accurate reproductions of anatomical axes [50–52]. Extramedullary alignment systems are based on bony landmarks which may be obscured in obese patients or covered by bulky surgical drapes (Fig. 10.13). Therefore most authors suggest that the intramedullary systems are more accurate and reproducible, especially in obese patients and they also reduce surgical time [53–55]. However, in cases with bowed tibia or other extra articular tibial deformities, extramedullary systems are more accurate [56, 57]. The extramedullary tibial guide should be set to engage the ankle 3–6 mm medial of the center, as the center of the talus is medial to the line bisecting the distance between the malleoli [58] (Fig. 10.14). If a intramedullary guide is chosen (Fig. 10.15), the starting hole should be placed approximately one third the distance from anterior to posterior surface of the tibia and slightly medial to the midline [54] (Fig. 10.16). The significance of the entry point on the tibial surface has been emphasized while the deformity of the axis should be taken into consideration [55]. In severe varus knees, it is suggested that the entry point should be placed slightly externally in order to avoid the rod engaging the diaphyseal cortex. Simmons et al. [59] have suggested that the entry point of the rod is an important factor affecting the orientation of the tibial cut and they also found that the 8 mm rod could be inserted in nearly all tibias. In the same study, a 90° tibial component angle was achieved in 83 % of varus knees, but only in 37 % of the valgus knees. The authors conclude that the intramedullary system is less accurate in valgus than in varus knees. Reed et al. [60] has conducted a prospective randomized trial and found that the intramedullary system was more accurate in determining proximal tibial cut in both the coronal and sagittal plane, with a mean deviation of 1.6° only (no outliers were detected). Few other studies have addressed the issue of tibial cut accuracy on the sagittal plane. Most of these have concluded that intramedullary systems can accurately determine tibial cut in the sagittal plane, within 3° or less [16, 52, 61]. However,

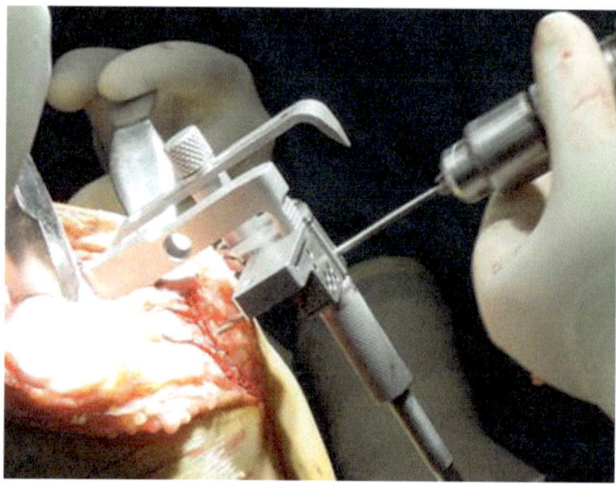

Fig. 10.13 Extramedullary tibial cutting jig is shown

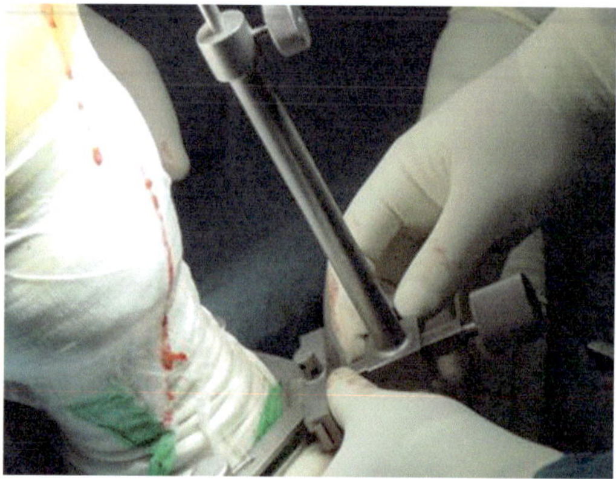

Fig. 10.14 Distal alignment of an extramedullary tibial cutting jig is shown

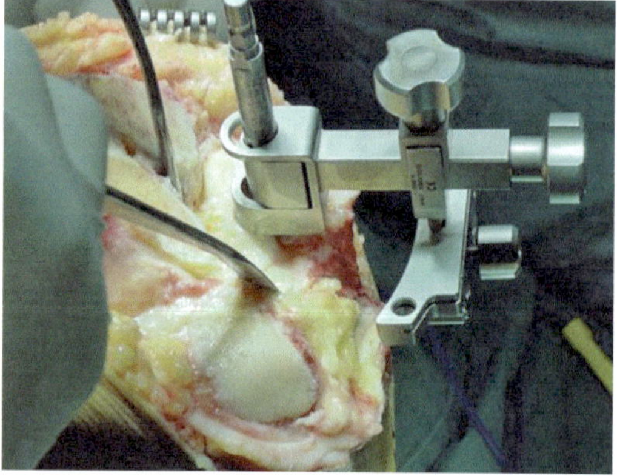

Fig. 10.15 Intramedullary tibial cutting jig is shown

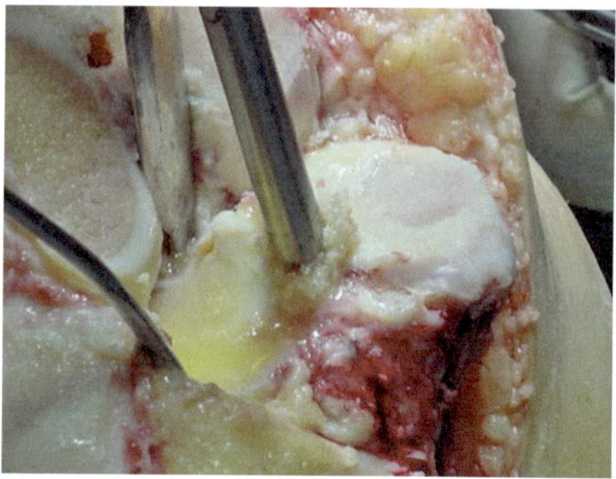

Fig. 10.16 The entrance point of an intramedullary cutting jig is shown

DeKroon et al. [63], in a prospective randomized study of intramedullary versus extramedullary instrumentation, reported better restoration of the posterior tibial slope with the extramedullary system. Finally, in a comparative study between intramedullary and extramedullary guiding systems, the intramedullary system was found to be more accurate for the coronal, while the extramedullary system was more reliable for the sagittal osteotomy, though the mean difference from the planned posterior slope was only 1° [64]. One should keep in mind that when the tibial guide is set to cut at some degrees of posterior slope, it should be set at the center of the tibia on the coronal plane, otherwise the cut will not be set to be horizontal, but in varus (with external rotation of the guide), or valgus (with internal rotation of the guide).

The association of the use of intramedullary systems with systematic effects such as embolism has been questioned (as the insertion of the rod increases medullary canal pressure) [65]. In order to avoid the high elevation of intramedullary pressure, contemporary rods are fluted to allow egress of the medullary material [54]. Transesophageal echocardiography during intramedullary instrumented TKA has demonstrated that a shower of fat or intramedullary embolic particles enter the right atrium of the heart, however, this is not clinically relevant [66]. The peak of the detectable embolization effect occurs shortly after tourniquet release, but no clinical

other authors have found wider deviations and have questioned the accuracy of intramedullary instrumentation [59, 62].

manifestation of fat embolism has been reported and the risk of venous embolism is not increased using intramedullary alignment techniques [67, 68].

The Clinical Relevance of Posterior Tibial Slope

There is great variability of the posterior slope of the native upper tibia in different populations and ethnic groups, often exceeding the conventional figure of 5–10° [69–71]. Tibial posterior slope angle affects flexion gap, tension of the posterior cruciate ligament and knee stability following TKA. Several authors suggest that increased posterior slope after TKA improves maximum knee flexion, but clinical studies have not always confirmed this, as it is well known that flexion achieved after TKA depends on several factors such as quadriceps length, capsular tightness, surgical technique, implant design and rehabilitation. Excessive posterior slope can lead to a slack posterior cruciate, anterior subluxation of the tibia, changes in the loading pattern of the knee and increased polyethylene wear, thus compromising the longevity of the TKA. In contrast, an inadequate posterior tibial slope, or even worse, creation of an anterior slope, is bound to concentrate high stresses on the weak anterior cancellous bone during weight bearing, increasing the possibility of anterior subsidence of the tibial tray. Flexion may also be compromised, due to the tight posterior cruciate and flexion gap [72].

Singh et al. [71] have shown that restoring the preoperative tibial slope to within a range of 2° maximizes the range of movement and flexion angle in posterior stabilized TKA. Bellemans et al. [73], observed an average gain of 1.7° for every degree of extra tibial slope in a cruciate retaining implant. Kim et al. [74] found no significant correlation between postoperative tibial slope and maximum flexion angle in a series of 79 patients, but Shi et al. [75] reported a 1.8° flexion increment with 1° increase of tibial slope in a cohort of 56 patients. Similarly, increased posterior slope was not correlated with increased

flexion angle in a comparative study between two groups of patients, one with tibial posterior slope of 5° and another of 0° [76]. An advantageous effect of posterior slope set at 10° compared to neutral is the improvement of the quadriceps lever arm, which might have a positive effect on postoperative mobilization [77]. Seo et al. [78] evaluated clinical outcomes in relation to the posterior tibial slope before and after the operation. Significant improvement was seen in all patients, but it was most notable when the change of the slope was within the range of +3° to −1° [78].

It seems it is important to determine the proper posterior slope angle, taking into consideration the preoperative inclination of the joint surface, but exact limits have not been established. It is recommended, though, that the slope should not exceed 10° [79]. Moreover, using a posterior stabilizing implant and sacrificing the posterior cruciate ligament leads to a slightly bigger flexion gap which, combined with excessive posterior tibial slope, may cause instability. Therefore, while using a cruciate retaining design, a posterior tibial slope of 6–9° is recommended, a maximum of 3° should be achieved in posterior substituting implants in order to avoid instability [80].

The Clinical Relevance of Restoration of Joint Line

Both incorrect femoral and tibial cuts and malpositioning of the components can alter the level of the joint line resulting (if it exceeds 5 mm) in malfunction of the extensor mechanism and anterior knee pain [36, 81]. Impingement of the inferior pole of patella against the tibial insert and impingement of the patellar tendon against the tibial component may occur (Fig. 10.17). Parrington et al. [82] have noted, in a study of 99 revision knee arthroplasties, a statistical difference in clinical scores when the elevation of the joint line was more than 8 mm. Midflexion instability is a relatively new concept, indicating symptomatic medio-lateral laxity in between 30° and 45° of flexion. Joint line elevation has been shown to contribute to the appearance of this form of instability [83, 84]. Removal of excessive bone from the distal part of femur is an important factor responsible for significant elevation of the joint line [85]. An attempt to replace bone loss using a thick polyethylene insert will cause significant elevation of the joint line with subsequent functional effect. Therefore correction of fixed flexion deformity should be attempted by elevation of the posterior capsule from the posterior part of the femoral condyles and not by excessive distal bone removal. During surgery, bony landmarks, like the medial epicondyle or fibular head, are used as guides for joint line calculation but it is not always easy to palpate and clearly see these landmarks. The use of a navigation system has been shown to enable surgeons to restore the joint line with more accuracy than conventional instrumentation systems [86].

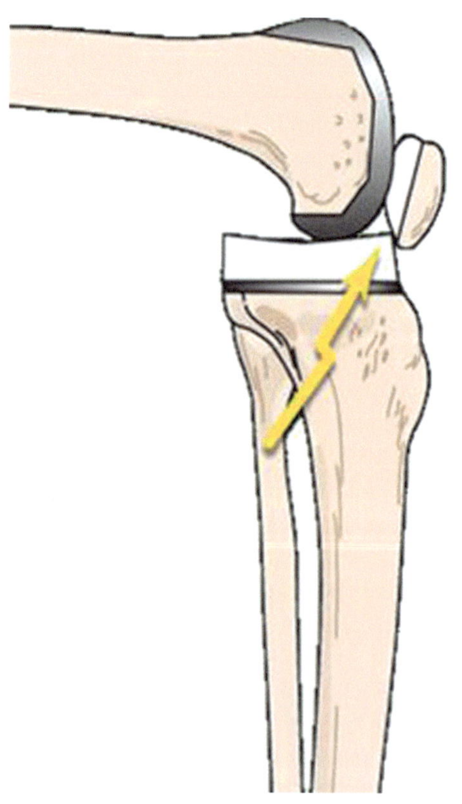

Fig. 10.17 Extensor mechanism impingement in flexion due to elevated joint line is shown

The Effect of Computer Assisted Surgery

Limb mechanical axis malalignment has been shown to have a negative effect on the long term stability of the implants [14, 87], while well aligned TKAs experience optimal mechanics and reduced stresses on the components and thus improved implant survivorship and functional outcome [88].

Computer assisted surgery (CAS) was introduced in the late 1990s, aiming to improve alignment of TKAs and optimize the clinical outcomes. Anatomic landmarks of the limb are used and with the help of infrared camera and appropriate software the mechanical axis of the limb is determined. The contracted ligaments are released to a stage of correction of axis. Size and position of the components are also guided by the system. However, the anatomic landmarks have to be indicated by the surgeon's hand.

A meta-analysis performed on this topic confirmed accurate restoration of mechanical axis to within 3° [89]. Bawens et al. [89] has reported that CAS offered a few advantages compared to conventional surgery. It did not significantly improve the mean mechanical axis alignment, though it decreased the risk for outliers with a deviation more than 2–3° from normal. At the same time it increased the time of surgery by 23 %. The improvement of axis correction using CAS was also confirmed by Novicoff et al. [90] who performed a systematic review of the literature, but superiority of the clinical outcome and survivorship of the implant has not been proved and thus further quality studies are required. Kim et al. [91] reported on a prospective randomized study including 520 patients with bilateral posterior cruciate retaining, mobile bearing, TKAs. On one side a navigation system was used, but on the other conventional instrumentation. At a mean follow up of 10.8 years, WOMAC, Knee Society score, radiographic assessments of component orientation and activity levels did not reveal significant differences between the two sides. It was concluded that navigation did not improve alignment or clinical outcome. The effect of CAS is important in cases with deformities of the femur or tibia which preclude the use of intramedullary alignment systems. Congenital deformities, extrarticular angulation of the femur or tibia, and the presence of implants with a long stem may preclude the use of alignment systems. In these cases the navigation system has proved successful [92]. A prospective double blind randomized study compared cardiac embolic load during computer assisted and intramedullary aligned TKA, using transesophageal echocardiography, and showed significantly fewer systemic emboli being released during the CAS procedure compared to conventional arthroplasty [93].

The Effect of Patient Specific Guides

Patient specific guides have been developed in order to improve the accuracy of bone cuts, implant orientation and the restoration of the axis. Patient specific cutting guides are manufactured based on three dimensional imaging in order to accurately capture the true anatomy of individual knees. Two guides are manufactured to match the patient's distal femur and proximal tibia. All cuts are made with the use of these guides focusing on the appropriate orientation and placement of the components and the restoration of normal limb axis. However, so far no significant superiority has been shown in comparison with conventional instrumentation [94].

References

1. Kurtz S, Ong K, Lau E, Mowat F, Halpern M. Projections of primary and revision hip and knee arthroplasty in the United States from 2005 to 2030. J Bone Joint Surg Am. 2007;89A:780–5.
2. Vessely MB, Whaley AL, Harmsen WS, Schleck CD, Berry DJ. The Chitranjan Ranawat award: long-term survivorship and failure modes of 1000 cemented condylar total knee arthroplasties. Clin Orthop. 2006;452:28–34.
3. Kelly MA, Clarke HD. Long-term results of posterior cruciate-substituting total knee arthroplasty. Clin Orthop. 2002;404:51–7.
4. Thadani PJ, Vince KG, Ortaaslan SG, Blackburn DC, Cudiamat CV. Ten- to 12-year followup of the Insall-Burstein I total knee prosthesis. Clin Orthop. 2000;380:17–29.
5. Buehler KO, Venn-Watson E, D'Lima DD, Colwell CW. The press-fit condylar total knee system: 8- to 10-year results with a posterior cruciate-retaining design. J Arthroplasty. 2000;15:698–701.
6. Dixon MC, Brown RR, Parsch D, Scott RD. Modular fixed-bearing total knee arthroplasty with retention of the posterior cruciate ligament. A study of patients followed for a minimum of fifteen years. J Bone Joint Surg Am. 2005;87:598–603.
7. Gill GS, Joshi AB. Long-term results of kinematic condylar knee replacement. An analysis of 404 knees. J Bone Joint Surg (Br). 2001;83:355–8.
8. Ritter MA, Berend ME, Meding JB, Keating EM, Faris PM, Crites BM. Long-term followup of anatomic graduated components posterior cruciate-retaining total knee replacement. Clin Orthop. 2001;388:51–7.
9. Lachiewicz PF, Soileau ES. Fifteen-year survival and osteolysis associated with a modular posterior stabilized knee replacement. A concise follow-up of a previous report. J Bone Joint Surg Am. 2009;91:1419–23.
10. Sharkey PF, Hozack WJ, Rothman RH, Shastri S, Jacoby SM. Insall award paper. Why are total knee arthroplasties failing today? Clin Orthop. 2002;404:7–13.
11. Cameron HU, Hunter GA. Failure in total knee arthroplasty: mechanisms, revisions, and results. Clin Orthop. 1982;170:141–6.
12. Rand JA, Bryan RS. Revision after total knee arthroplasty. Orthop Clin N Am. 1982;13:201–12.
13. Fehring TK, Odum S, Griffin WL, Mason JB, Nadaud M. Early failures in total knee arthroplasty. Clin Orthop. 2001;392:315–8.
14. Berend ME, Ritter MA, Meding JB, et al. Tibial component failure mechanisms in total knee arthroplasty. Clin Orthop. 2004;428:26–34.
15. Ritter MA, Faris PM, Keating EM, Meding JB. Postoperative alignment of total knee replacement. Its effect on survival. Clin Orthop. 1994;299:153–6.
16. Maestro A, Harwin SF, Sandoval MG, Vaquero DH, Murcia A. Influence of intramedullary versus extramedullary alignment guides on final total knee arthroplasty component position: a radiographic analysis. J Arthroplasty. 1998;13:552–8.
17. Moreland JR. Mechanisms of failure in total knee arthroplasty. Clin Orthop. 1988;226:49–64.
18. Lotke P, Ecker ML. Influence of positioning of prosthesis in total knee replacement. J Bone Joint Surg Am. 1977;59A:77–9.
19. Windsor RE, Scuderi GR, Moran MC, Insall JN. Mechanisms of failure of the femoral and tibial component in total knee arthroplasty. Clin Orthop. 1989;248:15–20.
20. Mont MA, Urquhart MA, Hungerford DS, Krackow KA. Intramedullary goniometer can improve alignment in knee arthroplasty surgery. J Arthroplasty. 1997;12:332–6.
21. Delp SL, Stulberg SD, Davies B, Picard F, Leitner F. Computer – assisted knee replacement. Clin Orthop. 1998;354:49–56.

22. Bargren JH, Blaha JD, Freeman MA. Alignment in total knee arthroplasty. Correlated biomechanical and clinical observations. Clin Orthop. 1983;173:178–83.

23. Aglietti P, Buzzi R. Posteriorly stabilised total-condylar knee replacement. Three to eight years' follow-up of 85 knees. J Bone Joint Surg (Br). 1988;70B:211–6.

24. Green GV, Berend KR, Berend ME, Glisson RR, Vail TP. The effects of varus tibial alignment on proximal tibial surface strain in total knee arthroplasty: the posteromedial hot spot. J Arthroplasty. 2002;17:1033–9.

25. Whiteside LA. Soft tissue balancing: the knee. J Arthroplasty. 2002;17:23–7.

26. Whiteside LA, Saeki K, Mihalko WM. Functional medical ligament balancing in total knee arthroplasty. Clin Orthop. 2000;380:45–57.

27. Insall JN, Scott WN, editors. Surgery of the knee: surgical techniques and instrumentation in total knee arthroplasty. New York: Churchill Livingstone; 2001. p. 1593–4.

28. Karachalios T, Sarangi PP, Newman JH. Severe varus and valgus deformities treated by total knee arthroplasty. J Bone Joint Surg (Br). 1994;76:938–42.

29. Favorito PJ, Mihalko WM, Krackow KA. Total knee arthroplasty in the valgus knee. J Am Acad Orthop Surg. 2002;10:16–24.

30. Peters CL, Mohr RA, Bachus KN. Primary total knee arthroplasty in the valgus knee: creating a balanced soft tissue envelope. J Arthroplasty. 2001;16:721–9.

31. Miyasaka KC, Ranawat CS, Mullaji A. 10- to 20-year followup of total knee arthroplasty for valgus deformities. Clin Orthop. 1997;345:29–37.

32. Buechel FF. A sequential three-step lateral release for correcting fixed valgus knee deformities during total knee arthroplasty. Clin Orthop. 1990;260:170–5.

33. Keblish PA. The lateral approach to the valgus knee. Surgical technique and analysis of 53 cases with over two-year follow-up evaluation. Clin Orthop. 1991;271:52–62.

34. Nikolopoulos DD, Polyzois I, Apostolopoulos AP, Rossas C, Moutsios-Rentzos A, Michos IV. Total knee arthroplasty in severe valgus knee deformity: comparison of a standard medial parapatellar approach combined with tibial tubercle osteotomy. Knee Surg Sports Traumatol Arthrosc. 2011;19: 1834–42.

35. Brilhault J, Lautman S, Favard L, Burdin P. Lateral femoral sliding osteotomy lateral release in total knee arthroplasty for a fixed valgus deformity. J Bone Joint Surg (Br). 2002;84B:1131–7.

36. Porteous AJ, Hassaballa MA, Newman JH. Does the joint line matter in revision total knee replacement? J Bone Joint Surg (Br). 2008;90B:879–84.

37. Lombardi Jr AV, Berend KR, Aziz-Jacobo J, Davis MB. Balancing the flexion gap: relationship between tibial slope and posterior cruciate ligament release and correlation with range of motion. J Bone Joint Surg Am. 2008;90A(S4):121–32.

38. Feng EL, Stulberg SD, Wixson RL. Progressive subluxation and polyethylene wear in total knee replacements with flat articular surfaces. Clin Orthop. 1994;299:60–71.

39. Mitts K, Muldoon MP, Gladden M, Padgett DE. Instability after total knee arthroplasty with the Miller-Gallante II total knee: 5- to 7-year follow-up. J Arthroplasty. 2001;16:422–7.

40. Poilvache PL, Insall JN, Scuderi GR, Font-Rodriguez DE. Rotational landmarks and sizing of the distal femur in total knee arthroplasty. Clin Orthop. 1996;331:35–46.

41. Stiehl JB, Abbott BD. Morphology of the transepicondylar axis and its application in primary and revision total knee arthroplasty. J Arthroplasty. 1995;10:785–9.

42. Olcott CW, Scott RD. A comparison of 4 intraoperative methods to determine femoral component rotation during total knee arthroplasty. J Arthroplasty. 2000;15:22–6.

43. Hanada H, Whiteside LA, Steiger J, Dyer P, Naito M. Bone landmarks are more reliable than tensioned gaps in TKA component alignment. Clin Orthop. 2007;462:137–42.

44. Arima J, Whiteside LA, McCarthy DS, White SE. Femoral rotational alignment, based on the anteroposterior axis, in total knee arthroplasty in a valgus knee. A technical note. J Bone Joint Surg Am. 1995;77A:1331–4.

45. Insall JN, Scott WN, editors. Surgery of the knee: surgical techniques and instrumentation in total knee arthroplasty. New York: Churchill Livingstone; 2001. p. 1557–9.

46. Stiehl JB, Cherveny PM. Femoral rotational alignment using the tibial shaft axis in total knee arthroplasty. Clin Orthop. 1996;331:47–55.

47. Griffin FM, Insall JN, Scuderi GR. The posterior condylar angle in osteoarthritic knees. J Arthroplasty. 1998;13:812–5.

48. Hanssen AD, Rand J. A. Management of the chronically dislocated patella during total knee arthroplasty. Tech Orthop. 1988;3:49–56.

49. Cates HE, Ritter MA, Keating EM, Faris PM. Intramedullary versus extramedullary femoral alignment systems in total knee replacement. Clin Orthop. 1993;286:32–9.

50. Anand S, Harrison JW, Buch KA. Extramedullary or intramedullary tibial alignment guides: a randomised, prospective trial of radiological alignment. J Bone Joint Surg (Br). 2003;85B:1084.

51. Dennis DA, Channer M, Susman MH, Stringer EA. Intramedullary versus extramedullary tibial alignment systems in total knee arthroplasty. J Arthroplasty. 1993;8:43–7.

52. Han HS, Kang SB, Jo CH, Kim SH, Lee JH. The accuracy of intramedullary tibial guide of sagittal alignment of PCL-substituting total knee arthroplasty. Knee Surg Sports Traumatol Arthrosc. 2010;18: 1334–8.

53. Brys DA, Lombardi Jr AV, Mallory TH, Vaughn BK. A comparison of intramedullary and extramedullary alignment systems for tibial component

placement in total knee arthroplasty. Clin Orthop. 1991;263:175–9.

54. Laskin RS. Intramedullary instrumentation: safer and more accurate than extramedullary instrumentation. Orthopedics. 2001;24:739.

55. Lozano LM, Segur JM, Macule F, et al. Intramedullary versus extramedullary tibial cutting guide in severely obese patients undergoing total knee replacement: a randomized study of 70 patients with body mass index >35 kg/m². Obes Surg. 2008;18:1599–604.

56. Laskin RS. Instrumentation pitfalls: you just can't go on autopilot! J Arthroplasty. 2003;18:18–22.

57. Teter KE, Bregman D, Colwell CW. Accuracy of intramedullary versus extramedullary tibial alignment cutting systems in total knee arthroplasty. Clin Orthop. 1995;321:106–10.

58. Akagi M, Mori S, Nishimura S, Nishimura A, Asano T, Hamanishi C. Variability of extraarticular tibial rotation references for total knee arthroplasty. Clin Orthop. 2005;436:172–6.

59. Simmons Jr ED, Sullivan JA, Rackemann S, Scott RD. The accuracy of tibial intramedullary alignment devices in total knee arthroplasty. J Arthroplasty. 1991;6:45–50.

60. Reed MR, Bliss W, Sher JL, Emmerson KP, Jones SM, Partington PF. Extramedullary or intramedullary tibial alignment guides: a randomised, prospective trial of radiological alignment. J Bone Joint Surg (Br). 2002;84B:858–60.

61. Karade V, Ravi B, Agarwal M. Extramedullary versus intramedullary tibial cutting guides in megaprosthetic total knee replacement. J Orthop Surg Res. 2012;7:33.

62. Denis K, Van Ham G, Bellemans J, et al. How correctly does an intramedullary rod represent the longitudinal tibial axes? Clin Orthop. 2002;397:424–33.

63. de Kroon KE, Houterman S, Janssen RP. Leg alignment and tibial slope after minimal invasive total knee arthroplasty: a prospective, randomized radiological study of intramedullary versus extramedullary tibial instrumentation. Knee. 2012;19:270–4.

64. Cashman JP, Carty FL, Synnott K, Kenny PJ. Intramedullary versus extramedullary alignment of the tibial component in the triathlon knee. J Orthop Surg Res. 2011;6:44.

65. Fahmy NR, Chandler HP, Danylchuk K, Matta EB, Sunder N, Siliski JM. Blood-gas and circulatory changes during total knee replacement. Role of the intramedullary alignment rod. J Bone Joint Surg Am. 1990;72A:19–26.

66. Caillouette JT, Anzel SH. Fat embolism syndrome following the intramedullary alignment guide in total knee arthroplasty. Clin Orthop. 1990;251:198–9.

67. Walker P, Bali K, Van der Wall H, Bruce W. Evaluation of echogenic emboli during total knee arthroplasty using transthoracic echocardiography. Knee Surg Sports Traumatol Arthrosc. 2012;20:2480–6.

68. Parmet JL, Horrow JC, Pharo G, Collins L, Berman AT, Rosenberg H. The incidence of venous emboli during extramedullary guided total knee arthroplasty. Anesth Analg. 1995;81:757–62.

69. Jiang CC, Yip KM, Liu TK. Posterior slope angle of the medial tibial plateau. J Formos Med Assoc. 1994;93:509–12.

70. de Boer JJ, Blankevoort L, Kingma I, Vorster W. In vitro study of inter-individual variation in posterior slope in the knee joint. Clin Biomech (Bristol, Avon). 2009;24:488–92.

71. Singh G, Tan JH, Sng BY, Awiszus F, Lohmann CH, Nathan SS. Restoring the anatomical tibial slope and limb axis may maximise post-operative flexion in posterior-stabilised total knee replacements. Bone Joint J. 2013;95B:1354–8.

72. Jojima H, Whiteside LA, Ogata K. Effect of tibial slope or posterior cruciate ligament release on knee kinematics. Clin Orthop. 2004;426:194–8.

73. Bellemans J, Robijns F, Duerinckx J, Banks S, Vandenneucker H. The influence of tibial slope on maximal flexion after total knee arthroplasty. Knee Surg Sports Traumatol Arthrosc. 2005;13:193–6.

74. Kim KH, Bin SI, Kim JM. The correlation between posterior tibial slope and maximal angle of flexion after total knee arthroplasty. Knee Surg Relat Res. 2012;24:158–63.

75. Shi X, Shen B, Kang P, Yang J, Zhou Z, Pei F. The effect of posterior tibial slope on knee flexion in posterior-stabilized total knee arthroplasty. Knee Surg Sports Traumatol Arthrosc. 2013;21:2696–703.

76. Kansara D, Markel DC. The effect of posterior tibial slope on range of motion after total knee arthroplasty. J Arthroplasty. 2006;21:809–13.

77. Ostermeier S, Hurschler C, Windhagen H, Stukenborg-Colsman C. In vitro investigation of the influence of tibial slope on quadriceps extension force after total knee arthroplasty. Knee Surg Sports Traumatol Arthrosc. 2006;14:934–9.

78. Seo SS, Kim CW, Kim JH, Min YK. Clinical results associated with changes of posterior tibial slope in total knee arthroplasty. Knee Surg Relat Res. 2013;25:25–9.

79. Piazza SJ, Delp SL, Stulberg SD, Stern SH. Posterior tilting of the tibial component decreases femoral roll-back in posterior-substituting knee replacement: a computer simulation study. J Orthop Res. 1998;16:264–70.

80. Peters CL. Soft-tissue balancing in primary total knee arthroplasty. Instr Course Lect. 2006;55:413–7.

81. Figgie HE, Goldberg VM, Heiple KG, Moller HS, Gordon NH. The influence of tibial-patellofemoral location on function of the knee in patients with the posterior stabilized condylar knee prosthesis. J Bone Joint Surg Am. 1986;68A:1035–40.

82. Partington PF, Sawhney J, Rorabeck CH, Barrack RL, Moore J. Joint line restoration after revision total knee arthroplasty. Clin Orthop. 1999;367:165–71.

83. Vince KG, Abdeen A, Sugimori T. The unstable total knee arthroplasty: causes and cures. J Arthroplasty. 2006;21:44–9.

84. Yercan HS, Ait Si Selmi T, Sugun TS, Neyret P. Tibiofemoral instability in primary total knee replacement: a review part 2: diagnosis, patient evaluation, and treatment. Knee. 2005;12:336–40.

85. Parratte S, Pagnano MW. Instability after total knee arthroplasty. J Bone Joint Surg Am. 2008;90A: 184–94.
86. Liow MH, Xia Z, Wong MK, Tay KJ, Yeo SJ, Chin PL. Robot-assisted total knee arthroplasty accurately restores the joint line and mechanical axis. A prospective randomised study. J Arthroplasty. 2013. doi:10.1016/j.arth.2013.12.010. pii: S0883-5403(13) 00899-1.
87. Collier MB, Engh Jr CA, McAuley JP, Engh GA. Factors associated with the loss of thickness of polyethylene tibial bearings after knee arthroplasty. J Bone Joint Surg Am. 2007;89A:1306–14.
88. Longstaff LM, Sloan K, Stamp N, Scaddan M, Beaver R. Good alignment after total knee arthroplasty leads to faster rehabilitation and better function. J Arthroplasty. 2009;24:570–8.
89. Bauwens K, Matthes G, Wich M, et al. Navigated total knee replacement. A meta-analysis. J Bone Joint Surg Am. 2007;89A:261–9.
90. Novicoff WM, Saleh KJ, Mihalko WM, Wang XQ, Knaebel HP. Primary total knee arthroplasty: a comparison of computer-assisted and manual techniques. Instr Course Lect. 2010;59:109–17.
91. Kim YH, Park JW, Kim JS. Computer-navigated versus conventional total knee arthroplasty a prospective randomized trial. J Bone Joint Surg Am. 2012;94A:2017–24.
92. Klein GR, Austin MS, Smith EB, Hozack WJ. Total knee arthroplasty using computer-assisted navigation in patients with deformities of the femur and tibia. J Arthroplasty. 2006;21:284–8.
93. Church JS, Scadden JE, Gupta RR, Cokis C, Williams KA, Janes GC. Embolic phenomena during computer-assisted and conventional total knee replacement. J Bone Joint Surg (Br). 2007;89:481–5.
94. Chareancholvanich K, Narkbunnam R, Pornrattanamaneewong C. A prospective randomised controlled study of patient-specific cutting guides compared with conventional instrumentation in total knee replacement. Bone Joint J. 2013;95B:354–9.

Long Term Results of Total Knee Arthroplasty. The Effect of Surgical Approach

Dimitrios Giotikas and Theofilos Karachalios

In total knee arthoplasty (TKA) "Surgical technique" usually refers to the type of surgical approach and the technique utilized for osteotomies and ligament balancing. Since the beginning of the modern era of total knee arthropasty (TKA) in the early 1970s, continuous research and the evolution of technique have led to the point where TKA is an effective and reliable treatment for degenerative knee disorders. In this chapter we analyse the impact of these parameters on the outcome of TKA.

Minimally Invasive Approaches

Introduction

The conventional medial parapatellar approach has always been the workhorse when approaching the knee for TKA. Despite repeated excellent

D. Giotikas, MD, DSc
Department of Trauma and Orthopaedics,
Addenbrookes Hospital–Cambridge, University
Hospitals NHS Foundation Trust,
Hills Road Biomedical Campus, CB2 0QQ
Cambridge, UK

T. Karachalios, MD, DSc (✉)
Orthopaedic Department, Faculty of Medicine,
School of Health Sciences, Center of Biomedical
Sciences (CERETETH), University of Thessalia,
University General Hospital of Larissa,
Mezourlo Region, Larissa 41110, Hellenic Republic
e-mail: kar@med.uth.gr

long term results in the early literature [1, 2], later studies published in the 1990s based on subjective evaluation of outcome by patients suggested that there was potential for improvement of subjective clinical outcome and patient satisfaction. Trousdale et al. [3] reported that the two most important patient considerations are postoperative pain and length of functional recovery. Dickstein et al. [4] showed that one third of their elderly patients were not satisfied with the results of their operation at 6 and 12 months postoperatively, especially regarding pain and stair climbing. More recently, Noble et al. [5] found that 14 % of patients were "dissatisfied" or "very dissatisfied" with the result of their operation.

Against this background, the concept of minimally invasive surgery (MIS) was introduced to TKA following the MIS trend in many other surgical disciplines [6] and after its successful application in unicompartmental knee replacement [7–9]. The proposed advantages in the initial reported studies were less blood loss [10–12], less postoperative pain and opioid use [13], less hospitalization [13–15], faster functional recovery [15, 16], less need for postoperative rehabilitation [13], increased patient satisfaction [17], increased cost efficiency [18, 19] and increased range of motion [16, 20, 21].

At the same time the first reservations were expressed as MIS techniques were correlated with an increased risk of implant malalignment and

© Springer-Verlag London 2015
T. Karachalios (ed.), *Total Knee Arthroplasty: Long Term Outcomes,*
DOI 10.1007/978-1-4471-6660-3_11

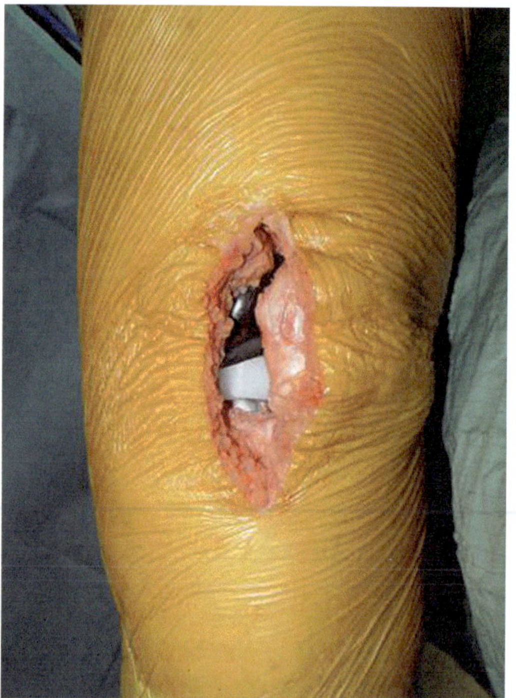

Fig. 11.1 Minimal but adequate knee exposure is shown

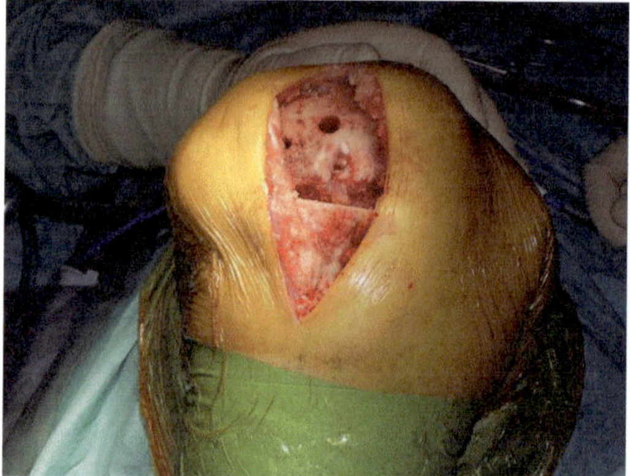

Fig. 11.2 Lateral displacement but not eversion of the patella is shown

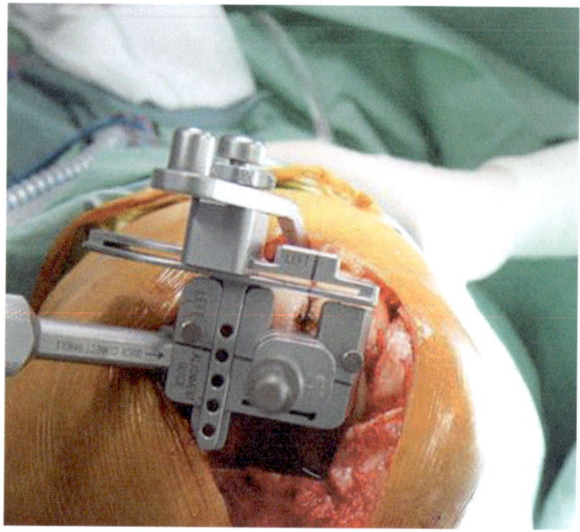

Fig. 11.3 Specially designed small instruments are necessary

possibly with increased early revision rates during the first 2 years from index surgery [22–24].

Despite the expressed scepticism, there was a vigorous promotion of the MIS concept in TKAR by the media and, as a consequence, a pressure on a surgeon's choice by well- informed patients [6]. This phenomenon was early recognized and raised many concerns and further investigations into the ways in which MIS related information is presented to the public [25–27].

Definition of MIS

Before proceeding with the impact of these techniques on the outcome of TKA it is worth clarifying what minimally invasive techniques actually are. A unanimous definition does not exist. Tenholder et al. [28] define incision length in MIS as being less than 14 cm, while Laskin et al. [29] describe it as the "least possible, barely adequate". Bonutti et al. [30] suggest the most complete definition as incision length of less than 14 cm, minimal involvement of the quadriceps tendon, avoidance of patella eversion and tibiofemoral dislocation (Fig. 11.1).

The concept of MIS generally involves: (1) smaller incisions of approximately 10–13 cm; (2) patella dislocation without eversion (Fig. 11.2); (3) minimal dissection of the quadriceps tendon; (4) preservation of the suprapatellar pouch; (5) utilization of specifically designed MIS instrument trays of reduced size (Fig. 11.3); and (6) performing the operation through a mobile soft tissue window with the appropriate use of retractors [31–33].

Based on these principles, five surgical approaches have been described, which are: the mini medial parapatellar, quadriceps-sparing, mini-midvastus, mini-subvastus, and the direct lateral approach [34]. It is not the goal of this chapter to extensively describe the technical details of

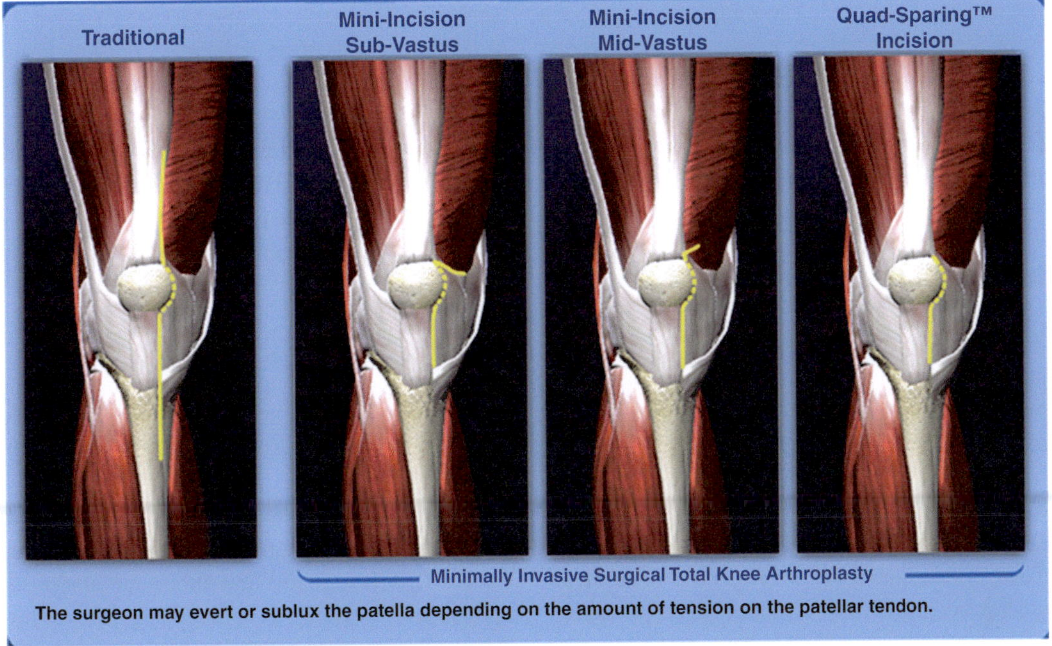

Fig. 11.4 A variety of popular MIS approaches is shown

each approach but it should be noted that they are basically variations of ways of handling the quadriceps tendon (Fig. 11.4).

The Various MIS Approaches

Some attempts have been made to compare effectiveness and safety among MIS approaches. Niki et al. [35] tested the lateral MIS approach in 26 valgus knees and found results comparable to medial MIS approaches in terms of clinical scores, postoperative pain, radiographic alignment and rates of complications. The fact, though, that a 1 cm snip of vastus lateralis had to be performed in five of their cases is indicative of the technical difficulties and the obstructed visibility of this approach. Lee et al. [36] report in their RCT that the mini midvastus and mini medial parapatellar (MMP) approaches gave comparable results in terms of pain, clinical scores and radiologic outcome in navigation assisted TKA's. Acknowledging the technical difficulties of MIS techniques, these authors favour the MMP approach because it is easier to convert to the conventional approach when necessary. After reviewing a total of 23 level I or II studies, Costa et al. [37] conclude that the lateral MIS approach had the highest rates of complications. The mini-midvastus had the best clinical results at 1 and 3 months postoperatively and the mini-subvastus had the lowest rate of complications.

Lin et al. [38] compares the quadriceps sparing approach (QS) with the mini medial parapatellar in their RCT and found that QS-TKA had more radiological outliers and longer operating times compared with the MMP approach even after adequate learning curve and with appropriately selected patients.

Based on this evidence and our personal experience we believe that for those surgeons who wish to perform an MIS-TKR, either the mini-midvastus or the mini-subvastus approach can most reasonably be expected to offer the proposed advantages of MIS, i.e. better short term clinical results without complications. These approaches have consistently shown good results with minimal complication rates. They are technically easier to perform compared to the QS and mini lateral approaches and they offer better intraoperative visibility. They are also easily extended to conventional approaches should the circumstances require. The mini lateral approach is an option for valgus knees but the surgeon should have gained extensive personal experience with the MIS conceptualization of TKA before deciding to proceed with MIS techniques in valgus knees.

MIS and Conventional Techniques

To date there have been more than 50 RCT's and approximately 16 systematic reviews and met-analyses investigating the difference between MIS and conventional approaches in TKA. From an overview of the literature we can see that up to now the majority of level I and II evidence reports short term results with follow up of 2–3 years. There is also significant heterogeneity between the studies because of the different MIS approaches, component choice or patient demographics.

Research during the past 10 years has focused on the investigation of the clinical efficiency of MIS techniques, the radiological alignment of the components and safety. Clinical efficiency was measured using clinical outcome scores, range of motion (ROM), the straight leg raise test (SLR), quadriceps strength, postoperative pain, and length of hospital stay. Radiological alignment was measured with alignment on the coronal plane and the rates of outliers. Safety was measured using blood loss, complication rates and revisions.

Clinical Scores

Costa et al. [37] reviewed 23 level I and II studies and found no significant difference in clinical scores between MIS and conventional techniques. In Li et al.'s [39] meta-analysis MIS-TKA has shown significantly improved results in objective and subjective outcome scores, VAS, ROM, knee flexion, flexion 90 day and straight leg rising day, all of which resulted in patients achieving faster recovery. In another study [40] results were analysed for measurements available at 6 weeks, 3 months and 6 months or more. The objective score at 3 months was just marginally significant in favour of the MIS group. In the same study the (VAS) was significantly improved in the MIS group.

Range of Motion

ROM is an important parameter of functional outcome. In control cohort studies, the MIS approach was found to be superior to the conventional approach in terms of ROM [41, 42]. Alcelic et al. [40] evaluated 507 MIS versus 513 conventional TKAs in a metanalysis. Knee flexion was significantly greater by 9.9° on average in the MIS group at 1 week postoperatively but not at 3 months.

Pain

Postoperative pain is an important parameter in terms of patient satisfaction and also greatly affects postoperative rehabilitation. Recently published meta-analyses report better results in VAS scores and postoperative pain [39, 40]. In our RCT [23] we report that during the first postoperative week pain was apparently greater in the minimally invasive group. In our opinion, pain management is a serious confounding factor in many published studies, and reduced pain levels should not be presented as a benefit of minimally-invasive TKA (Fig. 11.5).

Quadriceps Muscle Strength

The difficulty of consistently showing a definite clinical advantage of MIS techniques has led investigators to try to measure clinical outcome by other means. Bonutti et al. [43] used the contralateral knee as a control group and found that peak extensor muscle strength was significantly and consistently higher in the MIS group. Most patients preferred the knee treated with the MIS approach. Interestingly, these patients had different objective Knee Society Scores but similar Knee Function Scores. The authors conclude that this measure may not be sensitive enough to detect the improved outcomes of MIS techniques which are detectable with more specific measures, such as isokinetic muscle strength testing, ambulation and straight leg-raising time.

Costa et al. [37] concludes, in a systematic review, that the only significant difference observed was in the recovery of quadriceps muscle function (shorter in patients who had undergone a minimally invasive approach).

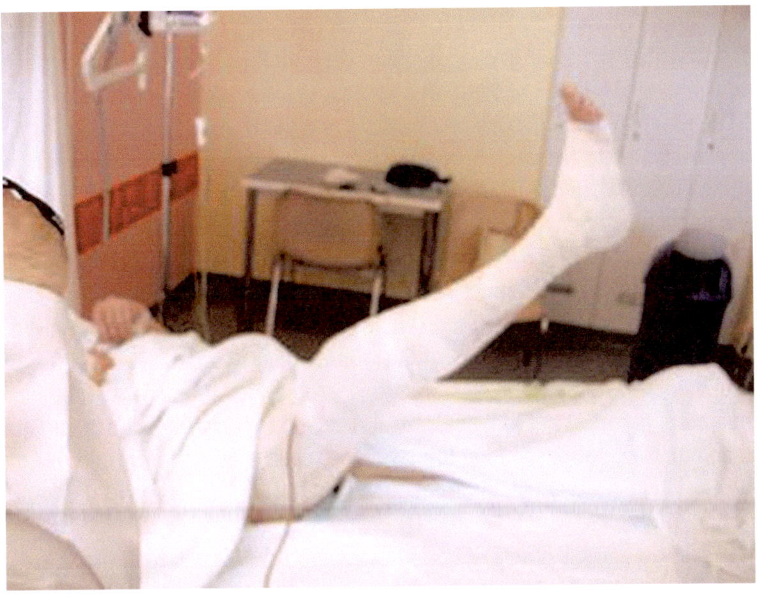

Fig. 11.5 Immediate post-operative straight leg raising, due (in our opinion) to patient controlled epidural anaesthesia

Alcelic et al. [40] also found a significant reduction in number of days to SLR in the MIS group.

Blood Loss

MIS techniques seem to offer the advantage of less total blood loss and early postoperative decrease of haemoglobin [39, 40].

Radiographic Alignment

Despite initial reservations, the fear of implant malposition does not seem to be confirmed. Most of the meta-analyses [37, 39, 44] did not find inferior radiological results in terms of component orientation and outliers with MIS techniques. Bonutti et al. [45] reviewed their first 1,000 MIS TKAs and their most important radiologic finding were 3 impending component failures, 2 tibial and 1 femoral. They raise the concern of potential tibial component loosening related to decreased exposure and possibly poor cement pressurization. In another study by there were more cement voids and more retained cement debris in the minimally invasive cohort. In our study a high incidence of wrong implant placement was found and we argue that femoral component malrotation is not detected by conventional radiography [23].

Complications

Costa et al. [37], after reviewing a total of 23 level I or II studies, conclude that there were no differences in complication rates between patients with various minimally invasive approaches compared with a standard approach. The minimally invasive lateral approach had more complications than the other minimally invasive approaches. Alcelic et al. [40], in a systematic review and metanalysis, analyzed four RCTs and quasi RCTs with a total of 296 MIS TKAs for complications. They did not find an increased risk of wound healing problems but MIS techniques showed a significantly increased risk of developing intraoperative complications with a risk ratio (RR) of 7.6. The most common complication was quadriceps tendon laceration (31 cases) and anterior femoral notching (5 cases). Other reported complications were patellar tendon rupture or partial avulsion (four cases), laceration of the popliteus (two cases), palsy of the deep peroneal nerve (two cases), one medial epicondylar avulsion fracture, one femoral condylar fracture, one tibial plateau fracture, one supracondylar fracture and the inability to displace the patella or achieve adequate exposure in four cases in the MIS group requiring conversion to the standard approach. This finding, in our opinion, reflects the technical difficulties that surgeons encounter when performing MIS techniques.

On the contrary, Li et al. [39] discovered significant differences in superficial wound healing problems and a risk of increased skin necrosis with MIS techniques but not in superficial wound infection, deep infection, DVT, fractures, femoral notching, peroneal nerve palsy, stiffness requiring manipulation, polities tendon injury, or knee instability. However, we do not feel that superficial wound problems, which are usually easily treated, should be regarded as severe complications.

Operative Time

MIS techniques are associated with longer operative and tourniquet times, especially during the learning curve period [40], but there are studies indicating that these parameters reduce to levels comparable with conventional techniques as experience is accumulated by the surgical team [24].

Length of Hospital Stay

Although there were some hopes that faster rehabilitation might result in shorter hospital stay, later level I and II evidence has not confirmed such a benefit [39, 40]. We also know that hospital stay is influenced by many parameters such as pre-operative preparation, nursing programs, discharge criteria and also by patient factors like age, co-morbidity, family status, financial situation and social insurance.

Revisions

Costa et al. [37] conclude, in a systematic review, that there were no differences in survivorship. It seems that the only study which has raised the issue of increased revision rate after MIS is that of Barrack et al. [24], in which 81.4 % of their revisions had previously been minimal incision surgery (MIS) primary TKA and 18.6 % had been standard primary TKA. Patients with MIS were younger (62.1 vs

66.2 years, P = 0.02). Most striking was the difference in time to revision, which was significantly shorter for the MIS group. We have noticed, though, that the time period for the cases involved in their study is from 2004 until 2006 which was actually the learning curve period and the time that the technique was introduced to the orthopaedic community So far there is no other evidence to our knowledge showing increased revision rates after MIS index TKA, although it needs to be emphasized that it is still too early to see the true influence of MIS techniques on survivorship.

Midterm or long term results are limited at the moment. The mid-term results of the author's study as well as Bonutti et al.'s [30, 43, 45] suggest that there are no significant differences in objective or subjective clinical and radiological outcomes in the mid-term period from 7 to 9 years. Complication rates are also comparable [45]. It is possible that the confinements of the current outcome measure scores are an obstructing factor in the detection of any modest advantage of MIS techniques.

Conclusion

Current evidence suggests that there is a modest advantage of MIS techniques during the first weeks or months after operation. Scepticism about the malpositioning of the implants does not seem to be confirmed by the studies mentioned. Currently, the initial enthusiasm for MIS techniques has abated. In 2012 Only 2 % of TKAs were performed with MIS techniques in the UK. It seems that the temporary advantage of MIS in combination with technical difficulties and suspected risks has not been considered adequate to change the practice of established surgeons. The truth is that performing a TKA with the MIS approach is technically challenging and requires the surgeon to re-learn how to judge during the procedure. Only the future will show whether there is a place for MIS techniques as part of enhanced recovery protocols (ERP) as we attempt to make the delivery of joint replacement services more cost efficient for health systems.

References

1. Ranawat CS, Flynn WF, Saddler S, Hansraj KK, Maynard MJ. Long-term results of the total condylar knee arthroplasty. A 15-year survivorship study. Clin Orthop. 1993;286:94–102.
2. Kelly MA, Clarke HD. Long-term results of posterior cruciate-substituting total knee arthroplasty. Clin Orthop. 2002;404:51–7.
3. Trousdale RT, McGrory BJ, Berry DJ, Becker MW, Harmsen WS. Patients' concerns prior to undergoing total hip and total knee arthroplasty. Mayo Clin Proc. 1999;74:978–82.
4. Dickstein R, Heffes Y, Shabtai EI, Markowitz E. Total knee arthroplasty in the elderly: patients' self-appraisal 6 and 12 months postoperatively. Gerontology. 1998;44:204–10.
5. Noble PC, Conditt MA, Cook KF, Mathis KB. The John Insall award: patient expectations affect satisfaction with total knee arthroplasty. Clin Orthop. 2006;452:35–43.
6. Lilikakis AK, Villar RN. Incisions great and small. J Bone Joint Surg Br. 2004;86B:781–2.
7. Romanowski MR, Repicci JA. Minimally invasive unicondylar arthroplasty: eight-year follow-up. J Knee Surg. 2002;15:17–22.
8. Price AJ, Webb J, Topf H, Dodd CA, Goodfellow JW, Murray DW. Rapid recovery after oxford unicompartmental arthroplasty through a short incision. J Arthroplasty. 2001;16:970–6.
9. Argenson JNA, Flecher X. Minimally invasive unicompartmental knee arthroplasty. Knee. 2004;11:341–7.
10. Tria AJ. Advancements in minimally invasive total knee arthroplasty. Orthopedics. 2003;26(8S):85963.
11. Tria AJ. Exploring the depths of minimally invasive quadriceps-sparing total knee arthroplasty. Orthopedics. 2006;29:214–5.
12. Tria AJ, Coon TM. Minimal incision total knee arthroplasty: early experience. Clin Orthop. 2003;416:185–90.
13. King J, Stamper DL, Schaad DC, Leopold SS. Minimally invasive total knee arthroplasty compared with traditional total knee arthroplasty. Assessment of the learning curve and the postoperative recuperative period. J Bone Joint Surg Am. 2007;89A:1497–503.
14. Kolisek FR, Bonutti PM, Hozack WJ, Purtill J, Sharkey PF, Zelicof SB, Ragland PS, Kester M, Mont MA, Rothman RH. Clinical experience using a minimally invasive surgical approach for total knee arthroplasty: early results of a prospective randomized study compared to a standard approach. J Arthroplasty. 2007;22:8–13.
15. Laskin RS. Mini-incision: occasionally desirable, rarely necessary in opposition. J Arthroplasty. 2006;21(1S):19–21.
16. Shankar NS. Minimally invasive technique in total knee arthroplasty. History, tips, tricks and pitfalls. Injury. 2006;37(5S):25–30.
17. Song EK, Seon JK, Yoon TR, Park SJ, Bae BH, Cho SG. Functional results of navigated minimally invasive and conventional total knee arthroplasty: a comparison in bilateral cases. Orthopedics. 2006;29(10S):145–7.
18. Bozic KJ, Beringer D. Economic considerations in minimally invasive total joint arthroplasty. Clin Orthop. 2007;463:20–5.
19. Coon TM. The economic impact of minimally invasive total knee arthroplasty. Am Orthop. 2006;35(7S):33–5.
20. Laskin RS. Minimally invasive total knee arthroplasty: the results justify its use. Clin Orthop. 2005;440:54–9.
21. Haas SB, Cook S, Beksac B. Minimally invasive total knee replacement through a mini midvastus approach: a comparative study. Clin Orthop. 2004;428:68–73.
22. Dalury DF, Dennis DA. Mini-incision total knee arthroplasty can increase risk of component malalignment. Clin Orthop. 2005;440:77–81.
23. Karachalios T, Giotikas D, Roidis N, Poultsides L, Bargiotas K, Malizos KN. Total knee replacement performed with either a mini-midvastus or a standard approach: a prospective randomised clinical and radiological trial. J Bone Joint Surg Br. 2008;90B:584–91.
24. Barrack RL, Barnes CL, Burnett RSJ, Miller D, Clohisy JC, Maloney WJ. Minimal incision surgery as a risk factor for early failure of total knee arthroplasty. J Arthroplasty. 2009;24:489–98.
25. Callaghan JJ, Warth LC, Liu SS, Hozack WJ, Klein GR. Internet promotion of MIS and CAOS in TKA by Knee Society members. Clin Orthop. 2006;452:97–101.
26. Warth LC, Callaghan JJ, Liu SS, Klein GR, Hozack WJ. Internet promotion of minimally invasive surgery and computer-assisted orthopedic surgery in total knee arthroplasty by members of American Association Of Hip And Knee Surgeons. J Arthroplasty. 2007;22:13–6.
27. Meena S, Palaniswamy A, Chowdhury B. Web-based information on minimally invasive total knee arthroplasty. J Orthop Surg. 2013;21:305–7.
28. Tenholder M, Clarke HD, Scuderi GR. Minimal-incision total knee arthroplasty: the early clinical experience. Clin Orthop. 2005;440:67–76.
29. Laskin RS, Beksac B, Phongjunakorn A, Pittors A, Davis J, Shim JC, Pavlov H, Petersen M. Minimally invasive total knee replacement through a mini-midvastus incision: an outcome study. Clin Orthop. 2004;428:74–81.
30. Bonutti RM, Mont MA, McMahon M, Ragland PS, Kester M. Minimally invasive total knee arthroplasty. J Bone Joint Surg Am. 2004;86A:26–32.
31. Laskin RS. Minimally invasive total knee replacement using a mini-mid vastus incision technique and results. Surg Technol Int. 2004;13:231–8.
32. Leopold SS. Minimally invasive total knee arthroplasty for osteoarthritis. N Engl J Med. 2009;360:1749–58.

33. Bonutti PM. Suspended leg approach and arthroscopic assisted techniques, in minimally invasive surgery in orthopaedics. New York: Springer; 2009.
34. Bonutti PM, Zywiel MG, McGrath MS, Mont MA. Surgical techniques for minimally invasive exposures for total knee arthroplasty. Instr Course Lect. 2010;59:83–91.
35. Niki Y, Matsumoto H, Hakozaki A, Kanagawa H, Toyama H, Suda Y. Clinical and radiographic outcomes of minimally invasive total knee arthroplasty through a lateral approach. Knee Surg Sports Traumatol Arthrosc. 2011;19:973–9.
36. Lee DH, Choi J, Nha KW, Kim HJ, Han SB. No difference in early functional outcomes for mini-midvastus and limited medial parapatellar approaches in navigation-assisted total knee arthroplasty: a prospective randomized clinical trial. Knee Surg Sports Traumatol Arthrosc. 2011;19:66–73.
37. Costa CR, Johnson AJ, Harwin SF, Mont MA, Bonutti PM. Critical review of minimally invasive approaches in knee arthroplasty. J Knee Surg. 2013;26:41–50.
38. Lin SY, Chen CH, Fu YC, Huang PJ, Lu CC, Su JY, Chang JK, Huang HT. Comparison of the clinical and radiological outcomes of three minimally invasive techniques for total knee replacement at two years. Bone Joint J. 2013;95B:906–10.
39. Li C, Zeng Y, Shen B, Kang P, Yang J, Zhou Z, Pei F. A meta-analysis of minimally invasive and conventional medial parapatella approaches for primary total knee arthroplasty. Knee Surg Sports Traumatol Arthrosc. 2014. [Epub ahead of print].
40. Alcelik L, Sukeik M, Pollock R, Misra A, Shah P, Armstrong P, Dhebar MI. Comparison of the minimally invasive and standard medial parapatellar approaches for primary total knee arthroplasty. Knee Surg Sports Traumatol Arthrosc. 2012;20:2502–12.
41. Rousseau MA, Lazennec JY, Catonné Y. Early mechanical failure in total knee arthroplasty. Int Orthop. 2008;32:53–6.
42. Dabboussi N, Sakr M, Girard J, Fakih R. Minimally invasive total knee arthroplasty: a comparative study to the standard approach. N Am J Med Sci. 2012;4:81–5.
43. Bonutti PM, Zywiel MG, Seyler TM, Lee SY, McGrath MS, Marker DR, Mont MA. Minimally invasive total knee arthroplasty using the contralateral knee as a control group: a case-control study. Int Orthop. 2010;34:491–5.
44. Smith TO, King JJ, Hing CB. A meta-analysis of randomised controlled trials comparing the clinical and radiological outcomes following minimally invasive to conventional exposure for total knee arthroplasty. Knee. 2012;19:1–7.
45. Bonutti PM, Zywiel MG, Ulrich SD, McGrath MS, Mont MA. Minimally invasive total knee arthroplasty: pitfalls and complications. Am J Orthop. 2010;39:480–4.

George A. Macheras and Spyridon P. Galanakos

Introduction

The debate over whether to preserve the posterior cruciate ligament (PCL) in total knee arthroplasty (TKA), so-called cruciate-retaining (CR), or to substitute for it, so-called posterior stabilized (PS), continues to engage orthopedic surgeons. Although multiple differing design philosophies have come and gone over the past several decades, no consensus has been reached as to which knee is preferable. Several factors account for this. First, no clear benefits or drawbacks are apparent for either type of implant to the extent that either is clearly superior. In addition, multiple confounding factors are present in the comparative evaluation of implant studies (e.g. function, patient satisfaction, implant longevity, complication rates etc.), as well as the influence of tradition in the implant choices of most surgeons, which makes comparison difficult.

The PCL in TKA functions to prevent posterior translation of the tibia and aids in femoral roll-back [1]. Roll-back allows for increased quadriceps lever arm and more efficient use of extensor musculature, permitting more normal stair climbing.

Potential advantages of a PS design include more predictable restoration of knee kinematics, improved range of motion, decreased polyethylene wear because of more congruent articular surfaces, easier correction of severe deformities, and easier ligament balancing [2]. While eliminating the reliance on a well-functioning PCL, a PS design introduces the risk of component dislocation with flexion instability, tibial post and femoral cam impingement creating polyethylene wear, patello-femoral problems, and increased bone resection of the distal femur [3–5].

However, good long-term data exist both radiographically and clinically for PCL sparing and PCL substituting types of implants [6, 7]. Some surgeons routinely sacrifice the PCL, and others routinely spare it. Some surgeons make an intraoperative decision based on intraoperative findings. The trends from the previous decade in which most knee arthroplasties were performed with CL designs have changed to a more recent trend of PS designs with a post and cam mechanism, or sacrificing and substituting with a highly conforming deep dish polyethylene [8]. It is important to realize that all PS TKAs are not the same. There are variations in the radii of curvature, patello-femoral articulation and the spine cam mechanism. The clinical results with one design cannot be readily extrapolated to a different design. An understanding of the history behind the current PS designs available, key design concepts, important surgical principles and techniques will aid surgeons in

G.A. Macheras, MD, DSc (✉)
S.P. Galanakos, MD, DSc
4th Orthopedic Department, KAT Hospital,
2 Nikis str, 14561 Athens, Greece
e-mail: gmacheras@gmail.com;
spgalanakos@gmail.com

© Springer-Verlag London 2015
T. Karachalios (ed.), *Total Knee Arthroplasty: Long Term Outcomes*,
DOI 10.1007/978-1-4471-6660-3_12

providing well-functioning, durable, TKAs. This chapter will first address the time line and progression of PS components, from the earliest years to the currently available designs. The advantages and disadvantages, complications, survival, clinical outcomes and the current trend will then be reviewed.

History, Rationale and the Need for PS Design

Although many TKA designs predate the total condylar prosthesis designed by Insall and others, its introduction in 1973 marked the beginning of the modern era of TKA. This implant design allowed mechanical considerations to outweigh the desire to reproduce anatomically the kinematics of normal knee motion. Influenced largely by the previous Imperial College/London Hospital design, both cruciate ligaments were sacrificed, with sagittal plane stability maintained by the articular surface geometry [9]. The design of TKA, since the concept of the total condylar implant was introduced, has yet to see another leap in advancement. The symmetrical femoral condyles had a decreasing sagittal radius of curvature posteriorly and were individually convex in the coronal plane. The double dished articular surface of the tibial polyethylene component was perfectly congruent with the femoral component in extension and congruent in the coronal plane in flexion. Translation and dislocation of the components were resisted by the anterior and posterior lips of the tibial component and the median eminence. The tibial component had a metaphyseal stem to resist tilting of the prosthesis during asymmetrical loading. The tibial component was originally all polyethylene, but metal backing was added later to allow more uniform stress transfer to the underlying cancellous metaphyseal bone and to prevent polyethylene deformation. The patella was resurfaced with a dome-shaped, all polyethylene patellar component with a central fixation lug. Many of these design characteristics are retained in current designs.

Concurrent with the development of the PS total condylar prosthesis, the duopatellar prosthesis was developed with the sagittal plane contour of the femoral component being anatomically shaped. This prosthesis included retention of the PCL. Originally, the medial and lateral tibial plateau components were separate, but this was soon revised to a one-piece tibial component with a cut-out for PCL retention.

Two early criticisms of the total condylar prosthesis were its tendency to subluxate posteriorly in flexion, if the flexion gap was not balanced perfectly with the extension gap and a smaller range of flexion compared with prosthetic designs that allowed femoral rollback to occur. By not being able to roll back, posterior femoral metaphysis in a total condylar knee impinged against the tibial articular surface at approximately 95° of flexion. The early clinical reviews of the total condylar prosthesis documented average flexion of only 90–100°. In order to correct these problems, the Insall-Burstein I posterior cruciate-substituting or posterior stabilized design was developed in 1978 by adding a central cam mechanism to the articular surface geometry of the total condylar prosthesis. The cam on the femoral component engaged a central post on the tibial articular surface at approximately 70° of flexion and caused the contact point of the femoral-tibial articulation to be posteriorly displaced, effecting femoral rollback and allowing further flexion [10]. The Insall-Burstein I posterior stabilized knee underwent significant modifications in the late 1980s to yield the Insall-Burstein II. Intramedullary instruments assisted the surgeon in obtaining appropriate alignment in a reproducible and accurate manner. The original tension device for determining equal and rectangular flexion and extension gaps was replaced with a technique using spacer blocks. The concept of modularity was expanded to include multiple sizes for the femoral and tibial components, different polyethylene thicknesses, intramedullary stems, and wedges in order to address defects. Additional changes were made to enhance femoral rollback, thereby improving flexion. Reports of component dislocation arose, especially in knees with preoperative valgus alignment or those that achieved a high degree of postoperative flexion. Consequently, additional modifications of the tibial insert included positioning the tibial post more anteriorly and increasing its height. This PS design proved to be a functionally sound concept that performed well for more than a decade before it evolved further. Most current total knee designs are derivatives of the Insall-Burstein and kinematic designs. Some total knee systems have incorporated a deep dish design as one of their available modular tibial polyethylene options. This design is similar to the original total condylar design that uses sagittal plane concavity or dishing alone to control anteroposterior stability. A comparison of deep-dish components with posterior-stabilized devices using the same femoral components found no difference at follow up in range of motion, ability to climb or descend stairs, or pain scores. This deep dish design incorporated many of the previously mentioned advantages of PS without the obligatory bone sacrifice in the intercondylar region of the femur, which may predispose to fracture. With proper flexion-extension gap balancing, posterior impingement in flexion was reported to be avoided, yielding flexion similar to the PS design. Many newer total knee designs have incorporated more complex post-cam interactions and even a dual-cam mechanism in which the anterior aspect of the post drives a screw-home mechanism as the knee is moved into full extension. The transverse plane rotation pattern in this type of design has been shown to be closer to normal knee kinematics than with older PS designs. Many manufacturers now change the positioning of the post and the cam, as well as their geometry, to guide a more normal tibiofemoral articulation pattern throughout the range of motion [11].

The increased desire of patients to pursue activities associated with greater degrees of knee flexion, as well as acknowledgment of the important cultural requirements in certain Asian populations, have driven the development of high-flexion TKA implants. These implants are designed to exceed 140–150° of flexion compared with the 120° permitted by traditional designs. To accommodate higher flexion, these design modifications include enhanced posterior condylar geometry of the femoral component, which improves contact areas in high flexion, thereby reducing the risk of polyethylene wear [12]. In addition, modifications to the anterior aspect of the tibial polyethylene insert

were made to reduce the potential for extensor mechanism impingement in high flexion. Finally the cam-post design of PS variants was optimized in order to reduce the risk of dislocation in high flexion. To date, studies of high-flexion TKAs have provided little data to support the theoretical advantages attributed to the optimized designs. In a recent meta-analysis, Ghandi and associates [13] have noted that high flexion designs were associated with improved ROM compared with traditional implants, but offered no clinical benefits. Meneghini and coworkers [14] have confirmed the lack of any functional benefit with flexion more than 125° after TKA.

The Medial Pivot TKA reflects contemporary data regarding knee kinematics. Magnetic resonance imaging (MRI) of knees from cadavers showed an absence of anteroposterior (AP) motion of the medial femoral condyle and posterior translation of the lateral femoral condyle during knee flexion. The Medial Pivot femoral component has a C curve design with a near constant radius of curvature of the distal and posterior femur. The tibial component is asymmetric with a highly conforming medial section. This design permits posterior rolling and sliding of the lateral femoral condyle around a stable spinning medial femoral condyle during knee flexion. The epicondylar axis of the femur serves as the axis of rotation of the Medial Pivot implant. In theory, these design features lower the contact stresses on the tibial surface, providing for enhanced durability of the polyethylene [15]. Recently, a novel design, the GMK Sphere system, was created in order to replicate ROM in the medial compartment, freedom of movement in lateral compartment, no paradoxical motion between femur and tibia and to permit patient-appropriate motion rather than imposing an average. In addition, it replicates natural lateralized patella tracking and reduces patello-femoral joint pressure [16, 17].

Ligament Retaining/Substituting Designs. The Biomechanical Basis

PCL is considered to play a vital role in posterior roll back of the femur in flexion. As it is in tension with flexion, it draws back the femoral condyles. The orientation of the fibres with its attachment to the medial femoral condyle leads to a rotational movement along the vertical axis, resulting in the lateral femoral condyle being drawn back more posteriorly. Retaining the PCL helps preserve this movement as long as its function is preserved by adequately balancing the knee in flexion and extension. As this ligament is normally under tension in flexion and lax in extension, this relationship needs to be maintained while performing bone cuts and choosing the size of the polythene insert. The tibial surface has to be relatively flat when the PCL is retained, to allow femoral roll back and prevent excessive tension in the PCL. The PCL in some cases may be incompetent due to injury or degeneration. Surgeons may also choose to sacrifice the PCL while performing a knee replacement in cases where flexion is tight, to prevent excessive stresses and wear of the polythene insert. There are prostheses that have been designed to substitute the function of the PCL by means of a central cam on the femoral implant, which is pushed back by the central post on the polythene insert [18]. This posteriorly stabilized (cruciate substituting) design helps reproduce femoral roll back. The centre post also provides anteroposterior stability in cases where there is a weak extensor mechanism. Furthermore, this design can have more congruent articulating surfaces, which helps decrease stress. The center of curvature of the femoral component was changed to improve ROM and the tibial spine was intended to prevent posterior subluxation of the tibia, improving the ability to perform activities such as stair climbing and rising from a chair. This type of design relies on a more conforming articular surface, as well as a polyethylene tibial post and femoral cam to provide restraint against posterior translation of the tibia and proper femoral rollback.

Both cruciate ligaments contain mechanoreceptors, and therefore advocates of PCL retention have proposed that preserving the natural ligament would lead to superior proprioception after TKA. However, the current literature has not demonstrated a clear advantage. Simmons and associates [19] were unable to identify any advantage in proprioception in patients who had aCR prosthesis versus those with a PS prosthesis. Warren and coworkers [20] noted slightly different results. After TKA, all patients experienced improved proprioception regardless of whether a CR or PS prosthesis had been used. However, the improvement was greater in patients with a CR prosthesis. The improved proprioception in both groups was due to elimination of pain, restoration of articular congruity, and retensioning of the collateral ligaments and soft tissues. These inconclusive results may be the result of structural integrity and functional quality of PCL in patients with arthritic knees. Kleinbart and colleagues [21] have observed significant degenerative changes in the PCLs of patients with arthritic knees that exceed those in age-matched controls. Therefore, a PCL which is preserved in a patient with a CR prosthesis is likely to be abnormal and should not be expected to have normal mechanical and proprioceptive function. The effects of PCL recession on the proprioceptive function of the ligament are not known. A review comparing retention or sacrifice of the PCL in a TKA with or without use of a PS implant did not find sufficient evidence to support decision making. The authors recommend interpreting these results with caution as the methodological quality of the studies was highly variable. As the normal configuration and tension of the PCL need to be reproduced accurately, performing a CR TKA can be difficult [6].

Indications and Contraindications for PS TKA

Specific indications for a PS TKA remain a topic of controversy. Proponents of PCL retention claim that correction of almost all deformities except severe flexion contracture is possible with a CR knee. However, the exact definition of severe flexion contracture is not well defined. Supporters of PS implants note easier extension and flexion gap balancing even with severe deformities. However, success of a CR TKA depends on a well-tensioned PCL, while that of a PS knee relies on equivalent extension and flexion spaces. Several preoperative conditions that may be more appropriate for PCL substitution include rheumatoid arthritis, previous patellectomy, prior proximal tibial or distal femoral osteotomy, or post-traumatic arthritis with disruption of the PCL. The synovitis associated with rheumatoid arthritis can lead to weakening of the PCL, which could result in instability or rupture after a CR TKA [22, 23]. A patellectomy places increased loads on the PCL by disrupting the normal four-bar linkage of the knee [24]. Since these abnormal forces can result in late PCL attenuation and instability, some investigators recommend a PS TKA in patients with prior patellectomy [24]. Previous osteotomies of the proximal tibia or distal femur often mandate bony resections or augmentations that affect the position of the joint line. In these situations, a PS knee provides more flexibility for soft tissue balancing. A CR TKA is contraindicated in cases where the PCL is found to be torn or incompetent such as with post-traumatic arthritis. A PS TKA is contraindicated when one or both of the collateral ligaments are significantly lax or disrupted. Failure to obtain balanced extension and flexion gaps after PCL resection necessitates conversion to a varus-valgus constrained implant.

Advantages and Disadvantages of PS TKA

There are several advantages with use of PS TKA designs. These include: (I) easier surgical exposure and ligament balancing, (II) predictable restoration of knee kinematics, (III) improved range of motion, (IV) less polyethylene wear, and (V) avoiding the possibility of PCL rupture. On the other hand, there are numerous of disadvantages such as: (I) tibial post wear and breakage, (II) excessive bone resection, (III) patellar clunk syndrome and (IV) tibio-femoral dislocations.

Advantages of PS TKA

Easier Surgical Exposure and Ligament Balancing

Adequate exposure of the tibia may not be possible with PCL retention. Excision of the PCL aids in exposing the tibia for adequate visualization

by releasing the tethering effect of a tightly contracted PCL. Moreover, the PCL can be excised from the femoral and tibial attachment in a reproducible way, making the ligamentous balancing and correction of the deformity more easily since it is not complicated by the tethering effect of the PCL. Abnormal PCL morphology is often encountered in the diseased knee making predictable gap balancing difficult in CR TKA. If the patient has a "tight", contracted PCL, the knee may be relatively tight in flexion with excessive femoral roll-back. On the other hand, if the PCL is lax or incompetent, the knee may experience posterior sag with no roll-back with knee flexion. Thus, the use of a PS TKA makes balancing more predictable, eliminating the reliance on abnormal PCL morphology and function.

Predictable Restoration of Knee Kinematics

In PS TKA, the tibial post predictably articulates with the transverse femoral cam with knee flexion, preventing posterior subluxation of the tibia while maintaining femoral roll back. Many studies report more normal kinematics with the use of posterior stabilized designs [10, 25]. Fluoroscopic kinematics have shown that PS TKAs experienced AP femoro-tibial translation more similar to the normal knee during normal gait and deep knee flexion [26]. Moreover, studies have shown no significant difference between PS TKA and normal knees with regard to spatiotemporal gait parameters, knee range of motion during stair climbing or in isokinetic muscle strength [27]. A study comparing CR, PS TKAs found that PS designs produced more roll back and better quadriceps efficiency than CR designs [28]. PS TKA predictably restores more normal knee kinematics when compared to either PCL substituting or PCL sacrificing designs.

Improved Range of Motion

Both CR and PS TKA designs can provide excellent range of motion. However, range of motion may be better when a PS TKA is used to maintain femoral roll back. It appears, according to most comparative studies, that PS designs may provide more predictable motion, with greater flexion under fluoroscopic visualization [29]. In a meta-analysis Jacobs et al. [6] analyzed eight randomized controlled trials comparing PS with CR TKA and found that the range of motion was 8° higher (105 versus 113°) in the PS group than in the CR group (P = 0.01, 95 % confidence interval 1.7–15).

Less Polyethylene Wear

Retention of the PCL requires that the prosthetic kinematics closely match that of the normal knee. This obligates the implant to have a "flat" polyethylene component relative to the radius of curvature of the femur. This "round on flat" design allows for minimal constraint on tibial component enabling roll back of the femur on tibia with knee flexion. This less conforming design can lead to excessive point contact pressure and increase polyethylene wear. In contrast, in posterior-stabilized design, it is possible to use more conforming polyethylene articulation with minimal point contact stress. Increasing the conformity of the implant increases the contact area and decreases the stress to which the polyethylene is subjected. This can potentially minimize polyethylene wear and increase the long-term survival of the TKA. Cases of severe polyethylene wear in CR implants with less conforming tibial inserts have been reported [27]. Additionally, technical issues may contribute to wear in CR TKA if the PCL is left too tight in flexion. This can lead to asymmetric posterior polyethylene wear from posterior femoral subluxation and may predispose to osteolysis.

Avoiding the Possibility of Posterior Cruciate Ligament Rupture

The PCL can rupture postoperatively with the use of CR TKA. This can occur after trauma or as inflammatory disease process. Late flexion instability can occur if the PCL fails over time. This complication can also occur iatrogenically when the PCL it is extensively recessed intraoperatively or when excessive proximal tibial resection is performed. When too much proximal tibia is resected, the PCL insertion site can be jeopardized. The PCL can also be weakened by synovitis

from inflammatory arthropathy, resulting in failure [28]. Thus, late PCL instability failures can be avoided with the use of PS TKA designs.

Disadvantages of PS TKA

Tibial Spine Wear and Breakage

There has been a recent focus on the spine-cam mechanism in some PS designs as a source of wear debris [30–32]. Callaghan et al. [33] have studied this phenomenon extensively. When they recognized osteolysis around IB II and PS PFC modular components, they began performing retrieval analyses. Their patients were able to hyperextend slightly and most had bilateral implants. They hypothesized that impingement on the anterior post by the femoral cam causes wear damage and transmits rotational stresses to the modular inserts, generating backside wear. Avoiding flexion of the femoral component and posterior slope in the proximal tibial resection should help eliminate the problem. In addition, cam-post designs should allow for hyperextension before impingement occurs. Pang et al. [34] investigated the relationship between limb alignment, implant position, joint line elevation and polyethylene damage in PS inserts. Damage was found in all the posts, and backside wear was demonstrated in most inserts. Damage scores were higher in TKA with suboptimal postoperative limb alignment and joint line elevation. In the same study wear was evident on the posts of all retrieved implants and the most prevalent location of wear was the posterior surface. The post acts as a contact guide for promoting femoral rollback and limiting tibial subluxation. It is therefore not surprising that most damage was found on the posterior surface. Hyperextension may lead to more damage on the anterior post. One of the postulated reasons for the decreased survival of PS TKA in comparison to the CR TKA is that of post-cam wear [36]. PS designs are subject to greater stress at the modular tibial interface because of shear forces transmitted directly to the post instead of the posterior cruciate ligament. Attempts have been made to reduce the incidence of backside wear to little avail. Rotating platform TKA has no surface damage advantage to fixed bearing ones and has reportedly greater backside wear as a result of third body debris scratching [35]. The concept of highly polished baseplate was applied to fixed bearing prostheses in the hope of reducing surface roughness. Backside wear persists despite these efforts. Improved locking designs may reduce relative micromotion and seal off third body debris from the modular interface.

Dislocations

As increasingly deep flexion was experienced with PS designs, there have been cases of the tibial spine riding underneath the femoral cam with subluxation of the flexed knee and painful locking of the joint. A knee with a dislocated implant normally presents acutely with inability to extend. In many cases, patients are unable to explain the exact mechanism, or the position of the knee, when the actual dislocation occurred. In fact, this problem can occur during sleep, causing the patient to awaken with an acute inability to extend the knee. On physical examination, an obvious knee deformity is commonly found. Radiographs reveal that femoral cam is translated anterior to the polyethylene tibial spine. Often, the spine can be reduced by hyperflexion of the knee and application of an anterior drawer. Lombardi et al. [37] have analyzed the incidence of dislocations in 3,032 primary knees implanted with the Insall-Burstein prosthesis. The incidence of this problem was rare with the original Insall-Burstein PS implant (0.2 %, or 1 in 494). However, with the advent of the IB II implant, the problem became more apparent (2.5 %, or 1 in 40). Knees that dislocated were found to have achieved statistically significant higher average flexion (118°) compared with control knees (105°; P<0.001). In addition, they tended to reach high flexion angles rapidly in the postoperative period. In response to this problem, the tibial plastic was modified by raising the tibial spine and moving it anteriorly. This increased the inherent stability of the component and decreased the incidence of dislocation (0.2 %, or 1 in 656).

A computer analysis of this phenomenon analyzed the propensity of PS components to dislocate in the sagittal plane. Kocmond et al. [38] have defined a dislocation safety factor (DSF) as the jump distance between the bottom of the femoral cam and the top of the tibial spine. The DSF was found to vary with the knee flexion angle. For knees with the PS Insall-Burstein mechanism, the DSF increases as knee flexion increases and peaks at about 70°. Knee flexion beyond this angle causes the DSF to decrease and theoretically increases the risk of dislocation. Many contemporary designs have attempted to minimize the risk of dislocation by ensuring a DSF equal to or greater than that of the original PS Insall-Burstein at high flexion angles.

Intercondylar Fractures

Femoral fractures, although a relatively rare occurrence, can occur at the time of TKA. Because PS components require the removal of extra bone from the intercondylar region, the possibility of distal femoral fracture with this technique is increased. Risk factors for fractures include inadequate, as well as excessive, intercondylar bone notch resection. Although it is self-evident that excessive bone removal results directly in stress risers and deficient bone, the risks associated with incomplete bone resection are not as clear-cut. Nonetheless, if insufficient notch bone is removed, the intercondylar region of the femoral component (or trial) can act like a wedge during insertion and induce a distal femoral fracture. It is imperative to remove enough bone to allow full seating of the cam. When placing the trial femoral component, forceful impaction should never be used. To ensure adequate bony resection, never undercut the femoral condyles. Although this complication has been reported, the exact incidence of this phenomenon has not been well defined. Lombardi et al. [39] have described the risk factors, which include osteopenic bone, improper bone cuts, an eccentric box cut for the posterior stabilized prosthesis, over impaction of the femoral component, and misplacement of the trial component. The same group also reported on this complication in comparing two large series of PS TKA [39]. In this report, 898 nonconsecutive primary PS TKAs were compared to a second nonconsecutive series of 532 PS TKAs. In the second series, an intercondylar sizing guide was used to confirm the intercondylar resection size. In the initial series, 40 distal femoral fractures were noted (approximate rate, 1:22; nondisplaced, 35; displaced, 5). In contrast, in the second series, only one displaced fracture was noted (rate, 1:532). The rate difference between the two series was statistically significant. The authors advocated careful resection technique and inter-condylar notch size verification to minimize this complication. Of note, no change in postoperative rehabilitation was required for patients identified with a nondisplaced intercondylar fracture or those with an intercondylar fracture treated with intraoperative stabilization.

Patellar Fractures

The initial reports of the original PS Insall-Burstein demonstrated a prevalence of high patellar fracture. The AP dimensions and shape of the femoral component tended to be full to accommodate the spine-cam mechanism in this implant. This pushed the patella anteriorly and presumably increased forces, which may have been responsible for a relatively higher rate of patellar fractures. In ten cadaver knee specimens, Matsuda et al. [40] demonstrated significantly higher contact stresses in the unresurfaced patella when compared with the normal knee throughout the flexion arc for several implants, including the PS Insall-Burstein TKA. They note that when flexion exceeded 105° patellofemoral contact occurred in two small patches. They conclude that the forces could be normalized by extending the trochlear groove farther posteriorly and were less concerned with the anterior prominence of the component. The groove of the IB II was deepened potentially to decrease patella fractures and other patella problems. Larson and Lachiewicz [41] suggested that many patellar complications with the PS Insall-Burstein could be avoided by a careful surgical technique. This includes appropriate rotation of the femur and tibia, adequate patellar resection, debridement of peripatellar

synovium, and proper evaluation of patellar tracking before wound closure. They studied arthroplasties at 2–8 years and found that no knee required reoperation for the patellofemoral joint. Mean flexion of 112° was comparable to other studies with this device, and they had no cases of patellar clunk syndrome and no subluxations. There were three patellar fractures (2.5 %) treated without surgery. Even this small number of fractures might be expected to improve with changes to the femoral prosthesis. It was concluded that the total patellofemoral complication rate in the series was 4.2 %. This was superior to the 11 % that has generally been described, of which 7 % were actually fractures. With improved design, surgical technique, and more favorable patellofemoral geometry, it is likely that the incidence of patellar fracture will continue to decrease. Ortiguera and Berry [42] found an incidence of periprosthetic fracture of the patella to be only 0.68 % following modern TKA. Additionally, when combining the 2 most recent articles on 323 knees treated with the PS NexGen Legacy, no patellar fractures were reported at 8 year follow-up [43, 44]. This is due to an improvement in implant design and better surgical technique.

Patellar Clunk Syndrome and Synovial Entrapment

The deeper flexion provided by the initial PS Insall-Burstein design enabled the quadriceps tendon to extend beyond the trochlear groove of the femoral component. If the anterior edge of the femoral component terminates abruptly, synovium or scar residing on the tendon falls into the intercondylar groove. If this has occurred, the same tissue must ride up out of the intercondylar area and "jump" back up onto the femoral trochlea as the patient extends his or her knee. Within a few months after the arthroplasty, the offending (or offended) tissue hypertrophies and becomes rubbery. This creates the painful and noisy complication that has been described as patellar clunk. Historically, a case of patellar catching was mentioned by Insall in his original report of PS TKAs. However, Hozack et al. [45] appear to be the first authors to define the term patellar clunk syndrome. They describe a prominent fibrous nodule at the junction of the proximal patellar pole and quadriceps tendon. They believe that during flexion, this fibrous nodule would enter the femoral component's inter-condylar notch but not restrict flexion. However, as the knee is extended, the nodule would remain within the notch while the rest of the extensor mechanism slid proximally. At 30–45° of flexion, the tension on the fibrous nodule would be sufficient to cause the nodule to jerk out of the notch as it returned to its normal position. This sudden displacement would cause the audible and palpable clunk found with this entity. Synovial entrapment or hyperplasia is a similar entity but less well-described syndrome [4]. It is caused by similar hypertrophy of soft tissue in the same location, but without a discrete nodule. Rather than a clunk or catch, the patient experiences pain and crepitus, typically with active knee extension from a 90° flexed position. This typically occurs during stair climbing or rising from a chair. Treatment recommendations for patellar clunk syndrome and synovial entrapment have included physical therapy, surgical removal of the nodule, patellar prosthesis revision, open resection through a limited lateral incision, and arthroscopic debridement [45]. Pollock et al. [4] have reviewed the prevalence of synovial entrapment with three different cam post designs. Those with proximally positioned or wide femoral boxes were more likely to have a higher prevalence of this problem.

Long Term Clinical Outcome and Survival of PS TKA Designs (Table 12.1)

Early PS designs of the total condylar TKA present excellent clinical outcomes. Insall et al. [46] report results of the first consecutive 200 TKAs performed in 183 patients at 3–5 years follow up. Although 93 % of knees were rated excellent or good, the complications, including four cases of posterior subluxation, highlighted the role for cruciate substitution. With evolution of the design, the Insall-Burstein TKA has incorporated posterior cruciate substitution. Stern and Insall [47] report on the 9- to 12-year results of the original Insall-Burstein prosthesis with an all-polyethylene tibial component. Of 289 TKAs implanted at the Hospital for Special Surgery, 180 knees in 139 patients were available for follow up, with excellent or good results found in 87 %. Fourteen knees required revision surgery; nine knees were revised

Table 12.1 Survival of posterior stabilized implants

Study	Type of prosthesis	Survivorship
Scuderi et.al. [55] (1989)	IB all poly tibia	97.34 % at 10 years
Scuderi et.al. [55] (1989)	IB metal back tibia	98.75 % at 10 years
Stern et.al. [47] (1992)	IB all poly tibia	94 % at 13 years
Colizza et al. [48] (1995)	IB metal back tibia	96.4 % at 11 years
Font-Rodriguez et.al. [56] (1997)	IB all poly tibia	94 % at 16 years
Font-Rodriguez et.al. [56] (1997)	IB metal back tibia	98 % at 14 years
Emmerson et.al. [57] (1996)	Kinematic stabilizer	95 % at 10 years
Ranawat et.al. [58] (1997)	PFC modular PS	97 % at 6 years
Ehrhardt et al. [59] (2011)	Optetrak® PS	97.2 % at 11.5 years
Lachiewicz and Soileau [60] (2014)	NexGen Legacy PS	95.5 % at 10 years, 88.8 % at 12 year
Lachiewicz and Soileau [61] (2009)	IB II PS	90.6 % at 15 years
Oliver et al. [54] (2005)	HA-coated IB II	93 % at 13 years
Thadani et al. [53] (2000)	IB I metal-backed	92 % at 12 years
Bozic et al. [44] (2005)	NexGen	100 % at 5 years, 94.6 % at 8 years
Mahoney and Kinsey [62] (2008)	Scorpio PS	With revision as an end point 95.8 %, with aseptic loosening as the end point, 98.6 % at 9.5 years

successfully for aseptic loosening of the femoral component (nine knees) or tibial component (nine knees), and five knees developed infection and were treated with a two-stage procedure. The average annual rate of failure was 0.4 %, with a 12 year survival rate of 94 %.

Modularity of the tibial component was introduced with the Insall-Burstein II prosthesis in 1987. The addition of modularity was attractive to surgeons because it simplified the procedure and allowed intraoperative fine tuning. However, concerns began to arise that polyethylene wear on the backside of the tibial component (backside wear) would lead to osteolysis. Colizza et al. [48] report on the long-term results of the PS Insall-Burstein TKA with a metal backed tibial component; 101 TKAs in 74 patients were examined at a mean follow up time of 10.8 years. Results were good to excellent in 96 % knees. In this cohort, with a monoblock metal backed tibial component, no cases of tibial component loosening were seen. Brassard et al. [49] have addressed the question of whether modularity affects clinical success with a long-term evaluation comparing the modular Insall-Burstein II prosthesis with the monoblock Insall-Burstein I. They compared the results of 101 Insall-Burstein I TKAs and 117 Insall-Burstein II TKAs. Excellent or good results were found in 96 % and 95 % of patients, respectively. The radiographic review demonstrated no cases of massive osteolysis, but the authors mentioned that three knees had local minimally progressive lesions, which were not clinically significant. This series of monoblock metal-backed tibial components had an overall incidence of tibial component radiolucent lines of 11 %, compared with 26 % seen with the modular tibial component. All radiolucent lines were nonprogressive and asymptomatic. Therefore, the introduction of modularity to this particular implant did not appear to raise concerns about osteolysis. In a recent study by Argenson et al. [12] a high postoperative range of motion has been shown to correlate well with improved patient rated outcomes. Interest, therefore, remains for improving knee flexion [12]. Finally, mobile bearings have been shown to improve knee kinematics and polyethylene wear,

but clinical performance and longevity appear equivocal [50]. Although these design changes seem to improve clinical outcomes, further studies are needed.

Aglietti et al. [51] have reviewed the outcome of 99 PS IB I TKAs, with 56 of them available for follow up at 12 years on average follow up. Results were excellent in 58 %, good in 25 %, fair in 7 %, and poor in 10 % of the knees. Knee flexion averaged 106°. Of the six (10 %) failures, four were due to aseptic component loosening; none was due to polyethylene wear. With revision as the end point, 10-year survival was 92 %. The same group then reviewed the outcome of 92 PS IB II TKAs at an average follow-up of 7.5 years [52]. Good to excellent Knee Society Scores were recorded in 97 % of the patients. The 8 years survival rates were at the level of 98.9 and 90.9 % (best and worst case scenarios).

Thadani et al. [53] have reviewed the outcome of PS IB I metal-backed TKAs at a minimum of 10 years; 100 TKAs were performed in 86 consecutive patients. At the latest follow-up, 64 % were rated as excellent, 18 % as good, 7 % as fair, and 11 % as poor, which included six failures. Flexion averaged 111°. Excluding the failures, the average Knee Society clinical score was 91.6. Of the six failures, two were due to infection, two to nonspecific pain, one due to patellar wear and fracture, and one because of aseptic tibial component loosening. Polyethylene wear was specifically examined in this study and no implant demonstrated significant polyethylene wear or failure. There were seven patellar fractures; four required additional surgery and the remaining three were asymptomatic and discovered incidentally at routine follow-up. Using revision as the end point, 12 year survival was 92 %.

Oliver et al. [54] report the clinical and radiographic outcomes of a consecutive series of 138 hydroxyapatite coated PS IB II TKAs with a mean follow up of 11 years (range, 10–13 years). Patients had entered into a prospective study and all living patients (76 knees) were evaluated. The HSS Knee Score was used in order to develop differences form baseline values. No patient was lost to follow-up. Radiographic assessment revealed no loosening. Seven TKAs were revised, giving a survival rate of 93 % at 13 years.

Posterior Cruciate Ligament Salvage or Sacrifice?

Whether the PCL is salvaged or sacrificed in a TKA has been debatable. Two recent meta-analyses have attempted to compare the outcomes of CR and PS TKAs [63, 64]. In the first study, the authors found 8 RCTs involving 888 patients with 963 TKAs which the met predetermined inclusion criteria. They conclude that CR and PS TKAs show similar clinical outcomes with regard to knee function and postoperative knee pain. A significant difference in flexion and range of motion in favor of PS TKAs was found, but no difference in complication rates. The clinical relevance of this finding is still unknown. The decision to use one design versus the other should rest on surgeon's preference and comfort with a particular design. Implant survival for both CR and PS TKAs is satisfactory and no differences were observed in short and mid-terms. Details and findings of the second study are shown in Table 12.2 [64].

Evidence suggests that PS TKAs present increased postoperative knee flexion. Perhaps this is due to more normal kinematics. Fluoroscopic studies demonstrate increased femoral rollback using the cam post articulation as compared with some CR designs [65]. Maruyama et al. [29] report the results of a RCT study comparing patients with bilateral TKA and suggest that the PS design shows greater range of movement as compared to the CR design at 2 years follow up [66]. A recent meta-analysis concludes that there was an average improvement in flexion of 8° in the PS when compared to the CR designs. However, improvement in flexion seemed limited and not associated with improved function. Other investigators have not detected improved flexion with PS TKAs [6]. A Cochrane review indicates no difference in clinical outcome when the PCL was retained or resected even when a PCL-stabilised knee was not used [67].

Concerns

PCL may be not functional in a CR TKA [65]. Moreover, an MRI study has shown that much of the tibial PCL insertion is resected in CR TKAs [66]. Additionally, problems with cam and post designs include the risk of wear at the cam-post interface, the need for additional bone resection to accommodate the design and the potential for 'cam over post' jump. A wear analysis study of PS TKAs concludes that cam post attrition may create polyethylene debris. Creation of a femoral box in these designs requires resection of significant bone and associated soft tissues from the femur. With younger patients undergoing TKA, a bias towards bone preservation might encourage alternative solutions for PCL insufficiency. Laskin et al. [68] have demonstrated that deeply dished inserts were as clinically effective as cam and post restraints in PCL deficient knees. Indeed, surface geometry is probably a more important determinant of tibiofemoral movement [69].

Current Practice

The question of which design of TKA produces a better outcome remains a controversial issue. Available studies are often small and surgeons' reported observational records often only represent early results. In 1997, 54 % of the 37 TKAs on the market had no reported data to support their use [70]. However, the choice of design obviously does matter. What is clear is that the consequences of using various designs are different. Despite possible superior kinematics in flexion, versions of PS TKAs involve greater bone loss and their cam-post articulations receive high loads. Regardless of their potential for self-alignment, mobile bearings have a greater potential to dislocate and may not demonstrate less wear. At present, HA-coated versions of PS TKAs remain more expensive than cemented alternatives. Results of TKA, however, are clearly not simply a function of prosthetic design. Indeed, patients declare themselves satisfied by most of the commonly available designs.

Table 12.2 The data of the eight randomized controlled trials comparing CR to PS TKA

Authors	Sample size			TKA		Mean age (years)		Male (%)		Mean BMI		Outcomes	Follow-up
	Patients	Knees	OA	CR	PS	CR	PS	CR	PS	CR	PS		
Aglietti et al. [71]	197	210	Not clear	103	107	71	69.5	14	19	27.5	27.5	ROM, KSS, KSFS, pain score, complication	4 years
Catani et al. [72]	40	40	100 %	20	20	70±6	71±7	35	25	Not clear	Not clear	ROM, KSS, KSFS, complication	2 years
Chaudhary et al. [73]	100	100	Not clear	51	49	69.2±9.1	70.2±8.4	47	55	32.4±5.7	30.9±4.3	Flexion/extension angle, KSFS, pain score, complication	22.7±5.2 months
Harato et al. [74]	222	222	100 %	99	93	68.3 (49–89)	66 (44–83)	34.3	34.4	29.8 (19.7–43.6)	31.4 (21.7–48.5)	Flexion/extension angle, KSS, KSFS, pain score, complication	5.0–7.3 years
Maruyama et al. [29]	20	40	100 %	20	20	74.3 (65–84)	74.3 (65–84)	40	40	Not clear	Not clear	ROM, flexion/extension angle, KSS, KSFS, complication	24–53 months
Tanzer et al. [75]	37	40	90.00 %	20	20	68 (51–86)	66 (52–77)	25	20	Not clear	Not clear	Flexion angle, KSS, KSFS, complication	2 years
Victor et al. [76]	44	44	100 %	22	22	70±7	70±3	22.7	18.2	34.4	32.7	Flexion angle, KSS, KSFS, pain score	2–5 years
Wang et al. [77]	228	267	91.00 %	157	110	54.5 (31–69)	55 (20–83)	19.7	19.8	27.9	27.5	Flexion/extension angle, KSS, KSFS, pain score	24–66 months

TKA total knee arthroplasty, *BMI* body mass index, *OA* osteoarthritis, *CR* posterior cruciate-retaining, *PS* posterior stabilized, *ROM* range of motion, *KSS* knee society score, *KSFS* knee society function score

Conclusion

The potential of the PS TKAs continues to evolve. In general, it has allowed the surgeon to perform a reproducible operation in almost all arthritic knees, no matter what the cause of the disease and how involved and complex the deformity of the knee. The recent modifications in prosthetic design and surgical technique have addressed most of the early concerns involving patellofemoral complication and tibiofemoral dislocation. Although many advances have been made, there is still potential for functional and clinical improvements in the current newer designs and those that will become available in the future.

References

1. Dorr LD, Ochsner JL, Gronley J, Perry J. Functional comparison of posterior curciate-retained versus cruciate-sacrificedot al knee arthroplasty. Clin Orthop. 1988;236:36–43.
2. Morgan H, Battista V, Leopold SS. Constraint in primary total knee arthroplasty. J Am Acad Orthop Surg. 2005;13:515–24.
3. Karrholm J, Saari T. Removal or retention. Will we ever know? The posterior cruciate ligament in total knee replacement. Acta Orthop Scand. 2005;76:754–6.
4. Pollock DC, Ammeen DJ, Engh GA. Synovial entrapment: a complication of posterior stabilized total knee arthroplasty. J Bone Joint Surg Am. 2002;84A:2174–8.
5. Beight JL, Yao B, Hozack WJ, Hearn SL, Booth Jr RE. The patellar "clunk" syndrome after posterior stabilized total knee arthroplasty. Clin Orthop. 1994;299:139–42.
6. Jacobs W, Clement DJ, Wymenga AB. Retention versus sacrifice of the posterior cruciate ligament in total knee replacement for treatment of osteoarthritis and rheumatoid arthritis. Cochrane Database Syst Rev. 2005;(19):CD004803.
7. NIH Consensus Panel. NIH consensus statement on total knee replacement, December 8–10, 2003. J Bone Joint Surg Am. 2004;86A:1328–35.
8. Mont M, Booth R, Laskin R, Stiehl JB, Ritter MA, Stuchin SA, Rajadhyaksha AD. The spectrum of prosthesis design for primary total knee arthroplasty. Instr Course Lect. 2003;52:397–407.
9. Scuderi GR, Pagnano MR. Review article: the rationale for posterior cruciate substituting total knee arthroplasty. J Orthop Surg. 2001;9:81–8.
10. Insall JN, Lachiewicz PF, Burstein AH. The posterior stabilized condylar prosthesis: a modification of the total condylar design. Two to four-year clinical experience. J Bone Joint Surg Am. 1982;64A:1317–23.
11. Nunley RM, Nam D, Berend KR, Lombardi AV, Dennis DA, Della Valle CJ, Barrack RL. New total knee arthroplasty designs: do young patients notice? Clin Orthop. 2015;473(1):101–8.
12. Argenson JN, Scuderi GR, Komistek RD, Scott WN, Kelly MA, Aubaniac JM. In vivo kinematic evaluation and design considerations related to high flexion in total knee arthroplasty. J Biomech. 2005;38:277–84.
13. Ghandi R, Tso P, Davey JR, Mahomed NN. High flexion implants in primary total knee arthroplasty: a meta-analysis. Knee. 2009;16:14–7.
14. Meneghini RM, Pierson JL, Bagsby D, Ziemba-Davis M, Berend ME, Ritter MA. Is there a functional benefit to obtaining high flexion after total knee arthroplasty? J Arthroplasty. 2007;22(2S):43–6.
15. Iwaki H, Pinskerova V, Freeman MA. Tibiofemoral movement 1: the shapes and relative movements of the femur and tibia in the unloaded cadaver knee. J Bone Joint Surg Br. 2000;82B:1189–95.
16. Pritchett JW. Patients prefer a bicruciate-retaining or the medial pivot total knee prosthesis. J Arthroplasty. 2011;26:224–8.
17. Freeman MAR, Pinskerova V. The movement of the normal tibio-femoral joint. J Biomech. 2005;38:197–208.
18. Joglekar S, Gioe TJ, Yoon P, Schwartz MH. Gait analysis comparison of cruciate retaining and substituting TKA following PCL sacrifice. Knee. 2012;19:279–85.
19. Simmons S, Lephart S, Rubash H, Pifer GW, Barrack R. Proprioception after unicondylar knee arthroplasty versus total knee arthroplasty. Clin Orthop. 1996;331:179–84.
20. Warren PJ, Olanlokun TK, Cobb AG, Bentley G. Proprioception after total knee arthroplasty: the influence of prosthetic design. Clin Orthop. 1993;297:182–7.
21. Kleinbart FA, Bryk E, Evangelista J, Scott WN, Vigorita VJ. Histologic comparison of posterior cruciate ligaments from arthritic and age-matched knee specimens. J Arthroplasty. 1996;11:726–31.
22. Hanyu T, Murasawa A, Tojo T. Survivorship analysis of total knee arthroplasty with the kinematic prosthesis in patients who have rheumatoid arthritis. J Arthroplasty. 1997;12:913–9.
23. Laskin RS, O'Flynn HM. The Insall Award. Total knee replacement with posterior cruciate ligament retention in rheumatoid arthritis. Problems and complications. Clin Orthop. 1997;345:24–8.
24. Paletta Jr GA, Laskin RS. Total knee arthroplasty after previous patellectomy. J Bone Joint Surg Am. 1995;77A:1708–12.
25. Scott WN, Rubinstein M, Scuderi GR. Results after knee replacement with a posterior cruciate-substituting prosthesis. J Bone Joint Surg Am. 1988;70A:1163–73.
26. Udomkiat P, Meng BJ, Dorr LD, Wan Z. Functional comparison of posterior cruciate retention and substitution knee replacement. Clin Orthop. 2000;378:192–201.

27. Wilson SA, McCann PD, Gotlin RS, Ramakrishnan HK, Wootten ME, Insall JN. Comprehensive gait analysis in posterior stabilized knee arthroplasty. J Arthroplasty. 1996;11:359–67.

28. Mahoney OM, Noble PC, Rhoads DD, Alexander JW, Tullos HS. Posterior cruciate function following total knee arthroplasty: a biomechanical study. J Arthroplasty. 1994;9:569–78.

29. Maruyama S, Yoshiya S, Matsui N, Kuroda R, Kurosaka M. Functional comparison of posterior cruciate retaining versus posterior stabilized total knee arthroplasty. J Arthroplasty. 2004;19:349–53.

30. Collier MB, Engh Jr CA, McAuley JP, Engh GA. Factors associated with the loss of thickness of polyethylene tibial bearings after knee arthroplasty. J Bone Joint Surg Am. 2007;89A:1306–14.

31. Puloski SK, McCalden R, Macdonald SJ, Rorabeck CH, Bourne RB. Tibial post wear in posterior stabilized total knee arthroplasty: an unrecognized source of polyethylene debris. J Bone Joint Surg Am. 2001;83A:390–7.

32. Mikulak SA, Mahoney OM, dela Rosa MA, Schmalzried TP. Loosening and osteolysis with the press-fit condylar posterior-cruciate-substituting total knee replacement. J Bone Joint Surg Am. 2001;83A:398–403.

33. Callaghan JJ, O'Rourke MR, Goetz DD, Schmalzried TP, Campbell PA, Johnston RC. Tibial post impingement in posterior-stabilized total knee arthroplasty. Clin Orthop. 2002;404:83–8.

34. Pang HN, Jamieson P, Teeter MG, McCalden RW, Naudie DD, MacDonald SJ. Retrieval analysis of posterior stabilized polyethylene tibial inserts and its clinical relevance. J Arthroplasty. 2014;29:365–8.

35. Stoner K, Jerabek SA, Tow S, Wright TM, Padgett DE. Rotating-platform has no surface damage advantage over fixed-bearing TKA. Clin Orthop. 2013;471:76–85.

36. Abdel MP, Morrey ME, Jensen MR, Morrey BF. Increased long-term survival of posterior cruciate-retaining versus posterior cruciate-stabilizing total knee replacements. J Bone Joint Surg Am. 2011;93A:2072–8.

37. Lombardi Jr AV, Mallory TH, Vaughn BK, Krugel R, Honkala TK, Sorscher M, Kolczun M. Dislocation following primary posterior-stabilized total knee arthroplasty. J Arthroplasty. 1993;8:633–9.

38. Kocmond JH, Delp SL, Stern SH. Stability and range of motion of Insall-Burstein condylar prostheses: a computer simulation study. J Arthroplasty. 1995;1:383–8.

39. Lombardi Jr AV, Mallory TH, Waterman RA, Eberle RW. Intercondylar distal femoral fracture: an unreported complication of posterior-stabilized total knee arthroplasty. J Arthroplasty. 1995;10:643–50.

40. Matsuda S, Ishinishi T, Whiteside LA. Contact stresses with an unresurfaced patella in total knee arthroplasty: the effect of femoral component design. Orthopedics. 2000;23:213–8.

41. Larson CM, Lachiewicz PF. Patellofemoral complications with the Insall-Burstein II posterior-stabilized total knee arthroplasty. J Arthroplasty. 1999;14:288–92.

42. Ortiguera CJ, Berry DJ. Patellar fracture after total knee arthroplasty. J Bone Joint Surg Am. 2002;84A:532–40.

43. Fuchs R, Mills EL, Clarke HD, Scuderi GR, Scott WN, Insall JN. A third-generation, posterior stabilized knee prosthesis: early results after follow-up of 2 to 6 years. J Arthroplasty. 2006;21:821–5.

44. Bozic KJ, Kinder J, Menegini M, Zurakowski D, Rosenberg AG, Galante JO. Implant survivorship and complication rates after total knee arthroplasty with a third-generation cemented system: 5 to 8 years follow-up. Clin Orthop. 2005;430:117–24.

45. Hozack WJ, Rothman RJ, Booth RE, Balderston RA. The patellar clunk syndrome: a complication of posterior stabilized total knee arthroplasty. Clin Orthop. 1989;241:203–8.

46. Insall J, Scott WN, Ranawat CS. The total condylar knee prosthesis. A report of two hundred and twenty cases. J Bone Joint Surg Am. 1979;61A:173–80.

47. Stern SH, Insall JN. Posterior stabilized prosthesis: results after follow- up of nine to twelve years. J Bone Joint Surg Am. 1992;74A:980–6.

48. Colizza W, Insall JN, Scuderi GR. The posterior stabilized total knee prosthesis: assessment of polyethylene damage and osteolysis: ten-year minimum follow-up. J Bone Joint Surg Am. 1995;77A:1713–20.

49. Brassard MF, Insall JN, Scuderi GR, Colizza W. Does modularity affect clinical success? A comparison with a minimum 10 year follow-up. Clin Orthop. 2001;388:26–32.

50. Delport HP, Banks SA, De Schepper J, Bellemans J. A kinematic comparison of fixed- and mobile-bearing knee replacements. J Bone Joint Surg Br. 2006;88B:1016–21.

51. Aglietti P, Buzzi R, Gaudenzi A. Patellofemoral functional results and complications with the posterior stabilized total condylar knee prosthesis. J Arthroplasty. 1988;3:17–25.

52. Indelli PF, Aglietti P, Buzzi R, Baldini A. The Insall-Burstein II prosthesis: a 5- to 9-year follow-up study in osteoarthritic knees. J Arthroplasty. 2002;17:544–9.

53. Thadani PJ, Vince KG, Ortaasian SG, Blackburn DC, Cudiamat CV. Ten- to 12-year followup of the Insall-Burstein I total knee prosthesis. Clin Orthop. 2000;380:17–29.

54. Oliver MC, Keast-Butler OD, Hinves BL, Shepperd JA. A hydroxyapatite-coated Insall-Burstein II total knee replacement: 11-year results. J Bone Joint Surg Br. 2005;87B:478–82.

55. Scuderi GR, Insall JN, Windsor RE, Moran MC. Survivorship of cemented knee replacements. J Bone Joint Surg Br. 1989;71B:798–803.

56. Font-Rodriguez DE, Scuderi GR, Insall JN. Survivorship of cemented total knee arthroplasty. Clin Orthop. 1997;345:79–86.

57. Emmerson KP, Moran CG, Pinder IM. Survivorship analysis f the kinematic stabilizer total knee replacement: a ten to fourteen year follow-up. J Bone Joint Surg Br. 1996;78B:441–5.

58. Ranawat CS, Luessenhop CP, Rodriguez JA. The press-fit condylar modular total knee system: four to six year results with a posterior-cruciate-substituting design. J Bone Joint Surg Am. 1997;79A: 342–8.

59. Ehrhardt J, Gadinsky N, Lyman S, Markowicz D, Westrich G. Average 7-year survivorship and clinical results of a newer primary posterior stabilized total knee arthroplasty. HSS J. 2011;7:120–4.

60. Lachiewicz PF, Soileau ES. Fixation, survival and osteolysis with a modern posterior-stabilized total knee arthroplasty. J Arthroplasty. 2014;29:66–70.

61. Lachiewicz PF, Soileau ES. Fifteen-year survival and osteolysis associated with a modular posterior stabilized knee replacement. A concise follow-up of a previous report. J Bone Joint Surg Am. 2009;91A:1419–23.

62. Mahoney OM, Kinsey TL. 5- to 9-year survivorship of single-radius, posterior stabilized TKA. Clin Orthop. 2008;4(66):436–42.

63. Bercik MJ, Joshi A, Parvizi J. Posterior cruciate-retaining versus posterior-stabilized total knee arthroplasty: a meta-analysis. J Arthroplasty. 2013;28:439–44.

64. Li N, Tan Y, Deng Y, Chen L. Posterior cruciate-retaining versus posterior stabilized total knee arthroplasty: a meta-analysis of randomized controlled trials. Knee Surg Sports Traumatol Arthrosc. 2014;22: 556–64.

65. Dennis DA, Komistek RD, Colwell Jr CE, Ranawat CS, Scott RD, Thornhill TS, Lapp MA. In vivo anterposterior femorotibial translation of the total knee arthroplasty: a multicentre analysis. Clin Orthop. 1998;356:47–57.

66. Clark CR, Rorabeck CH, MacDonald S, MacDonald D, Swafford J, Cleland D. Posterior-stabilised and cruciate-retaining total knee replacement – a randomised study. Clin Orthop. 2001;392:208–12.

67. Bassett RW. Results of 1,000 performance knees: cementless versus cemented fixation. J Arthroplasty. 1998;13:409–13.

68. Laskin RS, Maruyama Y, Villaneuva M, Bourne R. Deep-dish congruent tibial component use in total knee arthroplasty: a randomised prospective study. Clin Orthop. 2000;380:36–44.

69. Pandit H, Ward T, Hollinghurst D, Beard DJ, Gill HS, Thomas NP, Murray DW. Influence of surface geometry and the cam-post mechanism on the kinematics of total knee replacement. J Bone Joint Surg Br. 2005;87B:940–5.

70. Liow RYL, Murray DW. Which primary knee replacement? A review of currently available TKR in the United Kingdom. Ann R Coll Surg Engl. 1997;79: 335–40.

71. Aglietti P, Baldini A, Buzzi R, Lup D, De Luca L. Comparison of mobile-bearing and fixed-bearing total knee arthroplasty: a prospective randomized study. J Arthroplasty. 2005;20:145–53.

72. Catani F, Leardini A, Ensini A, Cucca G, Bragonzoni L, Toksvig-Larsen S, Giannini S. The stability of the cemented tibial component of total knee arthroplasty: posterior cruciate-retaining versus posterior-stabilized design. J Arthroplasty. 2004;19:775–82.

73. Chaudhary R, Beaupre LA, Johnston DW. Knee range of motion during the first two years after use of posterior cruciate stabilizing or posterior cruciate-retaining total knee prostheses. A randomized clinical trial. J Bone Joint Surg Am. 2008;90A:2579–86.

74. Harato K, Bourne RB, Victor J, Snyder M, Hart J, Ries MD. Midterm comparison of posterior cruciate-retaining versus-substituting total knee arthroplasty using the Genesis II prosthesis. A multicenter prospective randomized clinical trial. Knee. 2008;15: 217–21.

75. Tanzer M, Smith K, Burnett S. Posterior-stabilized versus cruciate-retaining total knee arthroplasty: balancing the gap. J Arthroplasty. 2002;17:813–9.

76. Victor J, Banks S, Bellemans J. Kinematics of posterior cruciate ligament-retaining and -substituting total knee arthroplasty: a prospective randomised outcome study. J Bone Joint Surg Br. 2005;87B:646–55.

77. Wang CJ, Wang JW, Chen HS. Comparing cruciate retaining total knee arthroplasty and cruciate-substituting total knee arthroplasty: a prospective clinical study. Chang Gung Med. 2004;27:578–85.

Long Term Clinical Outcome of Total Knee Arthroplasty. The Effect Posterior Cruciate Retaining Design

Irini Tatani, Antonios Kouzelis, and Panagiotis Megas

Introduction

Total knee arthroplasty (TKA) has provided high success rates (90 %), with many studies reporting survival rates over 95 % after 10 or more years [1–10]. As technology has evolved several different TKA designs, such as the PCL retaining TKA (CR TKA) the posterior stabilized TKA (PS TKA), and the anterior stabilized TKA (AS TKA or ultra-congruent TKA), have been utilized. There is still debate among surgeons over which knee arthroplasty design should be used for primary TKA. In order to further improve the procedure, debate has arisen regarding sources of failure in TKA, including thorough evaluation of the function and role of the posterior cruciate ligament (PCL).

The Role of the Posterior Cruciate Ligament

The PCL is the strongest ligament in the knee and an important stabilizing factor for flexion gap balancing in TKA. Along with the anterior cruciate ligament it forms part of the four-bar linkage system allowing normal knee function. In the healthy knee, PCL causes posterior translation of the femur onto the tibia when the knee is flexed. This is caused by the nature of its relative insertion sites posteriorly on the tibia and femur. As the knee is flexed the PCL is tensed because the femoral insertion site moves anteriorly. As a result, the femur is pulled posteriorly onto the tibia. This phenomenon is called "roll-back" and determines the AP contact points of the femur on the tibia. Also, the PCL is the primary constraint to the tibial posterior drawer at all angles of knee flexion. The posterolateral and posteromedial structures of the knee are responsible for posterior knee stability as the knee nears extension. This explains why isolated rupture of the posterior cruciate ligament does not lead to knee instability when walking [11, 12]. Furthermore, the PCL is the strongest ligament which prevents opening of the joint in flexion. Removal of the PCL results in an increase in the flexion gap of 5 mm [13]. Additionally, the PCL has a proprioceptive function. Studies using immunohistochemical stains specific for neural tissue have demonstrated the presence of mechanoreceptors in the PCL [14].

However, the function of the posterior cruciate ligament in patients with total knee arthroplasty is still controversial. The debatable issue is the integrity of the PCL during and after TKA. Rajgopal et al. [15] evaluated the status of the posterior cruciate ligament in 52 knees with a

I. Tatani, MD • A. Kouzelis, MD, DSc
P. Megas, MD, DSc (✉)
Department of Orthopaedics and Traumatology,
University Hospital of Patras, Rion GR-26504, Greece
e-mail: panmegas@gmail.com

© Springer-Verlag London 2015
T. Karachalios (ed.), *Total Knee Arthroplasty: Long Term Outcomes*,
DOI 10.1007/978-1-4471-6660-3_13

CR TKA and demonstrated the presence of a stable PCL in 94 % of them 11 years after surgery, raising an important argument for retaining the PCL rather than sacrificing one of the strongest ligaments in the body to achieve a near normal knee. On the other hand, contracture and fibrosis of the PCL is part of the arthritic process and may compromise its function. Albert et al. [16] performed histological analyses of 434 PCLs removed during total knee arthroplasty for osteoarthritis and found that 58 % of these ligaments presented histological lesions. They do not show a formal association between the histology and function of the PCL at the time of surgery, nor between its function and the long term clinical results of the arthroplasty. Sherif et al. [17] documented the status of the PCL during three stages of the TKA procedure and found that 94 % of PCL's were intact at initial presentation, 51 % of PCL's remained intact after the bone cuts were made and only 33 % of PCL's remained intact after knee balancing and all implants were in place. While current research does not show significant differences in outcome or function between PS and CR designs, it is usually the surgeon's preference to preserve the posterior cruciate ligament, when possible in primary TKA.

Mid and Long Term Survivorship of Cruciate Retaining TKA Designs

Above all, success of an arthroplasty is based on its ability to endure the course of time. Several factors can influence TKA survival rate: diagnosis, type of implant, type of fixation (cemented or cementless), the characteristics of the study population (age, sex, level of activity), the design of the patellar component as well as surgical technique (quality of placement, precision of bone cuts) [10, 18].

Studies performed on various cemented CR TKAs have shown a similar survival rate at 10 years of follow-up (Table 13.1): between 88 % and 98 % for the kinematic [20–22, 25, 26] (Fig. 13.1), 93.4–100 % for the PFC [5, 23, 34] (Fig. 13.2), 95–98 % for the AGC [19, 24], more

than 96 % for the Genesis [31, 32] (Fig. 13.3), and 97 % for the NexGen implants [39, 41]. Studies with longer follow up ($\geq$12 years), related to different CR designs, have shown survival rates which range from 77 % to 98.86 % [5, 10, 21, 25–29, 33–38, 40, 42–44]. The definition of failure of a TKA has not been consistent in the literature but revision for any reason has been the most commonly used criterion in order to determine the absolute survivorship of the implant. Some of the above studies include infections as failures, and others exclude infections recording aseptic loosening revision rates only. This may explain the variation of survival rates in different studies (Table 13.1).

Vessely et al. [37] evaluated the long term survival of 1,000 consecutive PFC (press fit condylar) CR TKAs with a modular tibial component and a cemented all polyethylene patellar component. Approximately one third of revisions were for aseptic loosening or tibial polyethylene wear, while infection and periprosthetic fractures accounted for a substantial proportion of revisions and reoperations. They conclude that, in addition to ongoing efforts to minimize long term reoperation rates after TKA for mechanical failure, efforts should also concentrate on the prevention and effective treatment of prosthetic infection and periprosthetic fractures. Patient's age at the time of surgery was the single most important determinant of implant survival. In those younger than 60 years, the 15 year survival free of revision for mechanical failure was 88.2 % (vs. 100 % for those over 80). In this study, survival at 15 years for revision for any reason was 95.9 similar to previously reported rates for CR PFC implants [5, 34]. Rodricks et al. [38] report the 14–17 year follow-up of the CR PFC in 160 consecutive TKAs. The overall survival rate was 91.5 % with revision for any reason as the endpoint and 97.2 % with revision for aseptic loosening as the endpoint. In this series, the patella was resurfaced in all cases and patella complications remained the most common problem (7 out of 11 revisions), supporting previous studies [23]. In a more recent study [43], survival over 17 years

Table 13.1 Review of the literature

Publication	Prosthesis (PCL-retaining)	Survivorship (Revision for any reason as end point except where noted)		
		5 years	10 years	≥12 years
Ritter (1995) [19]	AGC		98 %[a]	
Malkani (1995) [20]	Kinematic-I		96.0 %	
Weir (1996) [21]	Kinematic		92 %	87 % at 12 years
Abernethy (1996) [22]	Kinematic	94 %	88 %	
Buehler (2000) [23]	Press-fit condylar		93.4 % at 9 years	
Emerson (2000) [24]	AGC		95 %[a]	
Van Loon (2000) [25]	Kinematic		90 %	82 % at 14 years
Gill (2001) [26]	Kinematic	99.4 %	98.2 %	92.6 % at 17 years
Sextro (2001) [27]	Kinematic			88.7 % at 15 years[a]
Pavone (2001) [28]	Total Condylar knee			91 % at 23 years
Rodriguez (2001) [29]	Total Condylar knee			77 % at 21 years
Berger (2001) [30]	Miller-Galante II	100.0 %	100.0 %	
Laskin (2001) [31]	Genesis		96.0 %	
Chen (2001) [32]	Genesis I		97.0 %	
Ritter (2001) [33]	AGC			98.86 % at 15 years[a]
Fetzer (2002) [34]	Press-fit condylar		100.0 %	93.3 % at 12 years
Worland (2002) [35]	AGC			97 % at 14 years
Dixon (2005) [5]	Press-fit condylar	100.0 %	97.6 %	92.6 % at 15 years
Ma (2005) [36]	Total Condylar knee			83.2 % at 20 years
Vessely (2006) [37]	Press-fit condylar			95.9 % at 15 years
Rodricks (2007) [38]	Press-fit condylar			91.5 % at 17 years
Barrington (2009) [39]	NexGen	99.0 %	97.0 %	
Ritter (2009) [40]	AGC			97.8 % at 20 years[a]
Schwartz (2010) [41]	NexGen	98.7 %	97.7 %	
Mouttet (2011) [10]	EUROP	99.0 %	97.8 %	95.8 % at 12 years
Chalidis (2011) [42]	Genesis I			96.69 % at 13.6 years
Lin Guo (2012) [43]	Press-fit condylar			92.5 % at 17 years
Huizinga (2012) [44]	AGC			87 % at 20 years

[a]Revision for any reason excluding infection

using the CR PFC implant was 92.5 %. The authors conclude that varus and valgus deformity of the unoperated contralateral knee and tibial varus deformity of the operated knee could be important factors related to arthroplasty failure. Huizinga et al. [44] report 87 % survival rate, with failure defined as revision for any reason including infection, after 15–20 year follow-up in a study group of 211 CR AGC TKAs in 177 patients. In all but three (after prior patellectomy), the patella was resurfaced. Most of the patellae (71 %) were resurfaced with a polyethylene dome patella; (29 %) were resurfaced with a metal-backed patella. The main reasons for failure were infection and failure of the metal backed patellar component. The use of metal backed patellar components was suspended in 1991, because of a high incidence of aseptic loosening observed in the study published by Ritter et al. [45]. These rates were also confirmed by Emerson et al. [24]

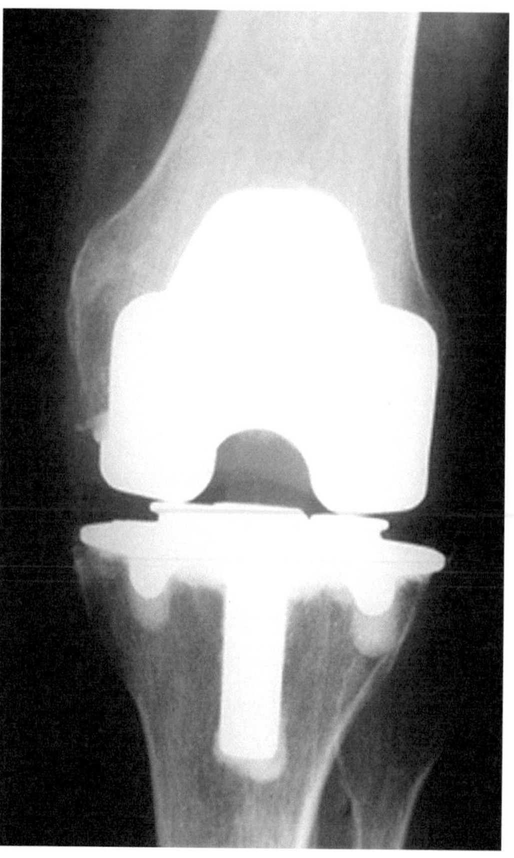

Fig. 13.1 Satisfactory AP radiograph of a Kinematic-KMS TKA at 18 years follow up is shown

who found a higher number of revisions in the metal backed patellar group at an average of 6.7 years after surgery. In another long-term follow-up study Ritter [40] reports a survival rate of 97.8 % after 20 years and attributes the success of the AGC implant to its relatively unconstrained articular geometry and the durability of a non-modular metal backed tibial component with compression molded polyethylene. Ritter's higher survival rate may be attributed to his correction for preoperative valgus deformity, which seemed to have a significant influence on survival. There are several other AGC outcome studies with shorter follow-up. Worland et al. [35] report 97 % survival at 14 years in a study group of 562 TKAs with revision for any reason as the end point. Emerson et al. [24] report survival rate of 95 % at 11.4 years in 62 TKAs with revision for any reason except infection. They only

included living patients. Ritter et al. [19] report 98 % survival at 10 years with revision for any reason except infection. In a different study, Ritter et al. [33] report survival of 98.86 % at 15 years in 4583 TKAs with revision for any reason except infection.

There are few studies of other TKA designs with a follow up of more than 12 years. Total Condylar TKAs have been performed for more than 35 years and several long term studies [28, 29, 36] report outcomes at 20 years. These studies have shown survival, with revision for any reason as the end point, of 83.2 % at 20 years [36], 77 % at 21 years [29], and 91 % at 23 years [28], respectively. Mouttet et al. [10] in a prospective, one center study of a series of 121 cemented CR, fixed bearing tibial plate EUROP TKAs, reports an overall survival rate of 95.8 % at 12 years with revision for any reason as an end point. Chalidis et al. [42] showed a 96.69 % survival rate, at an average of 13.6 year follow up, in a study of 393 primary CR Genesis I TKAs with non-resurfaced patellae.

PS Versus CR TKAs

Both CR (Table 13.1) and PS (Table 13.2) TKAs have shown excellent long term results in terms of implant survival and patient satisfaction. Studies comparing the clinical outcomes of the two designs have produced a wide range of results; some show no difference [53–56], some have favored CR designs [9, 10, 18, 42, 57], and others have questioned the importance of the PCL [58–60]. It is well understood that so far different TKA designs have shown satisfactory outcomes independent of the retaining or sacrificing of the PCL. While no current research shows a significant difference in survival between CR and PS implants, it is not well understood why surgeons are divided into cruciate retainers and cruciate substituters. The debate still continues today regarding the long term outcomes CR and PS designs. Two recent meta-analysis reports [61, 62] have attempted to throw light on the current debate. Jacobs et al. [61] undertook a systematic literature review and found and studied eight randomized control trials. Two of them compared

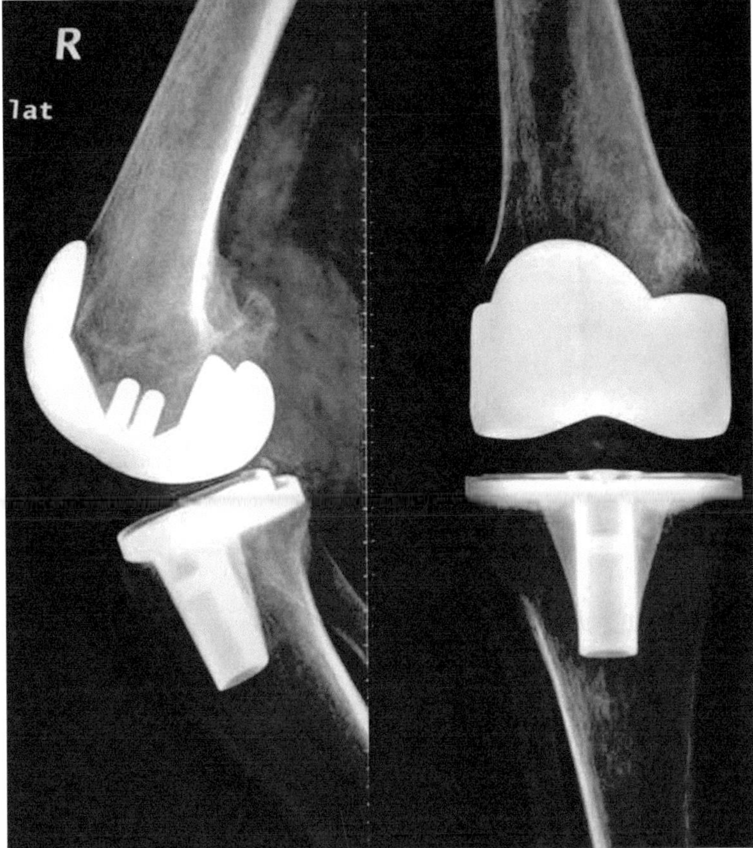

Fig. 13.2 AP and lateral radiograph of a PFC CR TKA with satisfactory clinical outcome (despite varus placement of the tibial tray) at 14 years follow up is shown

PCL retention against sacrifice, five against substitution and one had all three treatment options. The only statistical difference that could be found after analysis was that the PS group had 8° higher ROM when compared to the CR group. However, the study findings were heterogeneous at a level I^2 of 67 %. Bercik et al. [62], in a more recent meta-analysis, studied a total of 12 studies which included 1265 procedures (660 with CR designs and 605 with PS designs) after applying strict criteria. For knee flexion, the results of the study demonstrated a statistically significant difference between CR and PS implants in favor of PS by 2.4°. In terms of heterogeneity, I^2 was 40 % and no significant. ROM was also found to be statistically different, favoring PS implants by 3.33°, but heterogeneity was significant with an I^2 of 70 %. One can argue that these differences in ROM and knee flexion, although statistically significant, may not have actual clinical importance

for the patient. Thomsen et al. [63] found no association when comparing patients who had undergone bilateral TKA with high flex PS prosthesis in one knee and a standard CR prosthesis in the other knee. Besides the fact that the use of the high flex PS prosthesis resulted in significantly increased flexion compared to the standard CR prosthesis, this did not affect parameters such as pain and patient satisfaction. Two other studies performed by Padua et al. [64] and Ritter et al. [65] also found no significant correlation between increased postoperative flexion, either active or passive, and patient satisfaction.

It is widely accepted that the PCL cannot be preserved in a consistent fashion. For a number of reasons PCL resection is required including severe knee deformity requiring PCL release, PCL contracture due to the arthritic process requiring release, and PCL damage during surgical technique [16, 17, 66–69]. A surgeon using a CR

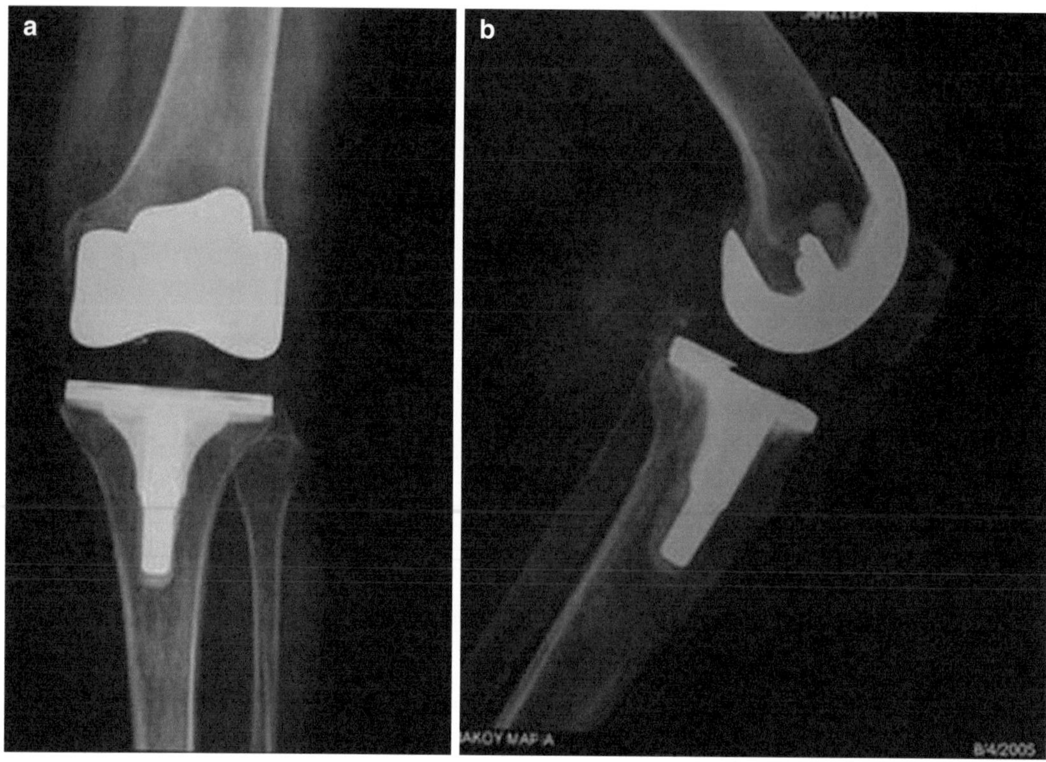

Fig. 13.3 AP (**a**) and lateral (**b**) radiograph of a Genesis II CR TKA with satisfactory clinical outcome at 15 years follow up is shown

Table 13.2 Review of the literature

Publication	Prosthesis (Posterior cruciate ligament substituting)		Survivorship
Scuderi (1989) [46]	Insall Burstein	All poly tibia	97.34 at 10 years
		Metal back tibia	98.75 at 7 years
Stern (1992) [1]	Insall Burstein	All poly tibia	94 at 13 years
Colizza (1995) [47]	Insall Burstein	Metal back tibia	96.4 at 11 years
Emmerson (1996) [48]	Kinematic stabilizer		95 at 10 years
Font-Rodriguez (1997) [49]	Insall Burstein	All poly tibia	94 at 16 years
		Metal back tibia	98 at 14 years
Nakamura (2010) [50]	Bisurface		97.4 at 10 years
Meftah (2012) [51]	LCS		97.7 at 10 years
Argenson (2012) [52]	LPS flex		98.3 at 10 years

TKA and retaining the PCL takes the risk of possible future ligament deficiency, which can happen before the TKA fails. Kleinbart et al. [59] harvested 24 PCLs from TKAs and compared them with 36 age matched PCLs collected from above the knee amputations. Sixty three percent of the arthritic knees that had undergone TKA had marked degenerative changes, compared to 0 % with marked changes from the control group. The study also showed that proprioception of the PCL had deteriorated in arthritic knee PCLs which, along with a deficiency, could partly explain the abnormal knee biomechanics in CR TKAs. For a young and active patient, retaining the PCL in a primary TKA seems logical, in order to keep knee anatomy as normal as possible. However, retaining and balancing the PCL is not as simple as it sounds. Balancing the PCL means choosing the insert thickness and component sizes so that the PCL is under adequate tension in the flexed position but relaxed in extension. Alternatively, a PCL release must be carried out in cases with a tight flexion gap. When PCL balancing has not been performed adequately, the patient has a PCL deficient TKA with pain and flexion instability [70, 71]. If the PCL is too tight, the patient suffers from limited flexion, and the polyethylene insert is subjected to high stresses and wear [70, 72]. All these issues make some surgeons to favor the removal of the PCL with routine conversion to a PS TKA.

Conclusion

Since both total knee designs have shown excellent long-term results, the factors that should influence the choice of either substitution or retention are the degenerative status of the PCL, the type of implant used, or the personal preference and experience of the surgeon. Lombardi et al. [73] have proposed a decision tree based on patient history, clinical examination, and intraoperative findings. However, more high-quality, randomized controlled studies are needed in the future to focus on clinical and functional outcome after CR and PS TKAs in order for surgeons to have a clearer idea about which prosthesis is superior.

References

1. Stern SH, Insall JN. Posterior stabilized prosthesis. Results after follow-up of nine to twelve years. J Bone Joint Surg Am. 1992;74:980–6.
2. Ritter MA, Herbst SA, Keating EM, Faris PM, Meding JB. Long-term survival analysis of a posterior cruciate-retaining total condylar total knee arthroplasty. Clin Orthop. 1994;309:136–45.
3. Meding JB, Keating EM, Ritter MA, Faris PM, Berend ME. Long-term follow-up of posterior-cruciate-retaining TKR in patients with rheumatoid arthritis. Clin Orthop. 2004;428:146–52.
4. Bozic KJ, Kinder J, Meneghini RM, Zurakowski D, Rosenberg AG, Galante JO. Implant survivorship and complication rates after total knee arthroplasty with a third-generation cemented system: 5 to 8 years followup. Clin Orthop. 2005;435:277.
5. Dixon MC, Brown RR, Parsch D, Scott RD. Modular fixed-bearing total knee arthroplasty with retention of the posterior cruciate ligament: a study of patients followed for a minimum of fifteen years. J Bone Joint Surg Am. 2005;87A:598–603.
6. Lachiewicz PF, Soileau ES. Ten-year survival and clinical results of constrained components in primary total knee arthroplasty. J Arthroplasty. 2006;21:803–8.
7. Bourne RB, Laskin RS, Guerin JS. Ten-year results of the first 100 Genesis II total knee replacement procedures. Orthopedics. 2007;30:83–5.
8. Attar F, Khaw FM, Kirk LM, Gregg PJ. Survivorship analysis at 15 years of cemented press-fit condylar total knee arthroplasty. J Arthroplasty. 2008;23:344–9.
9. Andriacchi TP, Galante JO, Fermier RW. The influence of total knee-replacement design on walking and stair-climbing. J Bone Joint Surg Am. 1982;64:1328–35.
10. Mouttet M, Louis L, Sourdet V. The EUROP total knee prosthesis: a ten-year follow-up study of a posterior cruciate-retaining design. Orthop Traumatol Surg Res. 2011;97:639–47.
11. Grood ES, Stowers SF, Noyes FR. Limits of movement in the human knee, effect of sectioning the posterior cruciate ligament and posterolateral structures. J Bone Joint Surg Am. 1988;70A:88–97.
12. Stiehl JB, Komistek RD, Dennis DA. A novel approach to knee kinematics. Am J Orthop. 2001;30:287–93.
13. Mihalko WM, Krackow KA. Posterior cruciate ligament effects on the flexion space in total knee arthroplasty. Clin Orthop. 1999;360:243–50.
14. Mihalko WM, Creek AT, Komatsu DE. Mechanoreceptors found in a posterior cruciate ligament from a well-functioning Total Knee Arthroplasty retrieval. J Arthroplasty. 2011;26:504.
15. Rajgopal A, Vasdev A, Dahiya V, Tyagi V. Evaluation of the posterior cruciate ligament in long standing cruciate retaining total knee arthroplasty. Acta Orthop Belg. 2011;77:497–501.
16. Albert A, Feoli F. Are lesions of the posterior cruciate ligament predictable before knee arthroplasty? A histological study of 434 ligaments in osteoarthritic knees. Acta Orthop Belg. 2008;74:652–8.
17. Sherif SM, Matthew V, Dipane BA, Edward J. McPherson MD. The fate of the PCL in cruciate retaining TKA A critical review of surgical technique. Joint Implant Surg Res Found Reconstr Rev. 2013;3(4).
18. Rand JA, Trousdale RT, Ilstrup DM, Harmsen WS. Factors affecting the durability of primary total knee prostheses. J Bone Joint Surg Am. 2003;85A:259–65.

19. Ritter MA, Worland R, Saliski J, Helphenstine JV, Edmondson KL, Keating EM, Faris PM, Meding JB. Flat-on-flat, nonconstrained, compression molded polyethylene total knee replacement. Clin Orthop. 1995;321:79–85.

20. Malkani AL, Rand JA, Bryan RS, Wallrichs SL. Total knee arthroplasty with the kinematic condylar prosthesis. A ten-year follow-up study. J Bone Joint Surg Am. 1995;77A:423–31.

21. Weir DJ, Moran CG, Pinder IM. Kinematic condylar total knee arthroplasty. 14-year survivorship analysis of 208 consecutive cases. J Bone Joint Surg Br. 1996;78B:907–11.

22. Abernethy PJ, Robinson CM, Fowler RM. Fracture of the metal tibial tray after kinematic total knee replacement. A common cause of early aseptic failure. J Bone Joint Surg Br. 1996;78B:220–5.

23. Buehler KO, Venn-Watson E, D'Lima DD, Colwell Jr CW. The press-fit condylar total knee system: 8- to 10-year results with a posterior cruciate-retaining design. J Arthroplasty. 2000;15:698–701.

24. Emerson Jr RH, Higgins LL, Head WC. The AGC total knee prosthesis at average 11 years. J Arthroplasty. 2000;15:418–23.

25. Van Loon CJ, Wisse MA, de Waal Malefijt MC, Jansen RH, Veth RP. The kinematic total knee arthroplasty. A 10- to 15- year follow-up and survival analysis. Arch Orthop Trauma Surg. 2000;120:48–52.

26. Gill GS, Joshi AB. Long-term results of kinematic condylar knee replacement. An analysis of 404 knees. J Bone Joint Surg Br. 2001;83:355–8.

27. Sextro GS, Berry DJ, Rand JA. Total knee arthroplasty using cruciate-retaining kinematic condylar prosthesis. Clin Orthop. 2001;388:33–40.

28. Pavone V, Boettner F, Fickert S, Sculco TP. Total condylar knee arthroplasty: a long-term followup. Clin Orthop. 2001;388:18–25.

29. Rodriguez JA, Bhende H, Ranawat CS. Total condylar knee replacement: a 20-year follow-up study. Clin Orthop. 2001;388:10–7.

30. Berger RA, Rosenberg AG, Barden RM, Sheinkop MB, Jacobs JJ, Galante JO. Long-term follow-up of the Miller-Galante total knee replacement. Clin Orthop. 2001;388:58–67.

31. Laskin RS. The Genesis total knee prosthesis: a 10-year followup study. Clin Orthop. 2001;388:95–102.

32. Chen AL, Mujtaba M, Zuckerman JD, Jeong GK, Joseph TN, Wright K, et al. Mid-term clinical and radiographic results with the genesis I total knee prosthesis. J Arthroplasty. 2001;16:1055–62.

33. Ritter MA, Berend ME, Meding JB, Keating EM, Faris PM, Crites BM. Long-term follow-up of anatomic graduated components posterior cruciate-retaining total knee replacement. Clin Orthop. 2001;388:51–7.

34. Fetzer GB, Callaghan JJ, Templeton JE, Goetz DD, Sullivan PM, Kelley SS. Posterior cruciate-retaining modular total knee arthroplasty: a 9- to 12-year follow-up investigation. J Arthroplasty. 2002;17:961–6.

35. Worland RL, Johnson GV, Alemparte J, et al. Ten to fourteen year survival and functional analysis of the AGC total knee replacement system. Knee. 2002;9:133–7.

36. Ma HM, Lu YC, Ho FY, Huan CH. Long-term results of total condylar knee arthroplasty. J Arthroplasty. 2005;20:580–4.

37. Vessely MB, Whaley AL, Harmsen WS, Schleck CD, Berry DJ. Long-term survivorship and failure modes of 1000 cemented condylar total knee arthroplasties. Clin Orthop. 2006;452:28–34.

38. Rodricks DJ, Patil S, Pulido P, Colwell Jr CW. Press-fit condylar design total knee arthroplasty. Fourteen to seventeen-year follow- up. J Bone Joint Surg Am. 2007;89A:89–95.

39. Barrington JW, Sah A, Malchau H, Burke DW. Contemporary cruciate-retaining total knee arthroplasty with a pegged tibial baseplate results at a minimum of ten years. J Bone Joint Surg Am. 2009;91A:874–8.

40. Ritter MA. The Anatomical Graduated Component total knee replacement: a long-term evaluation with 20-year survival analysis. J Bone Joint Surg Br. 2009;91B:745–9.

41. Schwartz AJ, Della Valle CJ, Rosenberg AG, Jacobs JJ, Berger RA, Galante JO. Cruciate-retaining TKA using a third-generation system with a four-pegged tibial component: a minimum 10-year follow up note. Clin Orthop. 2010;468:2160–7.

42. Chalidis BE, Sachinis NP, Papadopoulos P, Petsatodis E, Christodoulou AG, Petsatodis G. Long term results of posterior-cruciate-retaining Genesis I total knee arthroplasty. J Orthop Sci. 2011;16:726–31.

43. Guo L, Yang L, Briard JL, Duan XJ, Wang FU. Long-term survival analysis of posterior cruciate-retaining total knee arthroplasty. Knee Surg Sports Traumatol Arthrosc. 2012;20:1760–5.

44. Huizinga MR, Brouwer RW, Bisschop R, van der Veen HC, van den Akker-Scheek I, van Raay JAM. Long-term follow-up of anatomic graduated component total knee arthroplasty. A 15- to 20-year survival analysis. J Arthroplasty. 2012;27:1190–5.

45. Ritter MA, Lutgring JD, Davis KE, et al. Total knee arthroplasty effectiveness in patients 55 years old and younger: osteoarthritis vs. rheumatoid arthritis. Knee. 2007;14:9–11.

46. Scuderi GR, Insall JN, Windsor RE, Moran MC. Survivorship of cemented knee replacements. J Bone Joint Surg. 1989;71B:798–803.

47. Colizza W, Insall JN, Scuderi GR. The posterior stabilized knee prosthesis. Assessment of polyethylene damage and osteolysis after a minimum ten-year follow-up. J Bone Joint Surg Am. 1995;77A:1713–20.

48. Emmerson KP, Moran CG, Pinder IM. Survivorship analysis f the kinematic stabilizer total knee replacement: a ten to fourteen year follow-up. J Bone Joint Surg Br. 1996;78B:441–5.

49. Font-Rodriguez DE, Insall JN, Scuderi GR. Survivorship of cemented total knee arthroplasty. Clin Orthop. 1997;345:79–86.

50. Nakamura S, Kobayashi M, Ito H, Nakamura K, Ueo T, Nakamura T. The bi-surface total knee arthroplasty: minimum 10-year follow-up study. Knee. 2010;17:274–8.

51. Meftah M, Ranawat AS, Ranawat CS. Ten-year follow-up of a rotating-platform, posterior-stabilized total knee arthroplasty. J Bone Joint Surg Am. 2012;94A:426–32.

52. Argenson JN, Parratte S, Ashour A, Saintmard B, Aubaniac JM. The outcome of rotating-platform total knee arthroplasty with cement at a minimum of ten years of follow-up. J Bone Joint Surg Am. 2012;94A:638–44.

53. Kolisek FR, McGrath MS, Marker DR, Jessup N, Seyler TM, Mont MA, Barnes L. Posterior-stabilized versus posterior cruciate ligament-retaining total knee arthroplasty. Iowa Orthop J. 2009;29:23–7.

54. Becker MW, Insall JN, Faris PM. Bilateral total knee arthroplasty. One cruciate retaining and one cruciate substituting. Clin Orthop. 1991;271:122–4.

55. Ritter MA, Davis KE, Meding JB, Farris A. The role of the posterior cruciate ligament in total knee replacement. Bone Joint Res. 2012;1:64–70.

56. Tanzer M, Smith K, Burnett S. Posterior-stabilized versus cruciate-retaining total knee arthroplasty: balancing the gap. J Arthroplasty. 2002;17:813–9.

57. Abdel MP, Morrey ME, Jensen MR, Morrey BF. Increased long-term survival of posterior cruciate-retaining versus posterior cruciate-stabilizing total knee replacements. J Bone Joint Surg Am. 2011;93A:2072–8.

58. Misra AN, Hussain MR, Fiddian NJ, Newton G. The role of the posterior cruciate ligament in total knee replacement. J Bone Joint Surg Br. 2003;85B:389–92.

59. Kleinbart F, Bryk E, Evangelista J, Scott WN, Vigorita VJ. Histological comparison of posterior cruciate ligaments from arthritic and age-matched knee specimens. J Arthroplasty. 1996;11:726–31.

60. Swanik CB, Lephart SM, Rubash HE. Proprioception, kinesthesia, and balance after total knee arthroplasty with cruciate-retaining and posterior stabilized prostheses. J Bone Joint Surg Am. 2004;86A:328–34.

61. Jacobs WC, Clement DJ, Wymenga AB. Retention versus sacrifice of the posterior cruciate ligament in total knee replacement for treatment of osteoarthritis and rheumatoid arthritis. Cochrane Database Syst Rev. 2005;(4):CD004803.

62. Bercik MJ, Joshi A, Parvizi J. Posterior cruciate-retaining versus posterior-stabilized total knee arthroplasty: a meta-analysis. J Arthroplasty. 2013;28:439–44.

63. Thomsen MG, Husted H, Otte KS, Holm G, Troelsen A. Do patients care about higher flexion in total knee arthroplasty? A randomized, controlled, double-blinded trial. BMC Musculoskelet Disord. 2013;14:127.

64. Padua R, Ceccarelli E, Bondi R, Campi A, Padua L. Range of motion correlates with patient perception of TKA outcome. Clin Orthop. 2007;460:174–7.

65. Ritter MA, Campbell ED. Effect of range of motion on the success of a total knee arthroplasty. J Arthroplasty. 1987;2:95–7.

66. Arbuthnot JE, Wainwright O, McNicholas MJ. Dysfunction of the posterior cruciate ligament in the total knee arthroplasty. Knee Surg Sports Traumatol Arthrosc. 2001;19:893–8.

67. Chouteau J, Lerat JL, Testa R. Sagittal laxity after posterior cruciate ligament- retaining mobile-bearing total knee arthroplasty. J Arthroplasty. 2009;24:710–5.

68. Christen B, Heester beek PV, Wymenga A. Posterior cruciate ligament balancing in total knee replacement, the quantitative relationship between tightness of the flexion gap and tibial translation. J Bone Joint Surg Br. 2007;89B:1046–50.

69. Scuderi GR, Pagnano MW. Review article: the rationale for posterior cruciate substituting total knee arthroplasty. J Orthop Surg. 2001;9:81–8.

70. Pagnano MW, Hanssen AD, Lewallen DG, Stuart MJ. Flexion instability after primary posterior cruciate retaining total knee arthroplasty. Clin Orthop. 1998;356:39–46.

71. Waslewski GL, Marson BM, Benjamin JB. Early, incapacitating instability of posterior cruciate ligament-retaining total knee arthroplasty. J Arthroplasty. 1998;13:763–7.

72. Migaud H, Tirveilliot F. Preservation, resection or substitution of the posterior cruciate ligament in total knee replacement. In: Lemaire R, Horan F, Scott J, Villar R (eds.) Proceedings of the EFORT congress. European Instructional Course Lectures 2003;6:176–84.

73. Lombardi AV, Berend KR. Posterior cruciate ligament retaining, posterior stabilized, and varus/valgus posterior stabilized constrained articulations in total knee arthroplasty. Instr Course Lect. 2006;55:419–27.

Rationale and Long Term Outcome of Rotating Platform Total Knee Replacement

14

Vasileios S. Nikolaou and George C. Babis

Introduction

Rotating platform total knee replacements, were designed and introduced in the late 1970s aiming to more closely recreate normal knee kinematics and to minimize some of the problems (mainly wear and loosening) seen with earlier fixed bearing TKAs.

Instability, implant loosening and polyethylene wear are recognized as the major causes of failure in fixed-bearing knee prostheses. Hinged designs as well as designs with fixed high conformity bearing surfaces, failed due to transmission of extensive torque (torsional, coronal, and sagittal stresses) at bone-implant interface. Low conforming (flat-on-flat) bearing surfaces, on contrary, were more unstable and showed extensive polyethylene wear due to high contact stress [28, 36]. Indeed, early experience has shown that contact stresses experienced at the polyethylene surface are inversely proportional to the extent of conformity between the femoral condyle and tibial polyethylene insert [4, 11].

The rotating- platform designs provide both congruity and mobility in the tibio-femoral bearing surface. In most designs the polyethylene insert rotates around a central post on a flat, highly polished tibial tray [13]. This design has theoretical advantages that merit to be mentioned;

Firstly, mobile-bearing designs offer the advantage of allowing high conformity bearing surfaces without significantly increased stresses at the fixation interfaces [31, 37]. Kinematic studies have shown that in rotating platform TKRs, axial rotation of the polyethylene occurs onto the stable tibial tray in a predictable manner, following the rotation of the femoral condyles [13]. This has been shown to significantly decrease the torsional forces transmitted to the fixation interfaces [12, 40]. Additionally, in the sagittal plane, studies have shown that increased conformity results in more natural knee kinematics, decreasing phenomena such as paradoxical anterior femoral translation instead of the natural posterior femoral translation (femoral roll-back) [35].

Secondly, rotating platform total knees allows for self-alignment of the rotating polyethylene with the femoral component and correction of possible mistakes of tibial tray positioning. Usually the tibial tray is placed along anatomic landmarks, such as the medial third of the tibial tubercle and the second metatarsal bone of the foot. Other surgeons prefer the technique of "floated" tibial tray and fixation in a position parallel to the

V.S. Nikolaou, MD, PhD, MSc (✉)
G.C. Babis, MD, DSc
2nd Orthopaedic Department, School of Medicine,
Athens University, Konstantopouleio General
Hospital Nea Ionia, Athens, Greece
e-mail: vassilios.nikolaou@gmail.com;
george.babis@gmail.com

© Springer-Verlag London 2015
T. Karachalios (ed.), *Total Knee Arthroplasty: Long Term Outcomes*,
DOI 10.1007/978-1-4471-6660-3_14

135

femur, when the knee is in extension [1]. All these methods have been criticized regarding the accuracy and the effectiveness in positioning the tibial tray in proper rotation [19, 21, 30]. On the other hand, rotational malalignment may lead to patellar mal-tracking, anterior knee pain, instability and premature wear of the polyethylene [9, 40, 43]. Most rotating platform TKR designs allows for at least 10–20° of independent rotation of the polyethylene insert, in a way that it can be more forgiving to common surgeon-dependent mistakes [45].

Thirdly, the inherent ability to self-align, allows for positioning of the metal tibial tray in order to achieve the optimal tibial surface coverage. That means avoidance of medial or lateral tibial tray overhanging and also avoidance of popliteus tendon impingement [16].

Despite all these theoretical advantages, rotating platform TKRs were not initially accepted with enthusiasm from surgeons, and early as well as mid-term results failed to demonstrate significant advantages over the fixed bearing designs. Additionally, concerns raised regarding the polyethylene instability and dislocation and the possibility of extensive polyethylene wear due to the dual articulation (Figs. 14.1 and 14.2). On the other hand, the majority of well conducted randomized trials concluded that rotating platform TKRs perform at least as good as the well time–tested popular fixed bearing TKR designs [3, 10, 15, 17, 23, 26, 29, 33].

It is now almost three decades since the implantation of the first rotating platform TKR. Short and mid-term results were excellent and no difference with fixed bearing was found. However, nowadays, even more young and active patients require TKR. Additionally, patients who are candidates for TKR are more demanding and wish to remain active after surgery. Since one of the most commonly stated reason for using a mobile-bearing total knee arthroplasty was that it allows younger patients to be more active and it reduces both articular and backside wear of the tibial polyethylene bearing [14], it is logical to try to confirm this theory by examining the long term results of the RP TKR designs. Herein we

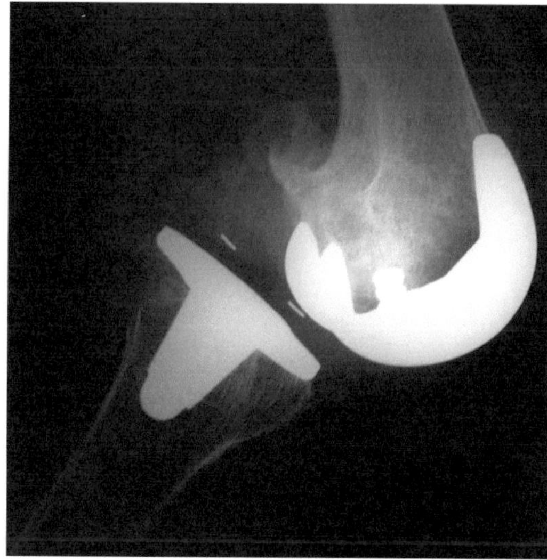

Fig. 14.1 Polyethylene spin-out, in a patient with LCS® RP TKR, 13 months after implantation. Dislocation and instability have been major concerns after the introduction of the RP TKR designs. However, after the initial few years of experience with these designs, the incidence of this complication has dropped to less than 1.5 %

present the best available evidence regarding the long term results of RP TKR from selected studies with minimum 10 years follow-up.

Selected Studies and Results of Long Term Follow Up of Rotating Platform TKRs

Buechel et al. in 2001 [5] presented the results of cemented and cementless New Jersey Low Contact Stress (LCS®) bicruciate sacrificing rotating platform TKRs after minimum 10 years follow up. The authors also compared results with a group of patients that had received the LCS, PCL retaining mobile bearing TKR. They reported excellent results for both cemented and uncemented RP TKRs at minimum follow-up of 10 years. More specifically, in the cemented RP primary TKR group (15 TKRs in 11 patients) the mean follow-up time was 173 months. In the cementless primary RP TKR group (47 TKRs in 35 patients) the mean follow-up time was 149 months. In the first group (cemented RP TKR) there was one patient with rotating platform

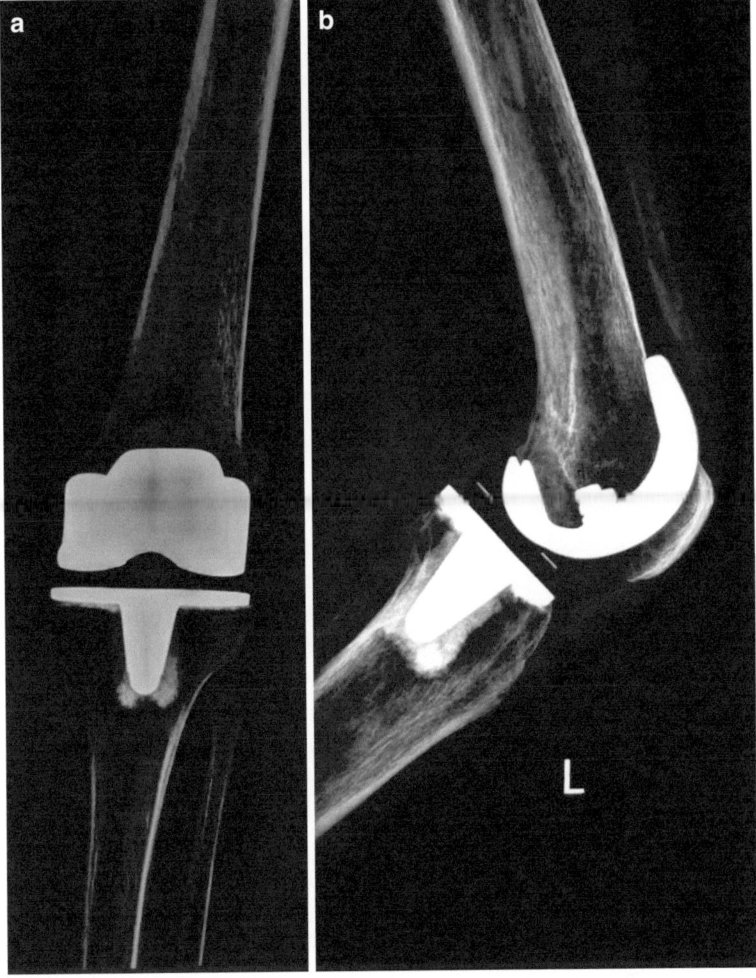

Fig. 14.2 (**a**, **b**) Twelve year follow-up AP and Lateral X-rays of a 80 years old patient with a hybrid LCS® TKA. There are no signs of loosening or polyethylene wear. The knee is stable with no pain and with a range of motion of 0–125°

dislocation. No bearing failures or component loosening were seen in patients of the second group (cementless RP TKR). Using as end point revision for any component loosening in patients with primary RP TKR the 20 year's survivorship was 95.8 % and 99.4 % for cemented and cementless prostheses respectively. Similar excellent results were obtained for the LCS® PCL retaining mobile bearing TKR.

In another study, Huang et al. [20] presented the results of LCS® RP TKR versus the LCS PCL retained meniscal-bearing prostheses (mixed cemented and cementless). The minimum follow-up was 10 years (range 10–15 years). There were 228 knees with the meniscal bearing prostheses and 267 knees with RP prostheses. Kaplan-Meier

survivorship analysis at 15 years gave 83 % survival rate for the meniscal bearing prostheses and 92.1 % survival rate for the RP prostheses. There were two early and five late (8–12 years after replacement) polyethylene dislocations in the RP TKR group. Osteolysis at the time of revision was seen in eight patients with RP TKR. The authors concluded that RP TKR performed better than the LCS meniscal bearing TKR. However, they mentioned that RP TKR results were not superior to the fixed bearing TKR designs.

In 2005, John Callaghan and colleagues [7], reported the results of the cemented LCS RP TKR with a minimum follow-up of 15 years (range 15–18 years). From an original study cohort of 86 patients (119 knees), 39 knees were available for clinical and radiological examination from 28 living patients. The authors reported excellent results, with no revision for component aseptic loosening or poor clinical results. They concluded that the cemented LCS RP is a durable TKR with results as good as those reported for fixed bearing TKR designs.

Few years later, in 2010, John Callaghan and colleagues reported results of the previous patient series at a minimum follow-up of 20 years [8]. Twenty patients (26 knees), had clinical and radiological follow-up at an average of 21 years (range 20–21 years). Authors reported that no knee required revision of any component at a minimum 20-year follow-up. One knee had radiological loosening of the femoral component. Six knees had osteolytic lesions. No knee demonstrated instability or polyethylene spin-out. The authors confirmed their previous findings regarding the durability of cemented LCS RP TKR at 20 years follow-up. They stated that these results are similar if not better than the 20 year results of other TKR devises. However, they acknowledge the fact that the average age of patients was 70 years, with only three patients under the age of 50 at the time of surgery.

Kim et al. [25] performed one-stage bilateral primary cemented TKRs in 160 patients using a fixed bearing PCL retaining TKR design (AMK; DePuy, Warsaw, Indiana) to the one side and the LCS (DePuy, Warsaw, Indiana) RP PCL sacrificing TKR at the other side of patients. 146 patients (292 knees) were available for clinical and radiological evaluation (including CT scan at the final follow-up) at a mean of 13.2 years (range 11–14.5 years). Results revealed that there was no statistical difference regarding the pre-op and post-op Hospital for Special Surgery scores, Knee society scores, range of movement or patients' preference regarding their prostheses. Also, there was no difference regarding the radiological findings, including evidence of radiolucent lines around any of the components and lateral tilting of the patella. In the LCS RP TKR group there were two revisions for instability and one for infection. Survival with revision for any reason defined as an end point at 14.5 years post-operatively was 97 % for the AMK prostheses and 98 % for the LCS RP

prostheses. Authors concluded that both prostheses yielded good results but provided no evidence to prove the superiority of the mobile-bearing over the fixed-bearing TKR.

Meftah et al. [32] presented the results of 10 years follow-up of cemented RP posterior stabilized TKR (PFC Sigma, DePuy, Warsaw, Indiana). Eighty-nine patients (106 knees) were followed-up for mean 10 years (range 9.5–11 years). They reported that at the latest follow-up 96 % had a good to excellent result according to the Knee Society pain score. Radiographic evaluation showed no mal-alignment, spin-out, aseptic loosening, or osteolysis. Survival of the prostheses with revision for any reason as an end point was calculated to 97.7 % at 10 years.

Argenson et al. [2] prospectively followed-up 104 patients (108 knees) that received a posterior-stabilized, rotating platform, total knee arthroplasty device (LPS- Flex Mobile; Zimmer, Warsaw, Indiana) for a minimum of 10 years (mean 10.6 years -range, 10–11.8 years). The authors reported no periprosthetic osteolysis and no evidence of implant loosening on follow-up radiographs. The average Knee Society knee and function scores improved from 34 to 94 points and from 55 to 88 points, respectively. Two knees were revised, one because of infection and one because of failure of the medial collateral ligament as the result of a fall. There was no spinout of polyethylene insert. The 10-year survival rate, with revision for any reason as the end point was calculated to be 98.3 %.

In another interesting prospective randomized trial, Kim et al. [24] evaluated the long-term clinical and radiographic results of fixed-bearing TKR (AMK; DePuy, Warsaw, Indiana) and mobile-bearing, rotating platform TKR (LCS RP; DePuy) in patients with osteoarthritis younger than 51 years of age. One hundred eight patients (216 knees) were included in the study. All patients had simultaneous bilateral sequential total knee arthroplasties and had a fixed-bearing implant in one knee and a mobile-bearing implant in the other. The mean follow-up period was 16.8 years (range, 15–18 years). At the latest follow-up there was no significant difference between the two groups to the studied parameters, including the Knee Society clinical score and Hospital for Special Surgery knee score, the range of movement and the alignment of the knee. Radiographic analysis and CT scans showed tibial osteolysis in two knees (2 %) in the fixed bearing TKR group, but no tibial osteolysis in the LCS RP group. There were five revisions in the fixed bearing TKR group (one for infection, two for wear of the polyethylene and two for aseptic loosening) and three revision in the LCS RP group (one for infection and two for instability). The rate of survival, at 16.8 years postoperatively, was 95 % for the AMK fixed bearing prosthesis and 97 % for the LCS RP prosthesis, when revision was defined as the end point. The authors concluded that no significant advantage could be demonstrated between fixed bearing and mobile bearing prostheses in this group of patients younger than 51 years old.

In a more recent study, Ulivi et al. [41] prospectively evaluated the long-term performance of a cemented posterior stabilized rotating platform TKR design (PFC Sigma, DePuy, Warsaw, Indiana). One hundred twelve knees were followed up for minimum 10 years (mean 11.5 ± 1.4 years). Five patients (3 %) had undergone revision; one for aseptic loosening, one due to infection and two patients due to anterior knee (patella) pain. These two patients underwent patella resurfacing. All patients had significant improvement to the tested clinical scores, including the Knee Society Score (KSS) and the Oxford Knee Score and the Visual Analogue Scale (VAS) score. Interestingly, the prevalence of anterior knee pain at final follow-up was 16.2 % (17 knees). Of note is that no patient had patella resurfacing during the initial surgery. Survivorship analysis revealed 96.6 % survival at 11.5 years when we consider revision for any cause and a 100 % survival with mechanical failure as endpoint.

There are several well conducted systematic reviews and meta-analyses published in the so far literature, comparing mobile –bearing versus fixed-bearing TKR designs [6, 22, 27, 34, 38, 39, 42, 44]. These studies have failed to show significant differences regarding the clinical scores, the radiological results, the prostheses related complications, the patient preference or the overall survivorship of the prostheses. Most of the studies, however, included mixed mobile bearing designs and short to mid-term follow-up time. On the other hand, Hopley et al. [18] recently published a well-designed meta-analysis, of papers reporting survivorship and clinical and function Knee Society Scores (KSS) of the LCS RP TKR. Outcomes were compared with non-LCS knees in the Swedish knee registry. Results revealed that the KSS scores were comparable for LCS RP and non-LCS RP knees at up to 15 years of follow-up. Excluding studies with less than mean 10 years follow-up, the authors reported incidence of osteolysis and loosening 1.4 % and incidence of instability (including spin-out) 1.4 % for the LCS RP group. Interestingly, the overall survivorship of the LCS RP TKR implanted between 1981 and 1997 and 1988 and 2005 was higher than that reported in the Swedish Knee Registry for knees implanted between 1991 and 1995 and 1996 and 2009, respectively.

Our personal (unpublished) experience with RP TKA designs the last 15 years has been excellent. We have not experienced complications, other than infections, and we have not revised any prostheses due to instability, loosening or wear.

Conclusions

In the long term, RP TKR designs have achieved excellent clinical results and survivorship rates. Initial concerns regarding stability and polyethylene dislocations have been proven basically unfounded. Similarly the possibility of higher osteolysis rates due to polyethylene wear has been proven wrong in the so far published long term studies. In the one study that has focused to the long term results of the RP TKRs in young and active patients (less than 51 years of age) [24], results were similarly excellent and promising. All authors have stressed the importance of the correct surgical technique and the meticulous soft tissue balancing, as a key factor to avoid early or late complications. As a matter of fact, many early failures of the first LR TKR designs, have been attributed to the luck of knowledge regarding the optimum surgical technique of implantation [18].

On the other hand, the vast majority of the studies, have failed to demonstrate significant advantages of the RP over the fixed bearing TKR designs. This finding is probably due to the fact that both RP and non-RP designs have excellent results in the up-to-date long term studies. Additionally, most of the long term results concern the well time-tested LCS RP TKR design. There is relatively paucity of evidence regarding the long term results of the newer RP TKR prostheses. Inevitably, more well conducted randomized trials and meta-analyses with longer than 20 years follow-up are needed to support or not the usage of RP TKRs in selected groups or subgroups of patients (i.e. young patients) in the future.

References

1. Akagi M, Mori S, Nishimura S, et al. Variability of extraarticular tibial rotation references for total knee arthroplasty. Clin Orthop Relat Res. 2005;436:172–6.
2. Argenson JN, Parratte S, Ashour A, et al. The outcome of rotating-platform total knee arthroplasty with cement at a minimum of ten years of follow-up. J Bone Joint Surg Am. 2012;94:638–44.
3. Ball ST, Sanchez HB, Mahoney OM, et al. Fixed versus rotating platform total knee arthroplasty: a prospective, randomized, single-blind study. J Arthroplasty. 2011; 26:531–6.
4. Bartel DL, Bicknell VL, Wright TM. The effect of conformity, thickness, and material on stresses in ultra-high molecular weight components for total joint replacement. J Bone Joint Surg Am. 1986;68: 1041–51.
5. Buechel Sr FF, Buechel Jr FF, Pappas MJ, et al. Twenty-year evaluation of meniscal bearing and rotating platform knee replacements. Clin Orthop Relat Res. 2001;388:41–50.
6. Callaghan JJ. Mobile-bearing knee replacement: clinical results: a review of the literature. Clin Orthop Relat Res. 2001;392:221–5.
7. Callaghan JJ, O'rourke MR, Iossi MF, et al. Cemented rotating-platform total knee replacement. a concise follow-up, at a minimum of fifteen years, of a previous report. J Bone Joint Surg Am. 2005;87:1995–8.
8. Callaghan JJ, Wells CW, Liu SS, et al. Cemented rotating-platform total knee replacement: a concise follow-up, at a minimum of twenty years, of a previous report. J Bone Joint Surg Am. 2010;92:1635–9.
9. Cheng CK, Huang CH, Liau JJ, et al. The influence of surgical malalignment on the contact pressures of fixed and mobile bearing knee prostheses–a biomechanical study. Clin Biomech. 2003;18:231–6.
10. Cheng M, Chen D, Guo Y, et al. Comparison of fixed- and mobile-bearing total knee arthroplasty with a mean five-year follow-up: a meta-analysis. Exp Ther Med. 2013;6:45–51.
11. D'lima DD, Chen PC, Colwell Jr CW. Polyethylene contact stresses, articular congruity, and knee alignment. Clin Orthop Relat Res. 2001;392:232–8.
12. Dennis DA, Komistek RD. Kinematics of mobile-bearing total knee arthroplasty. Instr Course Lect. 2005;54:207–20.
13. Dennis DA, Komistek RD, Mahfouz MR, et al. Mobile-bearing total knee arthroplasty: do the polyethylene bearings rotate? Clin Orthop Relat Res. 2005;440:88–95.
14. Duffy GP, Crowder AR, Trousdale RR, et al. Cemented total knee arthroplasty using a modern prosthesis in young patients with osteoarthritis. J Arthroplasty. 2007;22:67–70.
15. Gioe TJ, Glynn J, Sembrano J, et al. Mobile and fixed-bearing (all-polyethylene tibial component) total knee arthroplasty designs. A prospective randomized trial. J Bone Joint Surg Am. 2009;91:2104–12.
16. Goldstein WM, Branson JJ, Simmons C. Implant sizing of the P.F.C. sigma rotating-platform total knee system. Orthopedics. 2006;29:S30–5.
17. Hanusch B, Lou TN, Warriner G, et al. Functional outcome of PFC Sigma fixed and rotating-platform total knee arthroplasty. A prospective randomised controlled trial. Int Orthop. 2010;34:349–54.
18. Hopley CD, Crossett LS, Chen AF. Long-term clinical outcomes and survivorship after total knee arthroplasty using a rotating platform knee prosthesis: a meta-analysis. J Arthroplasty. 2013;28:68–77 e61–63.
19. Howell SM, Chen J, Hull ML. Variability of the location of the tibial tubercle affects the rotational alignment of the tibial component in kinematically aligned total knee arthroplasty. Knee Surg Sports Traumatol Arthrosc Off J ESSKA. 2013;21:2288–95.
20. Huang CH, Ma HM, Lee YM, et al. Long-term results of low contact stress mobile-bearing total knee replacements. Clin Orthop Relat Res. 2003;416:265–70.
21. Incavo SJ, Coughlin KM, Pappas C, et al. Anatomic rotational relationships of the proximal tibia, distal femur, and patella: implications for rotational alignment in total knee arthroplasty. J Arthroplasty. 2003; 18:643–8.
22. Jacobs W, Anderson P, Limbeek J, et al. Mobile bearing vs fixed bearing prostheses for total knee arthroplasty for post-operative functional status in patients with osteoarthritis and rheumatoid arthritis. Cochrane Database Syst Rev. 2004;(2):CD003130.
23. Kim YH, Kim JS. Comparison of anterior-posterior-glide and rotating-platform low contact stress mobile-bearing total knee arthroplasties. J Bone Joint Surg Am. 2004;86-A:1239–47.
24. Kim YH, Kim JS, Choe JW, et al. Long-term comparison of fixed-bearing and mobile-bearing total knee replacements in patients younger than fifty-one years of age with osteoarthritis. J Bone Joint Surg Am. 2012;94:866–73.

25. Kim YH, Yoon SH, Kim JS. The long-term results of simultaneous fixed-bearing and mobile-bearing total knee replacements performed in the same patient. J Bone Joint Surg Br. 2007;89:1317–23.
26. Ladermann A, Lubbeke A, Stern R, et al. Fixed-bearing versus mobile-bearing total knee arthroplasty: a prospective randomised, clinical and radiological study with mid-term results at 7 years. Knee. 2008;15:206–10.
27. Li YL, Wu Q, Ning GZ, et al. No difference in clinical outcome between fixed- and mobile-bearing TKA: a meta-analysis. Knee Surg Sports Traumatol Arthrosc Off J ESSKA. 2014;22:565–75.
28. Lonner JH, Siliski JM, Scott RD. Prodromes of failure in total knee arthroplasty. J Arthroplasty. 1999;14:488–92.
29. Luna JT, Sembrano JN, Gioe TJ. Mobile and fixed-bearing (all-polyethylene tibial component) total knee arthroplasty designs: surgical technique. J Bone Joint Surg Am. 2010;92(Suppl 1 Pt 2):240–9.
30. Lutzner J, Krummenauer F, Gunther KP, et al. Rotational alignment of the tibial component in total knee arthroplasty is better at the medial third of tibial tuberosity than at the medial border. BMC Musculoskelet Disord. 2010;11:57.
31. Matsuda S, White SE, Williams 2nd VG, et al. Contact stress analysis in meniscal bearing total knee arthroplasty. J Arthroplasty. 1998;13:699–706.
32. Meftah M, Ranawat AS, Ranawat CS. Ten-year follow-up of a rotating-platform, posterior-stabilized total knee arthroplasty. J Bone Joint Surg Am. 2012;94:426–32.
33. Pagnano MW, Trousdale RT, Stuart MJ, et al. Rotating platform knees did not improve patellar tracking: a prospective, randomized study of 240 primary total knee arthroplasties. Clin Orthop Relat Res. 2004;428:221–7.
34. Post ZD, Matar WY, Van De Leur T, et al. Mobile-bearing total knee arthroplasty: better than a fixed-bearing? J Arthroplasty. 2010;25:998–1003.
35. Ranawat CS, Komistek RD, Rodriguez JA, et al. In vivo kinematics for fixed and mobile-bearing posterior stabilized knee prostheses. Clin Orthop Relat Res. 2004;418:184–90.
36. Sharkey PF, Lichstein PM, Shen C, et al. Why are total knee arthroplasties failing today-has anything changed after 10 years? J Arthroplasty. 2014;29:1774.
37. Sharma A, Komistek RD, Ranawat CS, et al. In vivo contact pressures in total knee arthroplasty. J Arthroplasty. 2007;22:404–16.
38. Smith H, Jan M, Mahomed NN, et al. Meta-analysis and systematic review of clinical outcomes comparing mobile bearing and fixed bearing total knee arthroplasty. J Arthroplasty. 2011;26:1205–13.
39. Smith TO, Ejtehadi F, Nichols R, et al. Clinical and radiological outcomes of fixed- versus mobile-bearing total knee replacement: a meta-analysis. Knee Surg Sports Traumatol Arthrosc Off J ESSKA. 2010;18:325–40.
40. Stukenborg-Colsman C, Ostermeier S, Hurschler C, et al. Tibiofemoral contact stress after total knee arthroplasty: comparison of fixed and mobile-bearing inlay designs. Acta Orthop Scand. 2002;73:638–46.
41. Ulivi M, Orlandini L, Meroni V, et al. Survivorship at minimum 10-year follow-up of a rotating-platform, mobile-bearing, posterior-stabilised total knee arthroplasty. Knee Surg Sports Traumatol Arthrosc Off J ESSKA. 2014;1–7.
42. Van Der Bracht H, Van Maele G, Verdonk P, et al. Is there any superiority in the clinical outcome of mobile-bearing knee prosthesis designs compared to fixed-bearing total knee prosthesis designs in the treatment of osteoarthritis of the knee joint? A review of the literature. Knee Surg Sports Traumatol Arthrosc Off J ESSKA. 2010;18:367–74.
43. Van Jonbergen HP, Reuver JM, Mutsaerts EL, et al. Determinants of anterior knee pain following total knee replacement: a systematic review. Knee Surg Sports Traumatol Arthrosc Off J ESSKA. 2014;22:478–99.
44. Wen Y, Liu D, Huang Y, et al. A meta-analysis of the fixed-bearing and mobile-bearing prostheses in total knee arthroplasty. Arch Orthop Trauma Surg. 2011;131:1341–50.
45. Yang CC, Mcfadden LA, Dennis DA, et al. Lateral retinacular release rates in mobile- versus fixed-bearing TKA. Clin Orthop Relat Res. 2008;466:2656–61.

Mid to Long Term Clinical Outcome of Medial Pivot Designs

Nikolaos Roidis, Konstantinos Veltsistas, and Theofilos Karachalios

Introduction

Total Knee Arthroplasty (TKA) is the standard procedure for end stage osteoarthritis of the knee. Patients enjoy pain relief, improved function and quality of life. Advanced contemporary techniques, implants, minimally invasive and fast track surgery offer far more improved outcomes in regard to patient rehabilitation and return to every-day activities. More than 400,000 knee replacements are performed each year in the USA alone and numbers are increasing worldwide. Several factors influence long term survival and outcome of TKA. Patient, diagnosis, surgical technique and implant design related factors interact in order to provide satisfactory outcome. Over the last decades, progress in implant design has been impressive. New materials and implant designs in combination with refined surgical techniques have been responsible for improved implant survival with failure rates now being at the level of 5 % at 15 years [1].

Medial Pivot TKA designs (Advance, Wright Medical Technology, Arlington, Tennessee, USA and Medial Rotation Knee, MRK, Finsbury Orhtopaedics, Surrey, UK) were introduced into clinical practice in the late 1990s. They were both designed to address, for the first time in TKA, the reproduction of physiological anatomy, the patella friendly implant principle, stability in all planes and contemporary kinematics of the human knee. It is the editor's opinion, that medial pivot design outcomes, though not long term, deserve separate presentation.

N. Roidis, MD, DSc • K. Veltsistas, MD
3rd Orthopaedic Department, KAT Hospital,
Nikis 2, Kifisia, 14561 Athens, Hellenic Republic
e-mail: roidisnt@hotmail.com

T. Karachalios, MD, DSc (✉)
Orthopaedic Department, Faculty of Medicine,
School of Health Sciences, Center of Biomedical
Sciences (CERETETH), University of Thessalia,
University General Hospital of Larissa,
Mezourlo region, Larissa 41110, Hellenic Republic
e-mail: kar@med.uth.gr

Contemporary Human Knee Joint Kinematics

Recent work on normal knee kinematics including kinematics of cadaveric unloaded knees and unloaded and loaded knees in living subjects have shown that the knee does not work as a crossed four bar link as previously thought [2–4]. Rather, the normal knee moves with the medial side staying very nearly stable like a ball and socket joint while the lateral side moves front to back rotating around the centre of the medial side [5–17].

T. Karachalios (ed.), *Total Knee Arthroplasty: Long Term Outcomes*,
DOI 10.1007/978-1-4471-6660-3_15

The Advance Medial Pivot (AMP) TKA

AMP TKA was first introduced into clinical practice in 1998 (since then a number of papers have been published related to this implant) (Figs. 15.1 and 15.2). It was designed to replicate modern normal tibiofemoral joint kinematics. AMP implant geometry was designed to achieve stability in the antero-posterior direction [5, 6]. It was also designed to reduce complication rates seen with the use of conventional TKA cruciate retaining or cruciate substituting designs. These complications included irregular kinematics [18–20], abnormal patellar tracking [21, 22], polyethylene wear [23, 24] and poor range of motion [25, 26].

AMP Design Characteristics and Features

Restoration of Normal Knee Kinematics and Stability

For many decades it has been suggested that knee kinematics are controlled by a four-bar-link mechanism [2–4]. This mechanical link, with the cruciate ligaments acting as an almost rigid tensile element, describes a posterior "rollback" phenomenon demanding certain knee motions (the femur should roll back posteriorly in relation to the tibia). In the 1980s research confirmed that the knee is not controlled by the four-bar link, and does not "rollback". Rather, the medial side of the knee is more stable (less compliant or more constrained), and the lateral side is more mobile (more compliant and less constrained). Therefore, in the normal human knee, the tibia pivots about the medial femoral articular surface in flexion [5–17]. Thus, the knee is modeled as a shallow ball-in-socket on the medial side and two discs articulating convex to convex on the lateral side. AMP design followed this model and the principle that the kinematics and stability of a

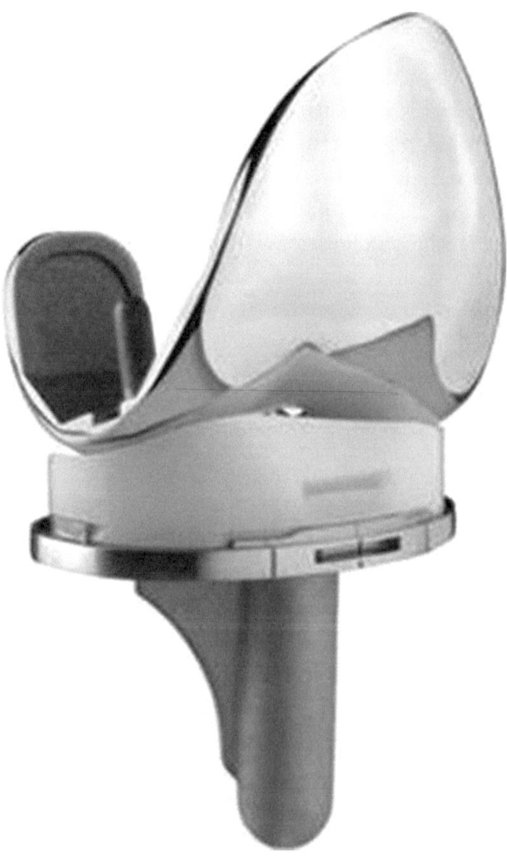

Fig. 15.1 The Advance Medial Pivot (AMP) total knee arthroplasty is shown (Reprinted with permission from Microport)

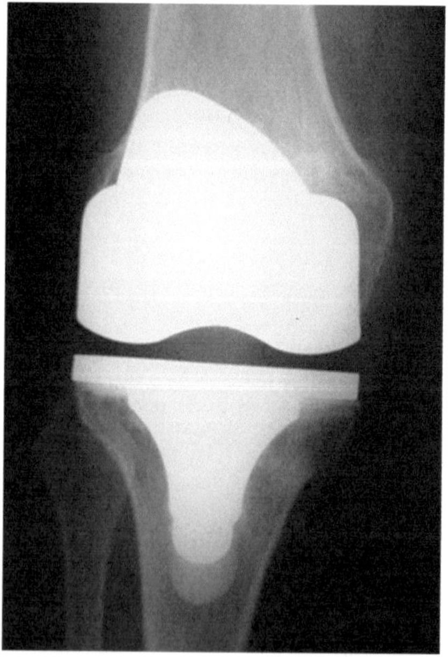

Fig. 15.2 Satisfactory radiological results of an AMP TKA at 10 years follow up is shown

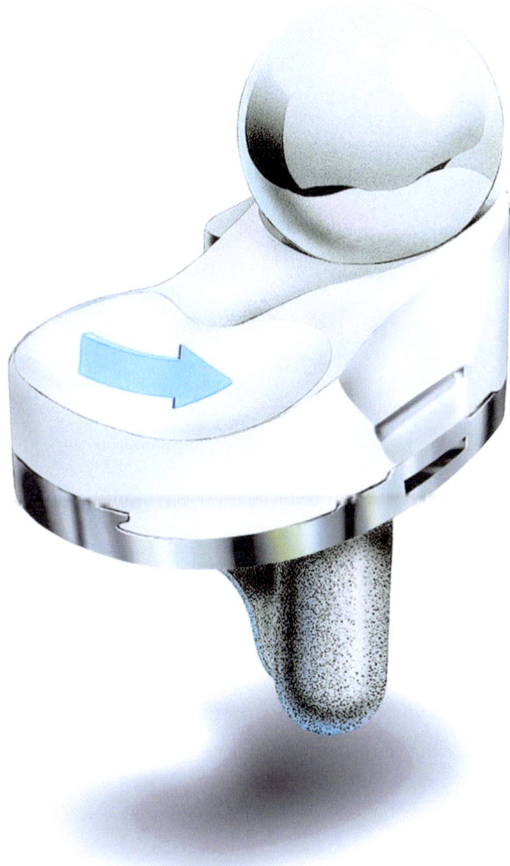

Fig. 15.3 The ball in socket medial compartment of the AMP design is shown (Reprinted with permission from Microport)

total knee prosthesis should be as close as possible to those of a normal knee, so that the arthroplasty would function more like the normal knee. Thus AMP is designed with medial femoro-tibial articulation comprised of a shallow ball-in-socket (creating stability), and the lateral side is an accurate trough (allowing mobility) (Fig. 15.3). This design more effectively recreates the kinematics of a normal knee than other implants. Studies have demonstrated that, after TKA, medial tibia pivoting is replaced by A/P sliding and rotation. This can significantly increase wear and reduce range of motion. The benefits of a ball-in-socket (medial-pivot) design are that it is stable to anterior/posterior loads and highly conforming, creating a large contact area allowing for low contact

stress. The rotation allowed by the arcuate lateral side allows rotational freedom and the combined medial and lateral articulations give stability while allowing rotational mobility [20].

Both static and dynamic knee joint stabilizers are responsible for knee joint stability (collateral ligaments, posterior capsule, anterior and posterior cruciate ligaments and medial compartment conformity). The stability and kinematics of the normal knee are created by the circular femoral condyles spinning in the cupped tibial surface on the medial side and rolling over the convex tibial surface on the lateral side. During TKA several stabilizing knee structures are sacrificed (e.g. meniscus, anterior cruciate ligament, tibial articular anatomic curvatures etc.). In order to ensure stability, surgeons attempt to equalize both the flexion and extension gaps, to balance the ligaments, and to achieve proper implant alignment and rotation. As a result, a reduction of TKA stability is often found. Conventional TKA designs (although designed to exhibit a posterior rollback in flexion) often slide anteriorly (paradoxical slide forward) due to loss of stabilizing structures and tibiofemoral congruity. As the knee flexes past 20°, body weight and force vectors slide the femur forward on the tibia (Fig. 15.4). This is termed "paradoxical motion" because normal knees are thought to roll-back as they flex [19, 20]. The raised anterior lip of the AMP polyethylene insert, coupled with the constant radius of the femoral component, resists this paradoxical motion by providing complete medial antero-posterior conformity throughout range of motion (Fig. 15.5) [5, 6, 20, 27].

Optimization of Range of Motion (ROM)

Clinical studies report that average flexion obtained after AMP TKA is 111°, while other authors report an average ROM from 115.4° to 123° after a primary TKA with the AMP TKA [28–30]. A multicenter study group compared the Range of Motion (ROM) data for the Medial-Pivot Implant with five contemporary knee designs (PROFIX®, LCS®, AXIOM®, NEXGEN® and

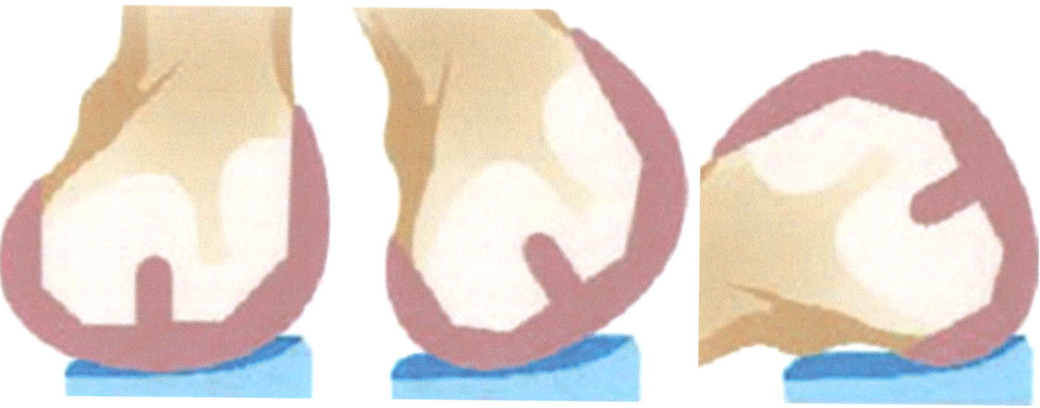

Fig. 15.4 The anterior roll back of the femoral component (paradoxical motion) is shown

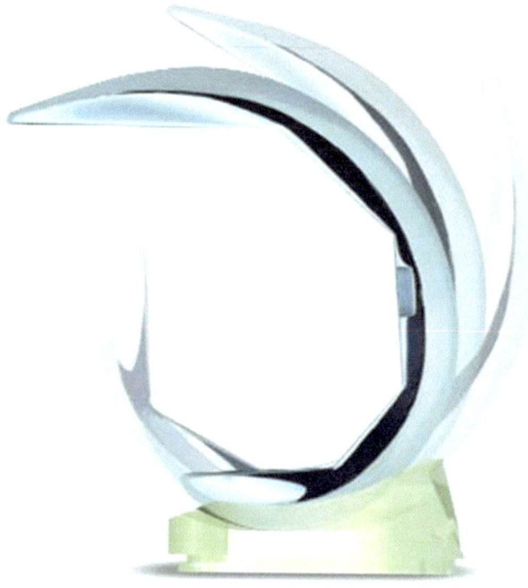

Fig. 15.5 The design feature for anteroposterior stability is shown

ethylene oxide instead of gamma radiation. Previous studies have shown gamma radiation sterilization increases stiffness and decreases polyethylene toughness [25]. Synovial fluid was obtained 1 year after knee arthroplasty from 17 patients (22 knees). Polyethylene particles were isolated and analyzed from the synovial fluid surrounding two knee designs: a PS and an AMP. The shape, size and number of the particles were compared. Particles were smaller and rounder in the AMP implants as compared to those of PS implants, but the differences in size and shape were not significant. In contrast, the difference in the amount of particles was significant. The Medial-Pivot Knee generated fewer particles than the traditional designs [32]. In an unpublished comparable dimensional study of retrieved AMP liners and intact unused AMP liners, satisfactory wear patterns were found in the mid-term (Fig. 15.6a–c).

ADVANTIM®). The data was collected at a 6-month and 1-year time period. Compared to the other five designs, the Medial-Pivot prosthesis delivers an average of 7.6° and 7.2° greater ROM at 6-months and 12-months respectively [31].

Improvement of Clinical Wear Rates

The ability of the AMP TKA to resist polyethylene wear has been verified in clinical studies. The polyethylene components are sterilized with

Restoration of Patellofemoral Joint Kinematics

High complication rates (pain, maltracking, subluxation and fractures) from the patellofemoral joint of conventional TKA designs have been reported [33, 34]. It has been shown in recent cadaveric studies that the average anatomic trochlear groove is oriented 3.6° related to the mechanical axis with small individual variations [35]. The AMP Femoral Component trochlear

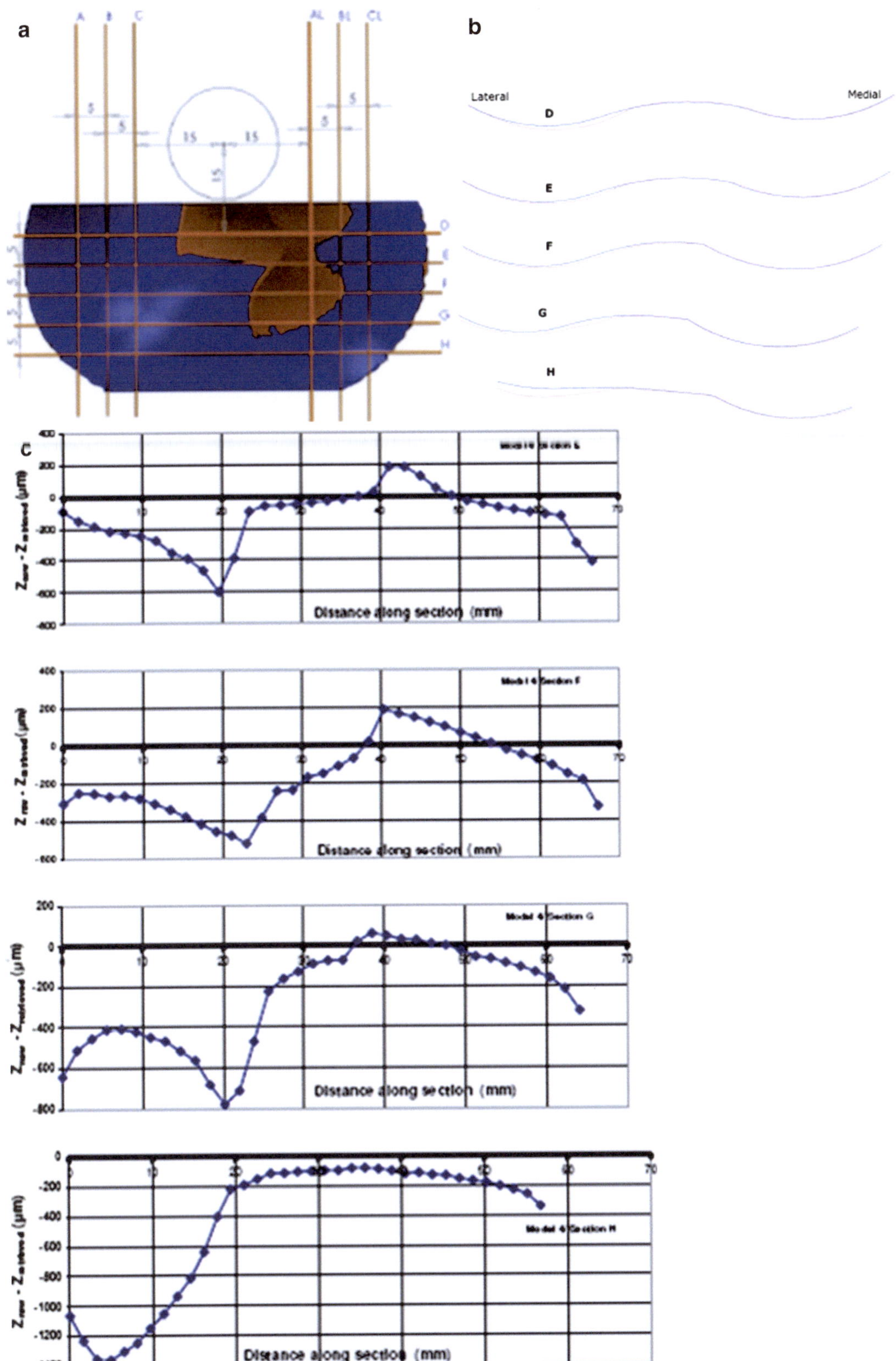

Fig. 15.6 Dimensional wear patterns of a AMP polyethylene retrieved insert at 7 years follow up: (**a**) the different dimensional sections studied, (**b**) mediolateral frontal sections studied, (**c**) satisfactory wear pattern of the retrieved insert compared to the intact one

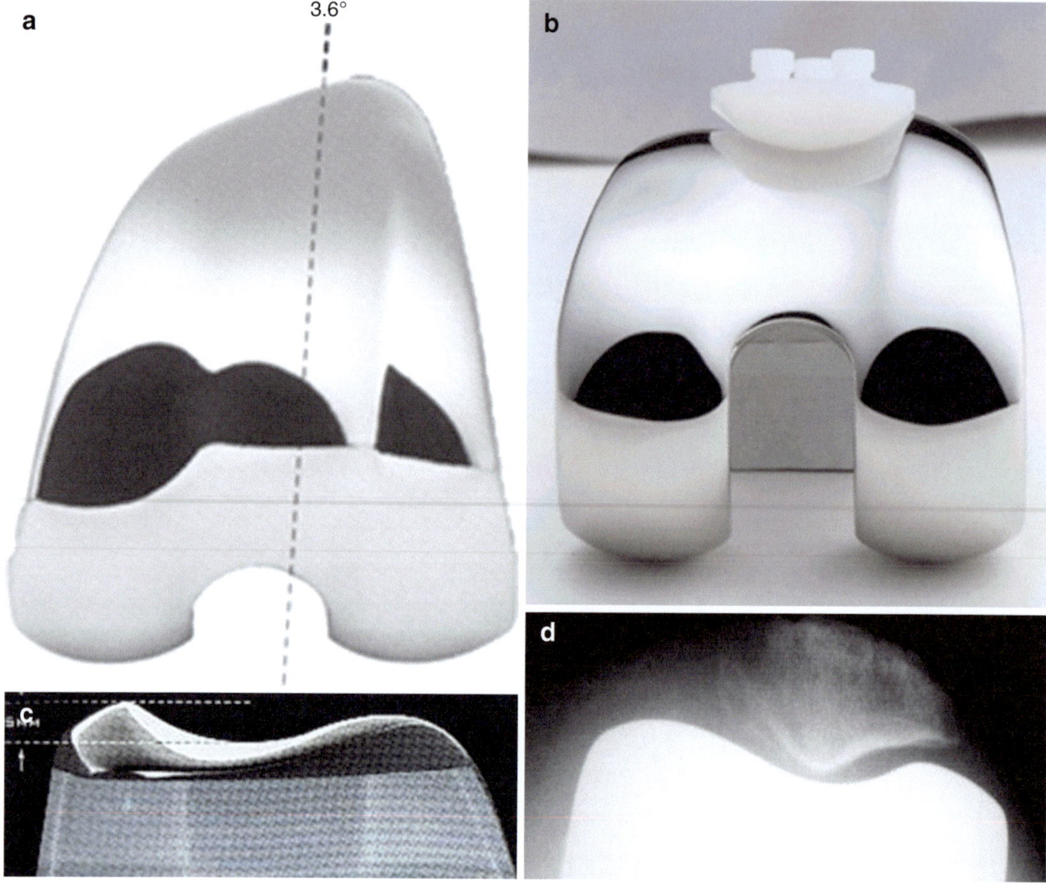

Fig. 15.7 AMP patellofemoral articulation design features are shown: (**a**) the orientation of the trochlear groove, (**b**) the length of the groove, and (**c**) the rise of the lateral anterior flange are shown, (**d**) skyline radiograph showing a congruent patellofemoral joint (Reprinted with permission from Microport)

groove is angled 3.6° to minimize strain in the lateral retinacular tissues. The trochlea is also long and deep. The lateral anterior flange rises 3–4 mm above the floor and provides resistance to lateral subluxation 9 (Fig. 15.7a–c).

Preservation of Bone Stock for Primary and Revision TKA

AMP femoral bone cutting instrumentation is designed in order to preserve bone. Additionally, the AMP revision system is a bone preserving design because no box cut is needed (60–80 % less bone removal is required [36]. In a study by Glasgow et al. [36], 29 patients who underwent revision TKA were tested for stability, ROM, extensor lag, leg alignment and clinical scores. Results showed that the medial pivot design provides AP stability of a PS insert without a need for extra bone removal [36].

Early Clinical Outcome

In a series of 440 patients who underwent a staged bilateral total knee arthroplasty with 5 different designs, using a different prosthesis on each side, Pritchett investigated patient satisfaction after a 2 year period [37]. The prostheses that were used were AMP, anterior and posterior cruciate retaining, posterior cruciate-retaining, posterior cruciate-substituting and mobile bearing [37]. Patients with bilateral TKA preferred retention of both cruciates with the use of the ACL-PCL retaining prosthesis or substituting with an MP prosthesis. When flexion was assessed in groups of patients with an AMP and a PS TKA no significant differences were found at 12 months follow up [38]. The same study showed that knees with a preoperative flexion up to 90° gained the most after the knee replacement (mean 19.6° for the AMP knee). On the other hand, knees with a preoperative flexion of 125° or greater, lost flexion (average 2.9°). This was attributed to patient factors such as pain, swelling and poor compliance with rehabilitation [38]. The hypothesis that the implication of increased constraint in the medial compartment of the TKA may lead to earlier aseptic loosening was tested by Amin et al. [39]. The authors compared (Freeman-Samuelson 1,000 Medial Pivot – Medial Rotation Knee-MRK and Freeman-Samuelson 1,000 modular TKA's) standard antero-posterior and lateral radiographs and studied radiolucent lines for component migration and signs of loosening. For a minimum follow-up period of 2 years, no sign of loosening was present in either group. Therefore, this early radiological survey concludes that the increased constraint of the medial pivot design did not result in an increased incidence of radiographic loosening [39].

In a Level I study conducted by Kim et al. [40], including 92 patients who had an AMP TKA implanted in one knee and a PFC Sigma mobile bearing TKA implanted in the other, the authors report that the early outcome of TKA is worse in the knees with the AMP compared to the PDC TKA. Knee scores and range of motion were worse in the AMP TKA, while a high infection rate was reported in the same group of patients [40]. The latter study has raised serious arguments in the literature with two letters to the Editor criticizing its methodology [41, 42].

Mid- and Long-Term Clinical Outcome

Several studies have shown favorable mid-term outcome of the Medial Pivot designs without records of implant related complications. In a multi-center study the clinical outcome of 298 AMP TKAs was reported after a minimum of 5 years follow up [43]. The 5 year survival rate was 97.2 %. Preoperative mean Knee Society Score and flexion were 33 points and 107° respectively, improving to 90 points and 121°. There was no sign of implant failure or migration. When compared to the average 6 year results of fixed INBS II and LCS TKA designs, AMP TKA showed superior flexion [43]. Satisfactory mid-term outcomes were also reported in another study of 55 consecutive patients who underwent 58 primary AMP TKAs [44]. The Knee Society Score improved from 30.5 to 91.1 and the functional score from 36.7 to 82.3. Few complications were found and most of the knees were found to be stable following thorough valgus–varus balancing [44]. Karachalios et al. [45] reports satisfactory outcomes for 284 AMP TKAs after a mean follow up of 7 years. Both objective and subjective clinical rating scales and serial radiographs were evaluated. All patients showed a statistically significant improvement in the Knee Society Score, Oxford knee score, SF-12 and WOMAC questionnaires. Range of motion improved from 101 to 117 on average. The majority of patients (93–95 %) experienced very good to excellent pain relief. This prospective clinical outcome study shows a cumulative success rate of 99.1 % at 5 years and 97.5 % at 9 years [45] (Figs. 15.8 and 15.9). More recently, Chinzei et al. [46] has retrospectively reported on 76 patients (85 knees) with AMP TKAs with a mean age at operation of 70.2 years and a mean follow-up period of 8 years (72–132 months). The survival rate at 8 years was 98.3 %. There was an improvement of knee extension angles (from 106.2 to 110.3°, p > 0.05) and of range of motion (from 94.2 to 110.6°, p < 0.05). All clinical evaluation scores (KSS, KSFS) improved significantly. According to the authors all AMP TKAs achieved excellent clinical and radiographic results without implant related failures at mid-term follow-up. Clinical and radiologic results of 172 AMP TKAs, at a mean follow-up period of 7 years, were presented by Vecchini et al. [47] showing a survival rate of 98.6 %. Satisfactory relief of pain was recorded in 90 % of patients, and 96 % of them were able to return to age-related daily life activities with 85 % of them showing excellent or good functional scores. Range of motion improved from a mean of 97.7° to a mean of 112.5° and Knee Society Score from a mean of 77.6 points to

a mean of 152.8 points. Patients also judged stability and comfort during walking as satisfactory. In another study, the outcome of 50 consecutive AMP TKAs was evaluated with pre and postoperative clinical scores (Knee Society score system, Western Ontario and McMaster Universities Arthritis Index Score). Patient satisfaction was also documented and standard radiographs were used in order to record signs of failure. The results were then compared with the results in the Australian Orthopaedic Association National Joint Replacement Registry [48]. It was found that, in the mid-term, the AMP TKA provided pain relief, functional improvement and complication and revision rates similar to reported registry data.

The AMP implant provides two different polyethylene liners, the conventional Medial pivot insert and the double high insert. The double-high tibial insert has been developed recently in order to provide high stability and high flexion. It has been designed with a 3 mm lower posterior lip, to allow posterior femoral rollback and get a better flexion angle. A comparison between the mid-term clinical results of the Medial Pivot insert and the double high insert, in combination with the same AMP TKA design, showed equally good results [49]. The authors suggest that improved range of motion cannot be

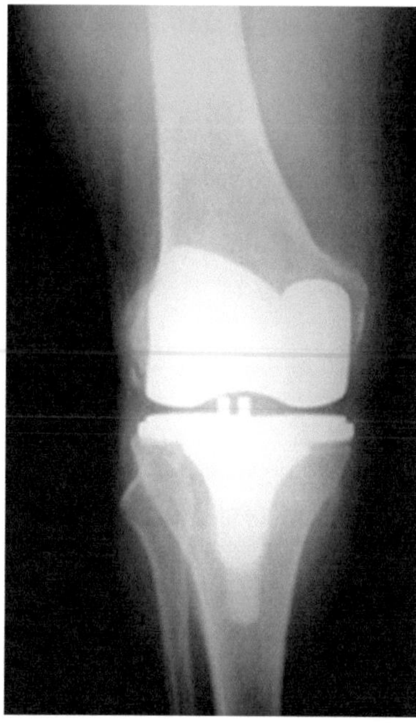

Fig. 15.8 Satisfactory radiological results of an AMP TKA (with the old version of PE insert locking mechanism) at 15 years follow up is shown

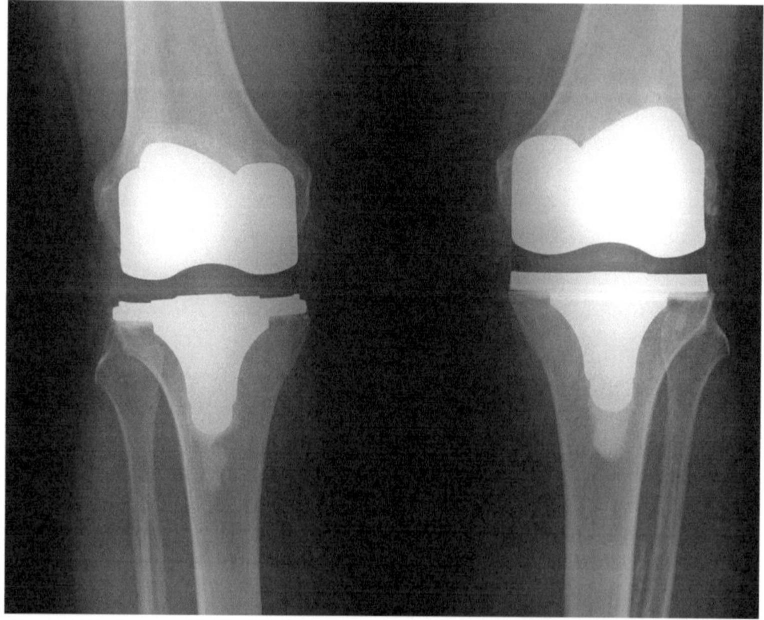

Fig. 15.9 Satisfactory radiological results of bilateral AMP TKA (right knee at 15 years and left knee at 14 years follow up) is shown

expected from changes in the design of the tibial insert only [49].

The medial pivot TKAs were initially designed as posterior cruciate sacrificing implants and anteroposterior stability is achieved with a raised anterior-lip of the polyethylene tibial insert. However, there is controversy as to whether the posterior cruciate ligament should be routinely retained or sacrificed in all patients. In a series of 137 knee replacements with an AMP TKA the posterior cruciate was retained in half of the patients and sacrificed in the rest. Knee and function scores did not vary significantly between the two groups, nor did the clinical results or femorotibial angles [50]. The authors suggest that there is a need for accurate balancing of the extension and flexion gaps. If such balance is not feasible, the posterior cruciate ligament should be resected [50]. No significant differences in the outcome of AMP TKAs were found when the posterior cruciate ligament was either retained or sacrificed in a study published by Karachalios et al. [45]. Satisfactory outcomes (Knee Society Score and Function Score) were also reported in a series with posterior cruciate retaining AMP TKAs [51]. Lateral radiographs in full extension and active flexion were taken and the magnitude of posterior femoral translation was recorded. The anteroposterior condylar contact point was consistently posterior to midline throughout the entire flexion range. No component migration or radiolucent line wider than 2 mm was reported, except for one case due to trauma [51].

Several surgeons warn against kneeling after TKA because kinematic data related to kneeling are scarce and its effect on the implant is still unknown. Nine AMP TKAs were evaluated radiographically at standing, mid-kneeling and full kneeling positions [52]. The contact point moved anteriorly from standing to mid-kneeling and posteriorly from mid- to full-kneeling. At all times it stayed within the articulation range of motion. It is thus suggested that kneeling is safe with AMP TKAs [52].

Clinical outcomes of AMP TKAs (80 patients, 107 knees) with alumina ceramic femoral component showed excellent mid-term results at 5-years follow up. Significant improvements in Knee Society Score, function score and post-operative range of motion were recorded [53]. Alumina ceramic femoral components have been associated with reduced polyethylene wear [53].

The relationship between patient reported outcomes and intraoperative knee kinematics patterns was studied in an AMP and a non AMP group of TKAs [54]. Functional activities, patient satisfaction and knee flexion angle of the AMP TKAs were significantly better than those of the non AMP TKAs. Postoperative varus deformity in the non AMP group tended to be greater than in the AMP group [54].

In Vivo Kinematic Analysis of the Medial-Pivot Knee

Advances in technology have now made it possible to precisely document kinematics in the laboratory setting. Kinematic of intact and AMP implanted cadaveric knees were tested by Barnes et al. [55]. The AMP medial compartment anteroposterior tibiofemoral translation did not prove to be greater than that of the intact specimens. In addition, the anteroposterior translation of the lateral compartment was less than the intact specimens. Extensor mechanism forces after the AMP implantation were no different from those of the same knee before implantation. In this open-chain model, intended kinematic goals of the AMP design were confirmed [55]. Fluoroscopic analysis of gait kinematics of the AMP TKA compared to a posterior cruciate retaining knee design showed that nine out of ten of the cruciate retaining TKAs had condylar lift-off averaging 1.7 mm whereas only one (out of five) AMP Medial TKAs had condylar lift-off measuring 1.1 mm. It has been shown that AMP knees show a medial pivot effect during the stance phase of gait with a lower frequency of condylar lift-off than conventional cruciate retaining designs. It was also suggested that this could lead to reduced polyethylene wear [30].

In vivo kinematics of a fixed-bearing, asymmetric, medial rotation knee arhtroplasty (Medial Rotation Knee, MRK, Finsbury Orhtopaedics, Surrey, UK) design were assessed in moderate and deep flexion. The participants were observed performing a weight-bearing activity to maximum comfortable flexion and kneeling on a padded bench from 90° to maximum comfortable flexion. The study concludes that the medial pivot rotation knee shows a medial pivot motion with tibial internal rotation during active weight bearing and deep knee flexion. The kinematics are similar in pattern to normal knees [56]. The same group of investigators studied the kinematics of the same design during weight-bearing activities through lateral fluoroscopy and model-image registration. It has been shown that during step activity there is a little anteroposterior translation or rotation from 0 to 100° flexion and a mean tibial internal rotation of 7° and condylar translation 3 mm medially and 5 mm laterally (pivot activity). It is suggested that the medial pivot design provides antero-posterior stability during demanding activities and exhibits a medial pivot motion pattern when subjected to twisting [57].

The patellofemoral kinematics of AMP TKAs has been studied with 2D–3D CT registration techniques. The results show that patellofemoral joint kinematics changed after surgery, mainly due to the design concepts for tibio-femoral joint motion, indicating the difficulty of reproducing normal patello-femoral kinematics. However, all patients in the series are clinically asymptomatic, despite an increment in patella tilt [58]. Favorable patellofemoral kinematics have also been shown in another study [59].

Conclusion

Published mid-term and unpublished long term clinical outcome data of medial pivot designs show satisfactory clinical outcomes with survival rates for revision for any reason above the level of 97 % at a mean follow up of 8 years. No serious implant related failure has been reported. Radiological evaluations and clinical wear data are also satisfactory. In vitro and in vivo kinematic data suggest that medial pivot designs actually do replicate contemporary human knee joint kinematics.

References

1. Ma HM, Lu YC, Ho FY, Huang CH. Long term results of total condylar knee arhtroplasy. J Arhtroplasty. 2005;20:580–4.
2. O'Connor J, Shercliff T, Fitzpatrick D, Goodfellow JW. Geometry of the knee in the saggital. Proc Inst Mech Eng [H]. 1989;203:223–33.
3. O'Connor J, Shercliff T, Fitzpatrick D, Goodfellow JW. Mechanics of the knee. In: Daniel D, Akeson W, O'Connor J, editors. Knee ligaments structure, function, injury and repair. New York: Raven Press, Ltd; 1990. p. 201.
4. Van Dijk R, Huiskes R, Selvik G. Roentgen stereogrammetric methods for the evaluation of the three dimentional kinematic behaviour and cruciate ligament length patterns of the human knee joint. J Biomech. 1979;12:27–31.
5. Blaha JD. The rationale for a total knee implant that confers anteroposterior stability throughout range of motion. J Arthroplasty. 2004;19:22–6.
6. Blaha JD. A medial pivot geometry. Orthopaedics. 2002;25:963–4.
7. Kurosawa H, Walker P, Abe S, Garg A, Hunter T. Geometry and motion of the knee for implant and orthotic design. J Biomech. 1985;18:487–99.
8. Iwaki H, Pinskerova V, Freeman MAR. Tibiofemoral movement 1: the shapes and relative movements of the femur and tibia in the unloaded cadaver knee. J Bone Joint Surg (Br). 2001;82B:1189–95.
9. Hill PF, Vedi V, Williams A, Iwaki H, Pinskerova V, Freeman MA. Tibiofemoral movement 2: the loaded and unloaded living knee studies by MRI. J Bone Joint Surg (Br). 2001;82A:1196–8.
10. Nakagawa S, Kadoya Y, Todo S, Kobayashi A, Sakamoto H, Freeman MA, et al. Tibiofemoral movement 3: full flexion in the living knee studies by MRI. J Bone Joint Surg (Br). 2000;82B:1199–200.
11. Karrholm J, Brandson S, Freeman MA. Tibiofemoral movement 4: changes of axial tibial rotation cause by forced rotation at the weight-bearing knee studied by RSA. J Bone Joint Surg (Br). 2001;82B:1201–3.
12. Martelli S, Piskerova V. The shapes of the tibial and femoral articular surfaces in relation to tibiofemoral movement. J Bone Joint Surg (Br). 2002;84B:607–13.
13. Freeman MA, Pinskerova V. The movement of the knee studied by magnetic resonance imaging. Clin Orthop. 2003;410:35–43.
14. Blaha JD, Mancinelli CA, Simons WH, Kish VL, Thyagarajan G. Kinematics of the human knee using an open chain cadaver model. Clin Orthop. 2003;410: 25–34.
15. Freeman MA, Pinskerova V. The movement of the normal tibio-femoral joint. J Biomech. 2005;38:197–208.
16. Pinskerova V, Maquet P, Freeman MA. Annotation: the anatomic literature relating to the knee between 1836–1917. Clin Orthop. 2003;410:13–8.

17. Pinskerova V, Johal P, Nakagawa S, Sosna A, Williams A, Gedroyc W, et al. Does the femur roll back with flexion? J Bone Joint Surg (Br). 2004;86B:925–31.

18. Andriacchi TP, Galante JO, Ferrier RW. The influence of total knee replacement design on walking and stair climbing. J Bone Joint Surg Am. 1982;64A:1328–35.

19. Stiehl JB, Kornistek RD, Dennis DA, Paxson RD. Fluoroscopic analysis of kinematics after posterior cruciate-retaining knee arthroplasty. J Bone Joint Surg (Br). 1995;77B:884–9.

20. Banks SA, Markovich GD, Hodge WA. In vivo kinematics of cruciate-retaining and –substituting knee arthroplasties. J Arthroplasty. 1997;12:297–304.

21. Beight JL, Yao B, Hozack WJ, Hearn SL, Booth RE. The patellar "clunk" syndrome after posterior-stabilized total knee arthroplasty. Clin Orthop. 1994;299:139–42.

22. Hozack WJ, Rothman RH, Booth RE, Balderston RA. The patellar "clunk" syndrome. A complication of posterior stabilized total knee arthroplasty. Clin Orthop. 1989;241:203–8.

23. Bartel DL, Bicknell VL, Wright TM. The effect of conformity, thickness and material on stresses in ultra-high molecular weight components for total joint replacement. J Bone Joint Surg Am. 1986;68A:1041–51.

24. Plante-Bordeneuve P, Freeman MAR. Tibial high-density polyethylene wear in conforming tibiofemoral prostheses. J Bone Joint Surg (Br). 1993;75B:630–6.

25. White SE, Paxson RD, Tanner MG, Whiteside LA. Effects of sterilization on wear in total knee arhtroplasty. Clin Orthop. 1996;331:164–71.

26. Maloney WJ, Schuman DJ. The effects of implant design on range of motion after total knee arthroplasty. Clin Orthop. 1992;278:147–52.

27. Miyazaki Y, Nakamura T, Kogame K, Saito M, Yamamoto K, Suguro T. Analysis of the kinematics of total knee prostheses with a medial pivot design. J Arthroplasty. 2011;26:1038–44.

28. Scuderi GR, Insall JN, Windsor RE, Moran MC. Survivorship of cemented knee replacements. J Bone Joint Surg (Br). 1989;71B:798–803.

29. Martin SD, McManus JL, Scott RD, Thornill TS. Press-fit condylar total knee arthroplasty. J Arthroplasty. 1997;12:603–14.

30. Schmidt R, Komistek RD, Blaha JD, Penenberg BL, Maloney WJ. Fluoroscopic analyses of cruciate-retaining and medial pivot knee implants. Clin Orthop. 2003;419:139–47.

31. 10-year clinical results of the ADVANCE® Medial-Pivot total knee prosthesis, "ADVANCE® Medial-Pivot Knee: 10 Years of Clinical Use" Symposium, Barcelona, June 8–9, 2008.

32. Minoda Y, Kobayashi A, Iwaki H, et al. Polyethylene wear particles in synovial fluid after total knee arhtroplasty. Clin Orthop. 2003;410:165–72.

33. Ortiguera CJ, Berry DJ. Patellar fracture after total knee arhtroplasty. J Bone Joint Surg Am. 2002;84A:532–40.

34. Mochizuki RM, Schurman DJ. Patellar complications following total knee arthroplasty. J Bone Joint Sur Am. 1979;61A:879–83.

35. Eckhoff DG, Burke BJ, Dwyer TF, Pring ME, Spitzer VM, VanGerwen DP. Sulcus morphology of the distal femur. Clin Orthop. 1996;331:23–8.

36. Glasgow D, Hennigar A, Ngan A, Gross M, Miller S, Amirault D. Bone-conserving revision TKA using the ADVANCE® Medial-Pivot implant. Unpublished data.

37. Pritchett JW. Patients prefer a bicruciate-retaining or the medial pivot total knee prosthesis. J Arthroplasty. 2011;26:224–8.

38. Shakespeare D, Ledger M, Kinzel V. Flexion after total knee replacement: a comparison between the medial pivot knee and a posterior stabilized implant. Knee. 2006;13:371–3.

39. Amin A, Al-Taiar A, Sanghrajka AP, Kang N, Scott G. The early radiological follow-up of a medial rotational design of total knee arthroplasty. Knee. 2008;15:222–6.

40. Kim YH, Yoon SH, Kim JS. Early outcome of TKA with a medial pivot fixed-bearing prosthesis is worse than with a PFC mobile-bearing prosthesis. Clin Orthop. 2009;467:493–503.

41. Pritchett JW. Early outcome of TKA with a medial pivot fixed-bearing prosthesis is worse than with a PFC mobile-bearing prosthesis. Letter to the editor. Clin Orthop. 2009;467:303.

42. Scott G. Early outcome of TKA with a medial pivot fixed-bearing prosthesis is worse than with a PFC mobile-bearing prosthesis. Letter to the editor. Clin Orthop. 2009;467:855–6.

43. Anderson MJ, Kruse RL, Leslie C, Levy LJ, Pritchett J, Hodge J. Medium-term results of total knee arthroplasty using a medially pivoting implant: a multicenter study. J Surg Orthop Adv. 2010;19:191–5.

44. Fan CYF, Hsieh JTS, Hsieh MS, Shih YC, Lee CHL. Primitive results after medial-pivot knee arhtroplasties. J Arthroplasty. 2010;25:492–6.

45. Karachalios T, Roidis N, Giotikas D, Bargiotas K, Varitimidis S, Malizos KN. A mid-term clinical outcome study of the advance medial pivot knee arthroplasty. Knee. 2009;16:484–8.

46. Chinzei N, Ishida K, Tsumura N, Matsumoto T, Kitagawa A, Iguchi T, Nishida K, Akisue T, Kuroda R, Kurosaka M. Satisfactory results at 8 years mean follow-up after ADVANCE® medial-pivot total knee arthroplasty. Knee. 2014;21:387–90.

47. Vecchini E, Christodoulidis, Magnan B, Ricci M, Regis D, Bartolizzi. Clinical and radiologic outcomes of total knee arthroplasty using the advance medial pivot prosthesis. A mean 7 years follow-up. Knee. 2012;19:851–5.

48. Brinkman JM, Bubra PS, Walker P, Walsh W, Bruce WJM. Midterm results using a medial pivot total knee replacement compared with the Australian National Joint Replacement Registry data. ANZ J Surg. 2014; 84:172–6.

49. Ishida K, Matsumoto T, Tsumura N, Iwakura T, Kubo S, Iguchi T, Akisue T, Nishida K, Kurosaka M, Kuroda R. No difference between double-high insert and medial-pivot insert in TKA. Knee Surg Sports Traumatol Arthrosc. 2014;22:576–80.

50. Bae DK, Song SJ, CHO SD. Clinical outcome of total knee arhtroplasty with medial pivot prosthesis. J Arthroplasty. 2011;26:693–8.

51. Cho SH, Cho HL, Lee SH, Jin HK. Posterior femoral translation in medial pivot total knee arhtroplasty of posterior cruciate ligament retaining type. J Orthop. 2013;10:74–8.

52. Barnes CL, Sharma A, Blaha JD, Nambu SN, Carroll BS. Kneeling is safe for patients implanted with medial-pivot total knee arhtroplasty designs. J Arthroplasty. 2011;26:549–54.

53. Iida T, Minoda Y, Kadoya Y, Matsui Y, Kobayashi A, Iwaki H, Ikebuchi M, Yoshida T, Nakamura H. Mid-term clinical results of alumina medial pivot total knee arhtroplasty. Knee Surg Sports Traumatol Arthrosc. 2012;20:1514–9.

54. Nishio Y, Onodera T, Kasahara Y, Takahashi D, Iwasaki N, Majima T. Intraoperative medial pivot affects deep knee flexion angle an patient-reported outcomes after total knee arhthroplasty. J Arthroplasty. 2014;29:702–6.

55. Barnes CL, Blaha JD, DeBoer D, Steminski P, Obert R, Caroll M. Assessment of a medial pivot total knee arthroplasty design in a cadaveric knee extension test model. J Arthroplasty. 2012;27:1460–8.

56. Moonot P, Mu S, Railton T, Field RE, Banks SA. Tibiofemoral kinematic analysis of knee flexion for a medial pivot knee. Knee Surg Sports Traumatol Arthrosc. 2009;17:927–34.

57. Moonot P, Shang M, Railton G, Field R, Banks S. In vivo weight-bearing kinematics with medial rotation knee arthroplasty. Knee. 2012;17:33–7.

58. Ishida K, Matsumoto T, Tsumura N, Chinzei N, Kitagawa A, Kubo S, Chin T, Iguchi T, Akisue T, Nishida K, Kurosaka M, Kuroda R. In vivo comparisons of patellofemoral kinematics before and after advance medial pivot total knee arthroplasty. Int Orthop. 2012;36:2073–7.

59. Chinzei N, Ishida K, Matsumoto T, Kuroda Y, Kitagawa A, Kuroda R, Akisue T, Nishida K, Kurosaka M, Tsumura N. Evaluation of pateloofemoral joint in ADVANCE® Medial-Pivot total knee arhtroplasty. Int Orthop. 2014;38:509–15.

Theofilos Karachalios and Ioannis Antoniou

Introduction

Total knee arthroplasty (TKA) is one of the most successful operations performed with 95–98 good to excellent results reported at 10–15 years follow up [1]. When it comes to fixation of components the technique can be cemented, cementless or hybrid (cementless femoral and cemented tibial components) [2, 3]. Cemented fixation has resulted in satisfactory long term outcome with low revision rates (Fig. 16.1) [2–5]. However, osteolysis often appears and the long term durability of the interface is questionable, especially in young patients [6, 7].

Cementless fixation was developed in order to achieve a more physiological bond between implants and bone and to improve longevity of the interface, especially in young patients. It has been available for more than three decades (Figs. 16.2 and 16.3) [3, 8–12]. However, due to less than optimal outcomes with the old generation of prostheses, cementless fixation in TKA has never gained popularity [3, 11, 12]. Osteolyis is still seen and RSA studies have shown early migration of the tibial plate, which is a long term determinant of implant failure [13–15]. A critical review of initial studies has shown that early cementless

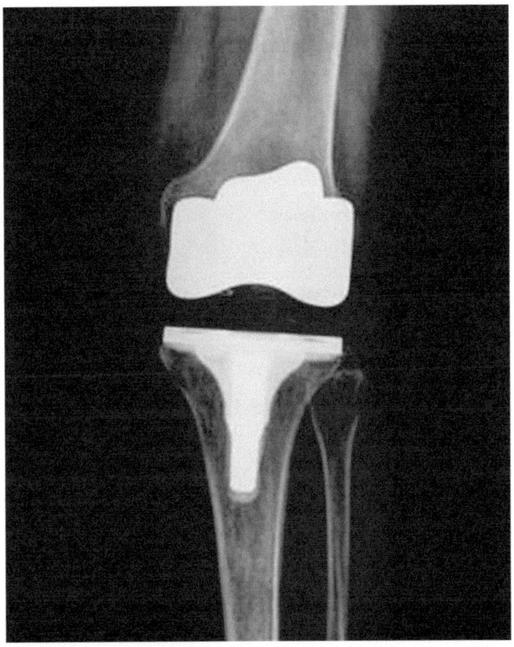

T. Karachalios, MD, DSc (✉)
Orthopaedic Department, Faculty of Medicine,
School of Health Sciences, University of Thessalia,
CERETETH, University General Hospital of Larissa,
Mezourlo region, Larissa 41110, Hellenic Republic
e-mail: kar@med.uth.gr

I. Antoniou, MD
Orthopaedic Department,
Center of Biomedical Sciences (CERETETH),
University of Thessalia, Larissa, Hellenic Republic

Orthopaedic Department,
Center of Biomedical Sciences (CERETETH),
University General Hospital of Larissa,
Larissa, Hellenic Republic

Fig. 16.1 Satisfactory clinical and radiological outcome of a cemented Genesis II TKA at 16 years follow up

© Springer-Verlag London 2015
T. Karachalios (ed.), *Total Knee Arthroplasty: Long Term Outcomes*,
DOI 10.1007/978-1-4471-6660-3_16

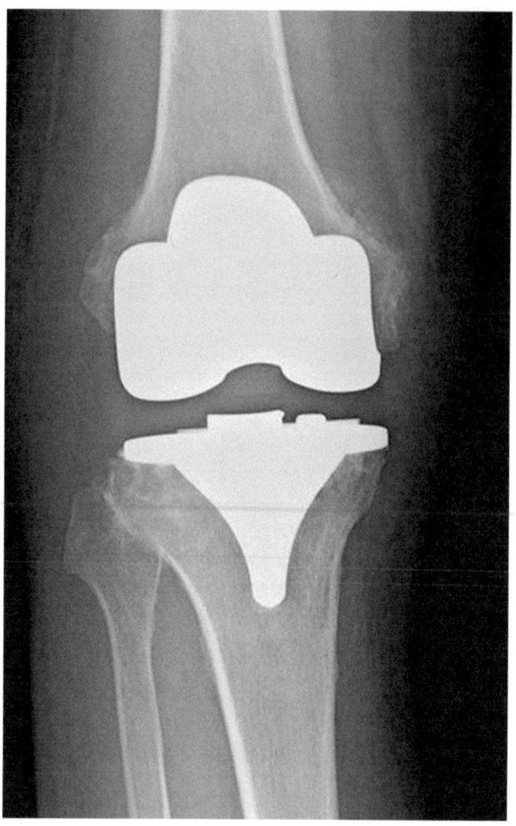

Fig. 16.2 Satisfactory clinical and radiological outcome of an cementless design at 17 years follow up

implants were used in young patients with higher demands and level of activity. Aseptic loosening, more common in the young, varied between 5 and 30 % at 5 years follow up and it was associated mainly to tibial tray failure [16–20].

As the indication and numbers of TKA continue to increase [12], younger and more active patients are undergoing the procedure and since new technologies for cementless fixation are available [11], we present, in this chapter, a review of old and new cementless TKA clinical outcomes and we critically evaluate future perspectives.

Old Designs

Old designs were developed based on the assumption that a more physiological bond between the implant and the bone can result in improved survival from the problem of aseptic loosening, due to the ability of the interface to respond to stresses in a physiological way [11, 21]. However, the long term durability of cemented fixation has come into question in young and active patients because cement has shown poor resistance to shear and tensile forces which may result in deformation and degradation over time [3, 11, 12, 22].

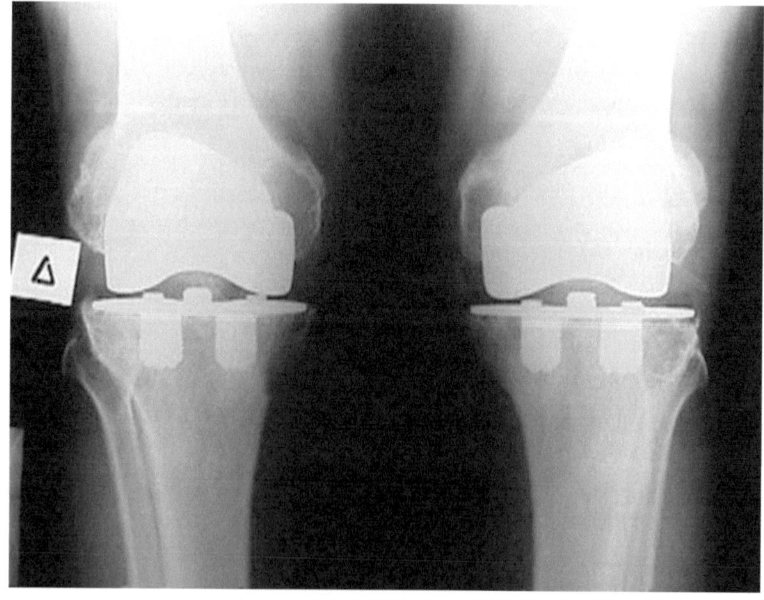

Fig. 16.3 Satisfactory clinical and radiological outcome of an early HA coated design (Goeland, Landos) at 24 years follow up

A critical evaluation of old studies with cementless implants reveals that inferior outcomes were produced due to screw track osteolysis, poor old polyethylenes, metal backed patella component failures, and poor tibial tray designs implanted inappropriately in cancellous bone instead on the cortical tibial rim [3, 11, 12, 23]. It also became apparent that cementless fixation is more sensitive to component tibial tray malalignment due to abnormal concentration of loads [11, 24, 25]. Failure of ingrowth, tibial tray radioluncencies and inferior survival curves (below 90 % at 10 years) were found in several studies (Miller Galante I, PFC designs etc.) [26–29]. Other newer designs (Natural Knee, Ortholoc, LCS etc.) showed survival rates over 90 % at 10 years [30–35]. In five prospective randomised studies which evaluated cemented and cementless old designs (PFC, Interax and NexGen) no statistically significant differences were found in clinical outcome between the two versions of the components with a follow up ranging from 10 to 17 years [1, 5, 36–38]. A meta-analysis by Gandhi et al. [39] evaluated the survivorship of cemented and cementless TKA in 11 studies (5 RCTs and 10 observational). It was found that the odds ratio for failure of the implant due to aseptic loosening and the cumulative success rates were in favour of cemented fixation. However, when the five randomised studies were isolated and evaluated, no differences in survivorship were detected between cemented and cementless implants. The authors conclude that the higher failure rate of the cementless implants in the observational studies was due to the younger age and increased activity levels of the patient population of these studies. In a more recent systematic review and meta-analysis by Mont et al. [23] 37 studies were evaluated comparing cemented to cementless TKA. It was found that cementless implants had comparable survivorship to cemented. The mean survival rate was 95.6 % and 95.3 % for cementless and cemented TKA respectively at 10 years. At 20 year follow up survival rates for cementless and cemented TKA decreased to 71 % and 76 % respectively. In more recent publications, with newer designs of implant, satisfactory outcomes have been reported in mid and long terms for cementless implants [10, 40–43]. Due to the fact that in old and new observational studies nearly all the failures for aseptic loosening were related to the tibial tray component several surgeons have suggested the use of hybrid fixation in TKA with satisfactory mid and long term results [44].

In a Cochrane database report evaluating cemented, cementless or hybrid fixation options in TKA for osteoarthritis and other non-traumatic diseases, there was a smaller displacement (assessed by radiostereographic analysis) of tibial components with cemented fixation in relation to cementless fixation in studies of patients with osteoarthritis and rheumatoid arthritis who underwent primary TKA with a follow-up of 2 years; however, cemented fixation presented a greater risk of future aseptic loosening than cementless fixation [45].

Hydroxyapaptite (HA) Coated Cementless Designs

Bioactive coatings have been used in order to enhance bone ingrowth on cementless component surfaces [46–48]. It has been suggested that HA transforms fibrous tissue to bone in loaded implant–bone interfaces [49]. Radiostereometric analysis has shown that cementless components sustain greater micromotion and early migration compared to cemented components which can lead to early migration [11, 15, 50, 51, 54]. Studies of similar design have shown equal early stability of the interface between HA coated cementless and cemented implants [50, 51, 53, 54]. In a systematic review study by Voigt and Moiser [52], early implant stability was evaluated by radiostereographic analysis in three groups of patients (HA coated, porous coated and cemented). It was found that the HA coated implants without screw fixation were less likely to be unstable at 2 years compared to the porous coated and cemented implants. In observational studies with old and new HA coated implants, survival rates above

90 % have been reported between 10 and 20 years follow up [3, 11, 20, 23, 55–57]. In a prospective randomised trial, at 5 years follow up, there was no difference between cementless tibial fixation with HA and cemented tibial fixation in terms of self-reported pain, function, health-related quality of life, postoperative complications, or radiographic scores [58].

New Technologies

Recently, cementless TKA have made a comeback with newer designs, improved materials and manufacturing techniques [3, 11, 12, 23, 30, 31, 59–61]. It has been strongly suggested that the longevity of fixation depends on: joint alignment (surgical technique and instrumentation), bone quality, patient factors (age, level activity, weight), implant features (stems, pegs) and implant surface characteristics (coating, material). Additionally, factors affecting bone ingrowth or ongrowth for implant coatings are related to the structure of the material, porosity of the structure and type and size of the porous. A series of new structures have been developed, tested in animals and applied to humans: tantalum trabecular metal technology (Zimmer) [61], Tritanium dimensionised matrix (Stryker), Regenerex (Biomet), and Titanium foam (Microport-Wright Medical) (Fig. 16.4). Table 16.1 summarises the basic characteristics of these structures. Trabecular metal technology tibial tray implants were the first to be used in humans. Satisfactory clinical and radiological results have been reported from different centers with a follow up ranging from 5 to 10 years [62–64]. Fernandez-Fairen et al. [65], in a prospective randomised trial, found comparable outcomes of tantalum cementless and cemented tibial implants at 5 years follow up.

Various Issues

Historically, the use of posterior stabilising designs in cementless TKA has been controversial. In theory the cam/post configuration of these implants could apply unpredictable stresses to

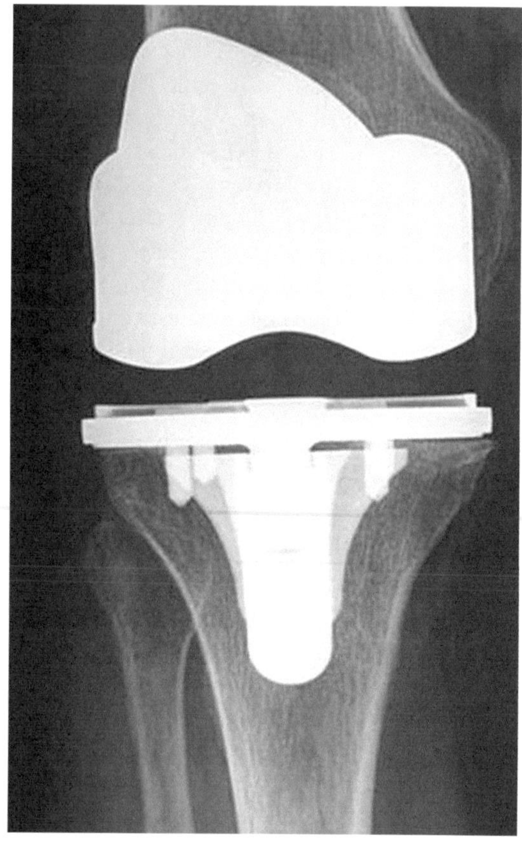

Fig. 16.4 Satisfactory clinical and radiological outcome of a titanium foam cementless advance medial pivot design at 6 years follow up

the tibial tray-bone cementless interface [66]. These reservations have been called into question in a recent publication [67]. Obesity in combination with young age are not negative predictive factors for implant survival in cementless TKA [68, 69]. Neither is rheumatoid arthritis is a negative factor for cementless TKA with patients enjoying satisfactory outcomes in mid and long term [70]. Both cemented and cementless TKAs present with areas of periprosthetic bone loss with the cementless fixation principle not preventing its appearance [71, 72]. Cementless TKA is not contraindicated in osteoarthritic knees with severe valgus or varus deformity [73]. Recent extensive research has been published evaluating tibial tray loading under different conditions in cementless TKA [74–81]. The methodology of older papers has been criticised, initial screw

Table 16.1 Structural and material characteristics of cementless TKA surfaces in use

Coating type	CsTi	Trabecular metal	Sintered beads	Fiber mesh	Ti foam	Spongiosa metal II
Company	Zimmer	Implex/Zimmer	WMT, Stryker, Depuy, S&N	Zimmer	WMT	ESKA
Porosity	52–58 %	80 %	30–40 %	50 %	65 and 75 %	60 %
Cell size[a]	480–560 µm	~500–550 µm[b]	N/A	N/A	~650 and 680 µm[b]	800–1,500 µm
Inter-connecting pore size[c]		~230 µm[b]	N/A	N/A	~280 and 300 um[b]	
Material	Ti	Ta	Ti, CoCr	Ti	Ti (CoCr)	Ti
Substrate	Ti, CoCr	Polymer, stand-alone, Ti	Ti, CoCr	Ti	Ti (CoCr)	Ti
Bioactive surface	N/A	N/A	Offered w. HA coating	N/A	TBD	N/A
Clinical history	15+ years	<5 years	20+ years	15+ years	N/A	20 years

[a]Cell size describes the average diameter of a pore cell
[b]Measured by WMT from a cross-section of the porous material
[c]Interconnecting pore size is the average diameter of the interconnection between pore cells

fixation has been withdrawn from the system, it has been suggested that peg fixation is preferable for tantalum trabecular metal tibial trays and that HA coated implants show a preferable initial mechanical environment.

Conclusion

Old cementless TKA designs produced unsatisfactory mid and long term outcomes for various reasons. The clinical outcomes of newer designs are comparable to those of cemented designs. The application of new materials and technologies in TKA designs shows promising early results [3, 11, 12, 23, 39, 82]. The cost-effectiveness of the use of such technology either in young or in all patients remains unclear since cementless TKA costs three times more than cemented TKA in most countries [58].

References

1. Kim YH, Park JW, Lim HM, Park ES. Cementless and cemented total knee arthroplasty in patients younger than fifty years. Which is better? Int Orthop. 2014;38:297–303.
2. Bauer TW, Schills J. The pathology of total joint arthroplasty. I: mechanisms of implant fixation. Skelet Radiol. 1999;28:423–32.
3. Lombardi Jr AV, Berasi CC, Berend KR. Evolution of tibial fixation in total knee arthroplasty. J Arthroplasty. 2007;22(4S1):25–9.
4. Scuderi GR, Insall JN. Total knee arthroplasty: current clinical perspectives. Clin Orthop. 1992;276:26–32.
5. Gicquel P, Kempf JF, Gastaud F, Schlemmer B, Bonnomet F. Comparative study of fixation mode in total knee arthroplasty with preservation of the posterior cruciate ligament. Rev Chir Orthop Reparatrice Appar Mot. 2000;86:240–9.
6. Naudie DD, Ammeen DJ, Engh GA, Rorabeck CH. Wear and osteolysis around total knee arthroplasty. J Am Acad Orthop Surg. 2007;15:53–64.
7. O'Rourke MR, Callaghan JJ, Goetz DD, Sullivan PM, Johnston RC. Osteolysis associated with a cemented modular posterior cruciate substituting total knee design: five to eight year follow up. J Bone Joint Surg Am. 2002;84A:1362–71.
8. Freeman MA, McLeod HC, Levai JP. Cementless fixation of prosthetic components in total arthroplasty of the knee and hip. Clin Orthop. 1983;176:88–94.
9. Freeman MA, Tennant R. The scientific basis of cement versus cementless fixation. Clin Orthop. 1992;276:19–25.
10. Bassett RW. Results of 1000 performance knees: cementless versus cemented fixation. J Arthroplasty. 1998;13:409–13.
11. Cherian JJ, Banerjee S, Kapadia BH, Jauregui JJ, Harwin SF, Mont MA. Cementless total knee arthroplasty: a review. J Knee Surg. 2014;27(3):193–7. Review.

12. Meneghini RM, Hanen AD. Cementless fixation in total knee arthroplasty: past, present, and future. J Knee Surg. 2008;21:307–14.

13. Nolan JF, Bucknill TM. Aggressive granulomatosis from polyethylene failure in an uncemented knee replacement. J Bone Joint Surg (Br). 1992;74B:23–4.

14. Berry DJ, Wold LE, Rand JA. Extensive osteolysis around septic, stable, uncemented total knee replacement. Clin Orthop. 1993;293:204–7.

15. Albrektsson BE, Carlsson LV, Freeman MS, Herberts P, Ryd L. Proximally cemented versus cementless Freeman-Samuelson knee arthroplasty: a prospective randomised study. J Bone Joint Surg (Br). 1992;74B:233–8.

16. Gioe TJ, Killeen K, Grimm K, Mehle S, Scheltema K. Why are total knee replacements revised? Analysis of early revision in a community knee implant registry. Clin Orthop. 2004;428:100–6.

17. Callaghan CM, Drake BG, Heck DA, Dittus RS. Patient outcomes following tricompartmental total knee replacement: a meta-analysis. JAMA. 1994;271:1349–57.

18. Sharkey PF, Hozack WJ, Rothman RH, Shastri S, Jacoby SM. Why are total knee arthroplasties failing today? Clin Orthop. 2002;404:7–13.

19. Fehring TK, Odum S, Griffin WL, Mason JB, Nadaud M. Early failures in total knee arthroplasty. Clin Orthop. 2001;392:315–8.

20. Epinette JA, Nanley MT. Hydroxyapatite coated total knee replacement: clinical experience at 10 to 15 years. J Bone Joint Surg (Br). 2007;89B:34–8.

21. Brown TE, Harper BL, Bjorgul K. Comparison of cemented and uncemented fixation in total knee arthroplasty. Orthopedics. 2013;36:380–7.

22. Efe T, Figiel J, Danek S, Tibesku CO, Paleta JR, Skwara A. Initial stability of tibial components in primary knee arthroplasty. A cadaver study comparing cemented and cementless fixation techniques. Acta Orthop Belg. 2011;77:320–8.

23. Mont MA, Pivec R, Issa K, Kapadia BH, Maheshwari A, Harwin SF. Long-term implant survivorship of cementless total knee arthroplasty: a systematic review of the literature and meta-analysis. J Knee Surg. 2014;27(5):369–76.

24. Drexler M, Dwyer T, Marmor M, Abolghasemian M, Sternheim A, Cameron HU. Cementless fixation in total knee arthroplasty: down the boulevard of broken dreams – opposes. J Bone Joint Surg (Br). 2012;94B(11SA):85–9.

25. Ranawat CS, Meftah M, Windsor EN, Ranawat AS. Cementless fixation in total knee arthroplasty: down the boulevard of broken dreams – affirms. J Bone Joint Surg (Br). 2012;94B(11SA):82–4.

26. Berger RA, Lyon JH, Jacobs JJ, Barden RM, Berkson EM, Sheinkop MB, Rosenberg AG, Galante JO. Problems with cementless total knee arthroplasty at 11 years follow up. Clin Orthop. 2001;392:196–207.

27. Duffy GP, Berry DJ, Rand JA. Cement versus cementless fixation in total knee arthroplasty. Clin Orthop. 1998;356:66–72.

28. Moran CG, Pinder IM, Lees TA, Midwinter MJ. Survivorship analysis of the uncemented porous coated anatomic knee replacement. J Bone Joint Surg Am. 1991;73A:848–57.

29. Whiteside LA. Effect of porous coating configuration on tibial osteolysis after total knee arthroplasty. Clin Orthop. 1995;321:92–7.

30. Hofmann AA, Evanich JD, Ferguson RP, Camargo MP. Ten to 14 year clinical follow up of the cementless natural knee system. Clin Orthop. 2001;388:85–94.

31. Whiteside LA. Cementless total knee replacement. Nine to 11 year results and 10 year survivorship analysis. Clin Orthop. 1994;309:185–92.

32. Watanabe H, Akizuki S, Takizawa T. Survival analysis of a cementless, cruciate-retaining total knee arthroplasty. Clinical and radiographic assessment 10 to 13 years after surgery. J Bone Joint Surg (Br). 2004;86A:824–9.

33. Buechel FF, Buechel FF, Pappas MJ, D'Alessio J. Twenty year evaluation of meniscal bearing and rotating platform knee replacements. Clin Orthop. 2001;388:41–50.

34. Ritter MA, Meneghini RM. Twenty-year survivorship of cementless anatomic graduated component total knee arthroplasty. J Arthroplasty. 2010;25:507–13.

35. Eriksen J, Christensen J, Solgaard S, Schrøder H. The cementless AGC 2000 knee prosthesis: 20-year results in a consecutive series. Acta Orthop Belg. 2009;75(2):225–33.

36. McCaskie AW, Deehan DJ, Green TP, et al. Randomised, prospective study comparing cemented and cementless total knee replacement: results of press fit condylar total knee replacement at five years. J Bone Joint Surg (Br). 1998;80B:971–5.

37. Khaw FM, Kirk LM, Morris RW, Gregg PJ. A randomised, controlled trial of cemented versus cementless press-fit condylar total knee replacement. Ten-year survival analysis. J Bone Joint Surg (Br). 2002;84B:658–66.

38. Baker PN, Khaw FM, Kirk LM, Esler CN, Gregg PJ. A randomised controlled trial of cemented versus cementless press-fit condylar total knee replacement: 15-year survival analysis. J Bone Joint Surg (Br). 2007;89B:1608–14.

39. Gandhi R, Tsvetkov D, Davey JR, Mahomed NN. Survival and clinical function of cemented and uncemented prostheses in total knee replacement: a meta-analysis. J Bone Joint Surg (Br). 2009;91B:889–95.

40. Efstathopoulos N, Mavrogenis AF, Lallos S, Nikolaou V, Papagelopoulos PJ, Savvidou OD, Korres DS. 10-year evaluation of the cementless low contact stress rotating-platform total knee arthroplasty. J Long-Term Eff Med Implants. 2009;19:255–63.

41. Chana R, Shenava Y, Nicholl AP, Lusted FJ, Skinner PW, Gibb PA. Five- to 8-year results of the uncemented Duracon total knee arthroplasty system. J Arthroplasty. 2008;23:677–82.

42. Hardeman F, Vandenneucker H, Van Lauwe J, Bellemans J. Cementless total knee arthroplasty with Profix: a 8- to 10-year follow-up study. Knee. 2006;13(6):419–21.

43. Choy WS, Yang DS, Lee KW, Lee SK, Kim KJ, Chang SH. Cemented versus cementless fixation of a tibial

component in LCS mobile-bearing total knee arthroplasty performed by a single surgeon. J Arthroplasty. 2014;29(12):2397–401.

44. Pelt CE, Gililland JM, Doble J, Stronach BM, Peters CL. Hybrid total knee arthroplasty revisited: midterm follow up of hybrid versus cemented fixation in total knee arthroplasty. Biomed Res Int. 2013;2013:854871.

45. Nakama GY, Peccin MS, Almeida GJ, Lira Neto Ode A, Queiroz AA, Navarro RD. Cemented, cementless or hybrid fixation options in total knee arthroplasty for osteoarthritis and other non-traumatic diseases. Cochrane Database Syst Rev. 2012;(10):CD006193. Review

46. Soballe K. Hydroxyapatite ceramic coating for bone implant fixation. Mechanical and histological studies in dogs. Acta Orthop Scand. 1993;255:S1–58.

47. Soballe K, Ovegaard S. The current status of Hydroxyapatite coating of prostheses. J Bone Joint Surg (Br). 1996;78B:689–91.

48. Gejo R, Akizuki S, Takizawa T. Fixation of the NexGen HA-TCP coated cementless, screwless total knee arthroplasty: comparison with conventional cementless total knee arthroplasty of the same type. J Arthroplasty. 2002;17:449–56.

49. Soballe K, Hansen ES, Brockstedt-Rasmussen H, Bunger C. Hydroxyapatite coating converts fibrous tissue to bone around loaded implants. J Bone Joint Surg (Br). 1993;75B:270–8.

50. Regnér L, Carlsson L, Kärrholm J, Herberts P. Tibial component fixation in porous- and hydroxyapatite-coated total knee arthroplasty: a radiostereometric evaluation of migration and inducible displacement after 5 years. J Arthroplasty. 2000;15:681–9.

51. Carlsson A, Björkman A, Besjakov J, Onsten I. Cemented tibial component fixation performs better than cementless fixation: a randomized radiostereometric study comparing porous-coated, hydroxyapatite-coated and cemented tibial components over 5 years. Acta Orthop Scand. 2005;76(3):362–9.

52. Voigt JD, Mosier M. Hydroxyapatite(HA) coating appears to be of benefit for implant durability of tibial components in primary total knee arthroplasty. Acta Orthop Scand. 2011;82:448–59.

53. Uvehammer J, Karrholm J, Carlsson L. Cemented versus hydroxyapatite fixation of the femoral component of the Freeman-Samuelson total knee replacement: a radiostereometric analysis. J Bone Joint Surg (Br). 2007;89B:39–44.

54. Nilsson KG, Karrholm J, Carlsson AS, Dalen T. Hydroxyapatite coating versus cemented fixation of the tibial component in total knee arthroplasty: prospective randomised comparison of hydroxyapatite coated and cemented tibial components with five year follow up using radiostereometry. J Arthroplast. 1999;14:9–20.

55. Cross MJ, Parish EN. A hydroxyapatite-coated total knee replacement: prospective analysis of 1000 patients. J Bone Joint Surg (Br). 2005;87B:1073–6.

56. Nilsson KG, Henricson A, Norgren B, Dalén T. Uncemented HA-coated implant is the optimum fixation for TKA in the young patient. Clin Orthop. 2006;448:129–39.

57. Tai CC, Cross MJ. Five- to 12-year follow-up of a hydroxyapatite-coated, cementless total knee replacement in young, active patients. J Bone Joint Surg (Br). 2006;88B:1158–63.

58. Beaupré LA, al-Yamani M, Huckell JR, Johnston DW. Hydroxyapatite-coated tibial implants compared with cemented tibial fixation in primary total knee arthroplasty. A randomized trial of outcomes at five years. J Bone Joint Surg Am. 2007;89A:2204–11.

59. Azboy I, Demitras A, Bulut M, Ozturkmen Y, Sukur E, Caniklioglu M. Long term results of porous coated cementless total knee arthroplasty with screw fixation. Acta Orthop Traumatol Turc. 2013;47:347–53.

60. Banerjee S, Kulesha G, Kester M, Mont MA. Emerging technologies in arthroplasty: additive manufacturing. J Knee Surg. 2014;27(3):185–91.

61. Bobyn JD, Stackpool GJ, Hacking SA, Tanzer M, Krygier JJ. Characteristics of bone ingrowth and interface mechanics of a new tantalum biomaterial J Bone Joint Surg (Br). 1999;81B:907–14.

62. Normand X, Pinçon JL, Ragot JM, Verdier R, Aslanian T. Prospective study of the cementless "New Wave" total knee mobile-bearing arthroplasty: 8-year follow-up. Eur J Orthop Surg Traumatol. 2015;25(2):349–54.

63. Helm AT, Kerin C, Ghalayini SR, McLauchlan GJ. Preliminary results of an uncemented trabecular metal tibial component in total knee arthroplasty. J Arthroplasty. 2009;24:941–4.

64. Kamath AF, Lee GC, Sheth NP, Nelson CL, Garino JP, Israelite CL. Prospective results of uncemented tantalum monoblock tibia in total knee arthroplasty: minimum 5-year follow-up in patients younger than 55 years. J Arthroplasty. 2011;26:1390–5.

65. Fernandez-Fairen M, Hernandez-Vaquero D, Murcia A, Torres A, Llopis R. Trabecular metal in total knee arthroplasty associated with higher knee scores: a randomised controlled trial. Clin Orthop. 2013;471:3543–53.

66. Mikulak SA, Mahoney OM, dela Rosa MA, Schmalzried TP. Loosening and osteolysis with the press fit condylar posterior cruciate substituting total knee replacement. J Bone Joint Surg Am. 2001;83A:398–403.

67. Harwin SF, Kester MA, Malkani AL, Manley MT. Excellent fixation achieved with cementless posteriorly stabilised total knee arthroplasty. J Arthroplasty. 2013;28:7–13.

68. Jackson MP, Sexton SA, Walter WL, Walter WK, Zicat BA. The impact of obesity on the mid-term outcome of cementless total knee replacement. J Bone Joint Surg (Br). 2009;91:1044–8.

69. Whiteside LA, Viganò R. Young and heavy patients with a cementless TKA do as well as older and light-weight patients. Clin Orthop. 2007;464:93–8.

70. Woo YK, Kim KW, Chung JW, Lee HS. Average 10.1-year follow-up of cementless total knee arthroplasty in patients with rheumatoid arthritis. Can J Surg. 2011;54(3):179–84.

71. Kamath S, Chang W, Shaari E, Bridges A, Campbell A, McGill P. Comparison of peri-prosthetic bone density in cemented and uncemented total knee arthroplasty. Acta Orthop Belg. 2008;74(3):354–9.

72. Abu-Rajab RB, Watson WS, Walker B, Roberts J, Gallacher SJ, Meek RM. Peri-prosthetic bone mineral density after total knee arthroplasty. Cemented versus cementless fixation. J Bone Joint Surg (Br). 2006;88B:606–13.

73. Sorrells RB, Murphy JA, Sheridan KC, Wasielewski RC. The effect of varus and valgus deformity on results of cementless mobile bearing TKA. Knee. 2007;14(4):284–8.

74. Cooke C, Walter WK, Zicat B. Tibial fixation without screws in cementless total knee arthroplasty. J Arthroplasty. 2006;21(2):237–41.

75. Ferguson RP, Friederichs MG, Hofmann AA. Comparison of screw and screwless fixation in cementless total knee arthroplasty. Orthopedics. 2008; 31(2):127.

76. Chong DY, Hansen UN, Amis AA. Analysis of bone-prosthesis interface micromotion for cementless tibial prosthesis fixation and the influence of loading conditions. J Biomech. 2010;43(6):1074–80.

77. Bhimji S, Meneghini RM. Micromotion of cementless tibial baseplates under physiological loading conditions. J Arthroplasty. 2012;27(4):648–54.

78. Stilling M, Madsen F, Odgaard A, Rømer L, Andersen NT, Rahbek O, Søballe K. Superior fixation of pegged trabecular metal over screw-fixed pegged porous titanium fiber mesh: a randomized clinical RSA study on cementless tibial components. Acta Orthop Scand. 2011;82(2):177–86.

79. Schepers A, Cullingworth L, van der Jagt DR. A prospective randomized clinical trial comparing tibial baseplate fixation with or without screws in total knee arthroplasty a radiographic evaluation. J Arthroplasty. 2012;27(3):454–60.

80. Galloway F, Kahnt M, Ramm H, Worsley P, Zachow S, Nair P, Taylor M. A large scale finite element study of a cementless osseointegrated tibial tray. J Biomech. 2013;46(11):1900–6.

81. Bhimji S, Meneghini RM. Micromotion of cementless tibial baseplates: keels with adjuvant pegs offer more stability than pegs alone. J Arthroplasty. 2014;29(7): 1503–6.

82. Maloney WJ. Cementless and cemented implants had similar survival in total knee replacement. J Bone Joint Surg Am. 2003;85-A(5):973.

Long Term Outcome of Total Knee Arthroplasty: The Effect of Polyethylene

Eduardo García-Rey, Enrique Gómez-Barrena, and Eduardo García-Cimbrelo

Introduction

Total knee arthroplasty (TKA) is the most common procedure for the surgical treatment of end-stage primary osteoarthritis of the knee joint and there are many different implants [1]. The use of TKA has been increasing during the last decade and projection shows even further increases [2]. Europe has confirmed the trend, although this increase may be influenced by cultural and socio-economic factors [3]. Recently, Gomez-Barrena et al. reported that the frequency of this procedure can vary strongly within the same country [4]. Although macroeconomic factors may influence these observations, which are also seen in other countries [5], part of this variability may be due to patient and surgeon decisions regarding the indication for TKA and this variation is even wider in revision TKA. The number of young patients undergoing primary TKA for obesity is rising, the indications are changing and knowledge is advancing, all of which may account for some differences between countries [1]. All these factors have led to an increase in rates of revision procedures, particularly in the long-term.

There are several important issues related to TKA nowadays. The different implant design options are controversial: although metal-backed modular components are the most frequent choice when selecting the tibial plate, the risk for revision is lower with monoblock all-polyethylene components [6]; mobile-bearing platforms have not improved the long term results presented by fixed-bearing designs in clinical or radiological scores [7]; despite different theoretical advantages between postero-stabilized (PS) and cruciate-retaining designs (CR), the clinical results seem similar [8]; and the use of the patellar button is increasing in most countries due to the associated lower revision risk, meanwhile reported risk of tibial component loosening is higher for resurfaced TKA [9]. To date, the influence of restoration of normal alignment at the long-term result after TKA has also been assessed, and although most authors agree on the associated better results, other reports provide some controversy [10].

The aim of this review is to present all current topics related to the long-term outcome of primary TKA with special interest in the performance of polyethylene bearing and its influence on revision rate and loosening.

E. García-Rey, MD, PhD, EBOT (✉)
E. Gómez-Barrena, MD, PhD
E. García-Cimbrelo, MD, PhD
Orthopaedics Department,
Hospital La Paz-Idi Paz, P° Castellana 261,
28046, Madrid, Spain
e-mail: edugrey@yahoo.es

Polyethylene Wear in TKA

Mechanisms

Sir John Charnley first introduced ultrahigh-molecular-weight polyethylene (UHMWPE) in

© Springer-Verlag London 2015
T. Karachalios (ed.), *Total Knee Arthroplasty: Long Term Outcomes*,
DOI 10.1007/978-1-4471-6660-3_17

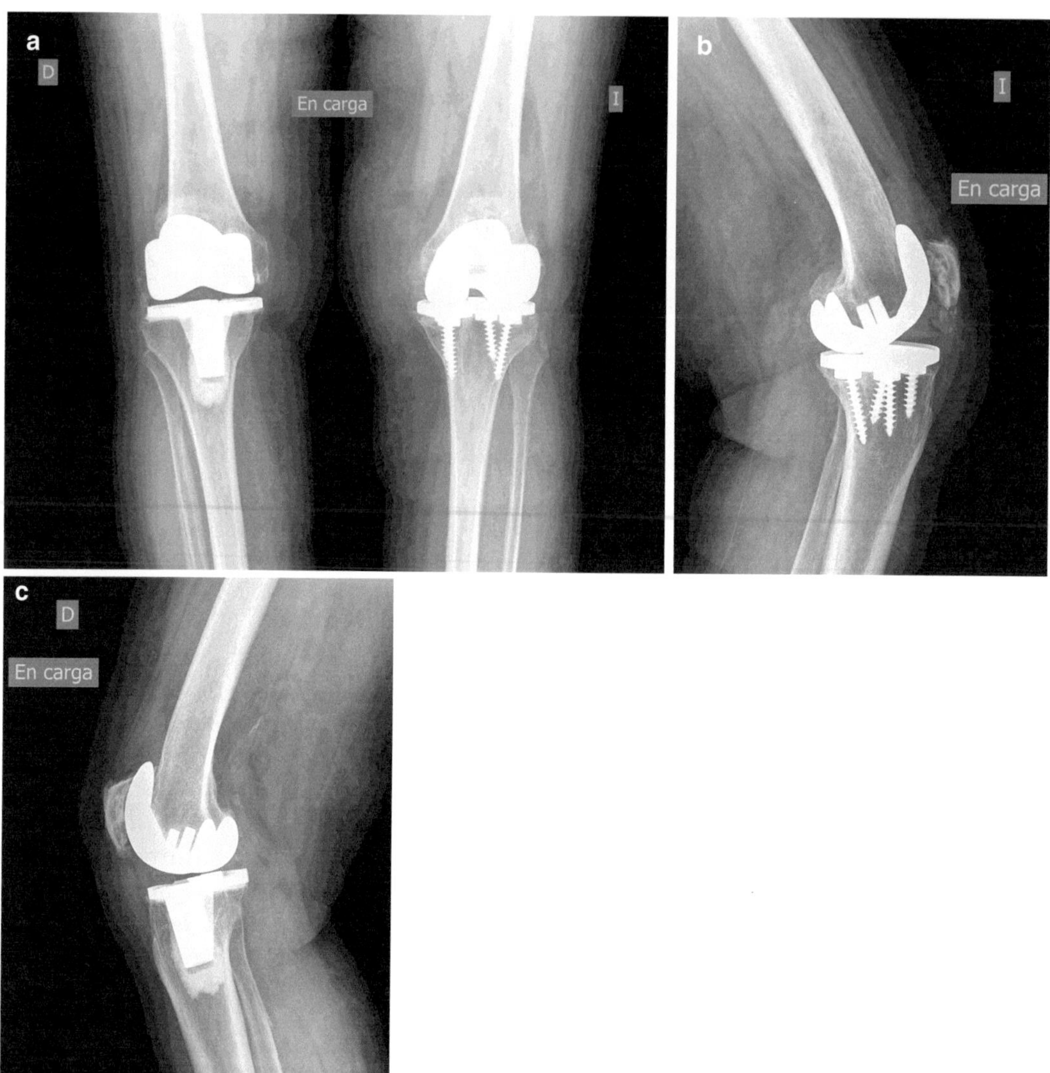

Fig. 17.1 Radiograph of a 76 year old female patient showing a right PS TKA 14 years after surgery and an uncemented TKA 18 years after surgery for the left knee (**a**) AP weight-bearing view, (**b**) Left lateral view, (**c**) Right lateral view

total joint arthroplasty. Despite the success of TKA, polyethylene wear and structural failures are some of the most important causes of revision in the mid and long term, with osteolysis always being a threat [11, 12]. Since the early reports from Freeman et al., the evolution of TKA has been linked to an optimal contact between surfaces [13]. The movement between a curved distal femur and a flat proximal tibia increases the stress forces on the polyethylene insert, so a higher conformity would theoretically decrease these forces and, consequently, wear [14].

However, femoro-tibial contact conditions are not the only factors that contribute to wear in primary TKA, with the quality of UHMWPE, the fabrication process and thickness of the insert being other factors reported to affect wear [15]. Delamination and third body wear may be more important after TKA than after total hip arthroplasty; to date it has been suggested that the greater physical demands by young rather than old patients, femoro-tibial alignment, choice of implant, mobile-bearing, and metal-backed tibial components can also affect wear (Fig. 17.1).

Almost one in every four revision TKAs may be due to polyethylene wear [16]. Causes for UHMWPE failure in TKA are: (1) oxidative degradation of polyethylene sterilized by gamma irradiation in the air, which increases surface wear producing wear particles that cause osteolysis; and (2) fatigue failure due to delamination [17]. Recently, a reduction in cross shear, observed in platform mobile-bearing designs, and low conforming fixed-bearing designs which reduce surface wear, contrary to previous findings for increased conformity designs which attempted to decrease delamination wear, are heralding new approaches for so-called low-wear TKAs for young and active patients [17]. Retrieval studies seem to confirm these data. Greater conformity can increase surface fatigue damage in TKA. Wimmer et al. compared 38 inserts made of the same polyethylene from the same manufacturer and observed higher delamination and pitting scores for the conforming posterior cruciate-substituting inserts than for the less conforming posterior cruciate-retaining inserts [18].

Long-Term Clinical Results

There is much controversy over different options available for TKA. The success of the Total Condylar knee has been explained by its higher conformity and lower stress on the insert, making it easier to correct deformity [19].

One of the most important sources for wear after primary TKA is the type of tibial plate. Modularity may have some advantages like insert exchange in case of wear [20] or infection. During the surgical procedure it may also be easier to test the flexion and extension gaps, However, there are more important consequences. Backside wear is a very well known cause of wear in TKA, and different UHMWPE protrusions have been reported with different brands and capture mechanisms of the TKA tibial tray [21]. The number of clinical reports supporting the use of all polyehylene tibial plates is rising (Fig. 17.2). The risk of revision is lower for monoblock tibial constructs, particularly in younger patients [6]. Other authors do not report better results with metal-backed components [22, 23] and the lower cost of the monoblock component is also an important issue when choosing these implants.

Mobile-bearing TKAs are supposed to improve wear performance and subsequently decease the rates of aseptic loosening in the long-term; however, this is another topic of controversy. Recently, Van der Voort et al. have reported that revision rates are similar for both fixed- and mobile-bearing inserts; thus, the clinical results did not improve with mobile-bearing TKAs [24]. Increased implant conformity and less transmission of forces to bone interface have not been confirmed clinically. Radiological and radiosteometric studies have shown similar radiolucency and osteolysis rates. Table 17.1 shows some randomized controlled trials for comparative studies between monoblock all-polyethylene tibial implants and metal backed components, and rotating platform and fixed-bearing tibial components. Finally, Kalisvaart et al. have reported similar results at 5 years for clinical outcome and durability in all three options for a single posterior-stabilized distal femoral implant in a randomized study involving 240 TKAs; to date the only revision for aseptic loosening was the metal-backed group [28].

New Polyethylenes and Designs

Highly cross linked polyethylenes are widely used due to their lower rates of wear in total hip arthroplasty at 10 years [29]; however, their use is not as frequent in primary TKA. Type of sterilisation has been studied as a possible factor for loss of medial compartment thickness [30]. This loss was higher with gamma-in-air polyethylene than with other types of UHMWPE sterilized with gamma radiation in an inert gas or with a non-irradiation method. In retrieval analysis, Medel et al. has reported lower oxidation and oxidation potential for tibial inserts sterilized in inert gas compared to those sterilized with gamma radiation in air; although wear resistance was similar between both types, there was a

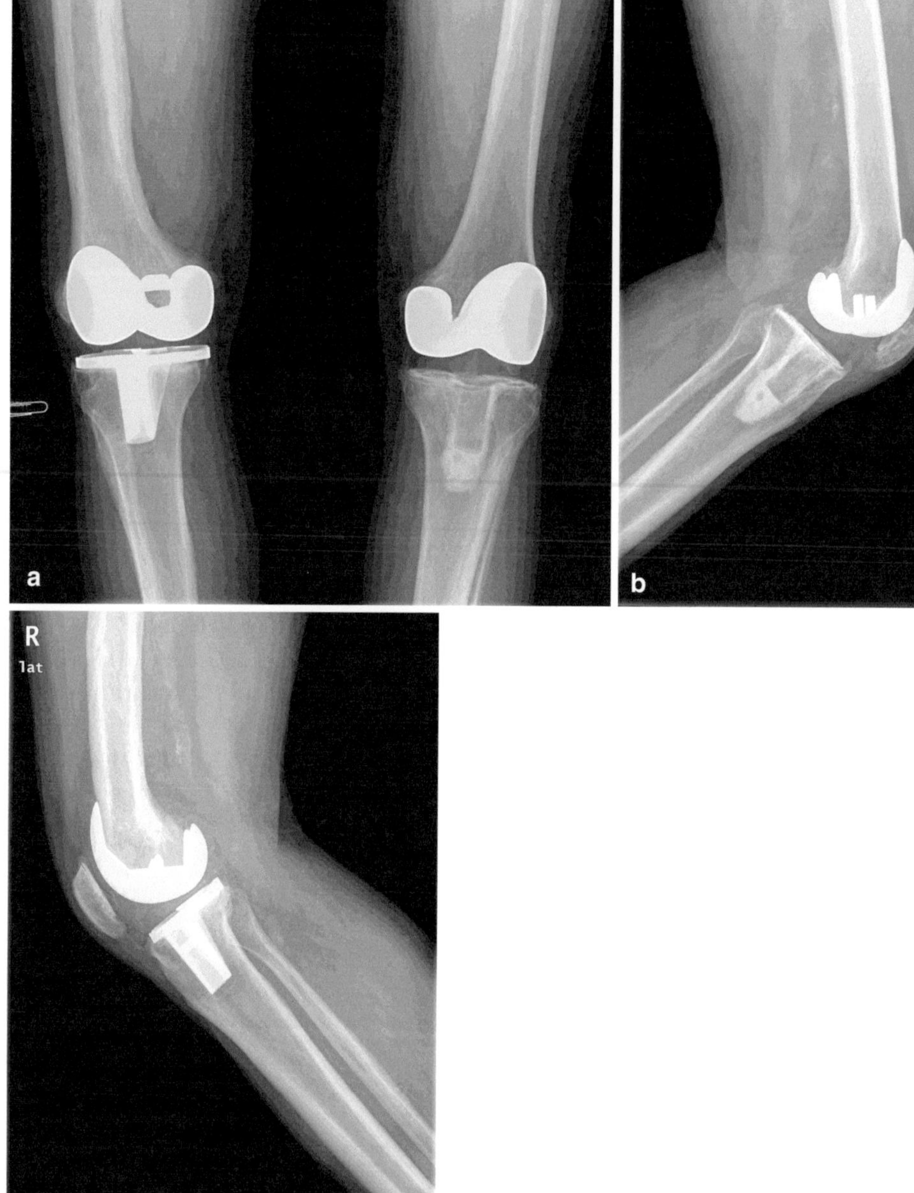

Fig. 17.2 Radiographs of a 82 year old male patient showing a right CR TKA 15 years after primary surgery and an all polyethylene tibial component TKA 14 years after surgery (**a**) AP weight-bearing view, (**b**) Right lateral view, (**c**) Left lateral view

lower delamination rate in the first decade of implantation for UHMWPE tibial inserts [31]. In vitro analyses report lower wear rates for highly cross-linked polyethylenes tested after aging [32]. Clinical studies with PS designs have shown good mid-term results and a lower incidence of radiolucent lines for these new tibial inserts [33]. The introduction of vitamin E to stabilized UHMWPE has produced better performance after aging and a reduction in wear rates [34].

Table 17.1 Randomized controlled trials with clinical long-term results for total knee arthroplasty according to tibial component

Authors	Tibial component	Number of patients	Follow-up	Survivorship for loosening
Bettinson et al. [22]	All-poly/metal backed	293	10	96.8 %/97 %
Gioe et al. [23]	All-poly/metal backed	147	10	100 %/94.3 %
Aglietti et al. [25]	MB/FB	103/107	3	
Woolson et al. [26]	RP/FB	60/47	11.4	2 MB knees
Kim et al. [27]	RP/FB	160/160	13.2	100 %/99 %

MB mobile bearing. *RP* rotating platform, *FB* fixed bearing

Other options rather than the type of UHMWPE have been assessed. Oxidized zirconium is used for the femoral component due to the low-friction oxide that is observed after oxygen diffusion, and in vitro studies have confirmed higher wear resistance with oxidized zirconium compared with cobalt-chromium (Co-Cr) alloys [35]. Clinical results also suggest that it is a safe implant, although there is a lack of long-term and comparative studies [36]. Finally, short term clinical studies show no benefit for these implants or highly cross-linked polyethylene when compared to traditional Co-Cr femoral components on conventional UHMPEs [37].

Conclusions

Variability and the age and physical activity of patients who undergo a TKA determine the different options available to surgeons nowadays. Long-term results show no benefit for any particular design and emphasize the importance of wear and osteolyis rather than other short- or mid-term failures; excellent long term results suggest that all polyethylene monoblock tibial components may be adequate despite the possibility of non-modular trays. The sterilization method for UHMWPE is one of the most important factors in choosing a particular TKA. Although new highly cross-linked polyethylenes are safe in primary TKA, there is a lack of studies to confirm the superior in vitro results in patients.

References

1. Robertsson O, Bizjajeva S, Fenstad AM, Furnes O, Lidgren L, Mehnert F, Odgaard A, Pedersen AB, Havelin LI. Knee arthroplasty in Denmark, Norway and Sweden. A pilot study from the Nordic Arthroplasty Register Association. Acta Orthop Scand. 2010;81:82–9.
2. Kurtz S, Ong K, Lau E, Mowat F, Halpern M. Projection of primary and revision hip and knee arthroplasty in the United States from 2005 to 2030. J Bone Joint Surg Am. 2007;89A:780–5.
3. Kurtz S, Ong K, Lau E, Widmer M, Maravic M, Gómez-Barrena E, et al. International survey of primary and revision total knee replacement. Int Orthop. 2011;35:1783–9.
4. Gómez-Barrena E, Padilla-Eguiluz NG, García-Rey E, Cordero-Ampuero J. Factors influencing regional variability in the rate of total knee arthroplasty. Knee. 2014;21:236–41.
5. Judge A, Welton NJ, Sandhu J, Ben-Shlomo Y. Equity in access to total joint replacement of the hip and the knee in England: cross-sectional study. BMJ. 2010; 341:c4092.
6. Mohan V, Inacio MC, Namba RS, Sheth D, Paxton EW. Monoblock all-polyethylene tibial components have a lower risk of early revision than metal backed modular components. Acta Orthop Scand. 2013;84:530–6.
7. Pijls BG, Vlastar ER, Kaptein BL, Nelissen RG. Differences in long-term fixation between mobile-bearing and fixed-bearing knee prostheses at ten to 12 years' follow-up: a single randomised controlled radiostereommetric trial. J Bone Joint Surg (Br). 2012;94B:1366–71.
8. Bercik MJ, Joshi A, Parvizi J. Posterior cruciate-retaining versus posterior-stabilized total knee arthroplasty: a meta-analysis. J Arthroplasty. 2013;28:439–44.
9. Lygre SH, Espehaug B, Havelin LI, Vollset SE, Furnes O. Failure of total knee arthroplasty with or without patella resurfacing. Acta Orthop Scand. 2011;82:282–92.
10. Parratte S, Pagnano MW, Trousdale RT, Berry DJ. Effect of postoperative mechanical axis alignment of the fifteen-year survival of modern, cemented total knee replacements. J Bone Joint Surg Am. 2010;92A:2143–9.
11. Sharkey PF, Hozack WJ, Rothman RH, Shastri S, Jacoby SM. Why are total knee arthroplasties failing today? Clin Orthop. 2002;404:7–13.
12. Gupta SK, Chu A, Ranawat S, Slamin J, Ranawat CS. Osteolysis after total knee arthroplasty. J Arthroplasty. 2007;22:787–99.

13. Freeman MAR, Swanson SAV, Todd RC. Total knee replacement of the knee using the Freeman-Swanson knee prosthesis. Clin Orthop. 1973;94:153.

14. Thatcher JC, Zhou XM, Walker PS. Inherent laxity in total knee prostheses. J Arthroplasty. 1987;2: 199–207.

15. Berend ME, Ritter MA, Meding JB, Faris PM, Keating EM, Redelman R, Faris GW, Davis KE. Tibial component failure mechanisms in total knee arthroplasty. Clin Orthop. 2004;428:26–34.

16. Hossain F, Patel S, Haddad FS. Midterm assessment of causes and results of revision total knee arthroplasty. Clin Orthop. 2010;468:1221–8.

17. Fisher J, Jennings LM, Galvin AL, Jin ZM, Stone MH, Ingham E. Polyethylene wear in total knee. Clin Orthop. 2010;468:12–8.

18. Wimmer MA, Laurent MP, Haman JD, Jacobs JJ, Galante JO. Surface damage versus tibial polyethylene insert conformity. Clin Orthop. 2012;470: 1814–25.

19. Ranawat CS, Flynn Jr WF, Saddler S, Hansrj KK, Maynard MJ. Long-term results of the total knee arthroplasty. A 15-year survivorship study. Clin Orthop. 1993;286:94–102.

20. Pijls BG, Van der Linden-Van der Zwang HMJ, Nelissen RGH. Polyethylene thickness is a risk factor for wear necessitating insert exchange. Int Orthop. 2012;36:1175–80.

21. Conditt MA, Stein JA, Noble PC. Factors affecting the severity of backside wear of modular tibial inserts. J Bone Joint Surg Am. 2004;86A:305–11.

22. Bettinson KA, Pindor IM, Moran CG, Weir DJ, Lingard EA. All-polyethylene compared with metal-backed tibial components in total knee arthroplasty at ten years. A prospective, randomized controlled trial. J Bone Joint Surg Am. 2009;91:1587–94.

23. Gioe TJ, Stroemer ES, Santos ER. All-polyethylene and metal-backed tibias have similar outcomes a 10 years: a randomized level I evidence study. Clin Orthop. 2007;455:212–8.

24. Van der Voort P, Pijls BG, Nouta KA, Valstar ER, Jacobs WC, Nelissen RG. A systematic review and meta-regression of mobile-bearing versus fixed-bearing total knee replacement in 41 studies. Bone Joint J. 2013;95B:1209–16.

25. Aglietti P, Baldini A, Buzzi R, Lup D, De LL. Comparison of mobile-bearing and fixed-bearing total knee arthroplasty: a prospective randomized study. J Arthroplasty. 2005;20:145–53.

26. Woolson ST, Epstein NJ, Huddleston JI. Long-term comparison between mobile-bearing and fixed-bearing total knee arthroplasty. J Arthroplasty. 2011; 26:1219–23.

27. Kim YH, Yoon SH, Kim JS. The long-term of simultaneous fixed-bearing and mobile-bearing performed in the same patient. J Bone Joint Surg (Br). 2007;89B: 1317–23.

28. Kalisvaart MM, Pagnano MW, Trousdale RT, Stuart MJ, Hanssen AD. Randomized clinical trial of rotating-platform and fixed-bearing total knee arthroplasty: no clinically detectable difference at five years. J Bone Joint Surg Am. 2012;94:481–9.

29. Garcia-Rey E, Garcia-Cimbrelo E, Cruz-Pardos A. New polyethylenes in total hip replacement: a ten- to 12- year follow-up study. Bone Joint J. 2013;95B:326–32.

30. Collier MB, Engh CAJR, Hatten KM, Ginn SD, Shells TM, Engh GA. Radiographic assessment of the thickness lost from polyethylene tibial inserts that had been sterilized differently. J Bone Joint Surg Am. 2008;90A:1543–52.

31. Medel FJ, Kurtz SM, Hozack WJ, Parvizi J, Purtill JJ, Sharkey PF, Mac Donald D, Kraay MJ, Golberg V, Rimnac CM. Gamma inert sterilization: a solution to polyethylene oxidation ? J Bone Joint Surg Am. 2009;91A:839–49.

32. Muratoglu OK, Bragdon CR, Jasty M, O'Connor DO, Von Knoch RS, Harris WH. Knee-simulator testing of conventional and cross-linked polyethylene tibial inserts. J Arthroplasty. 2004;19:887–97.

33. Hodrik JT, Severson EP, Mc Alister DS, Dahl B, Hofmann AA. Highly crosslinked polyethylene is safe for use in total knee arthroplasty. Clin Orthop. 2008;466:2806–12.

34. Haider H, Weisenburger JN, Kurtz SM, Rimnac CM, Freedman J, Schroeder DW, Garvin KL. Does vitamin E-stabilized ultrahigh-molecular weight polyethylene address concerns of cross-linked polyethylene total knee arthroplasty? J Arthroplasty. 2012;27:461–9.

35. Ezzet KA, Hermida JC, Colwell Jr CW, D'Lima DD. Oxidized zirconium femoral components reduce polyethylene wear in a knee wear simulator. Clin Orthop. 2004;428:120–4.

36. Hui C, Salmon L, Maeno S, Roe J, Walsh W, Pinczewski L. Five-year comparison of oxidized zirconium and cobalt-chromium femoral components in total knee arthroplasty: a randomized controlled trial. J Bone Joint Surg Am. 2011;93A:624–30.

37. Inacio MC, Cafri G, Paxton EW, Kurtz SM, Namba RS. Alternative bearings in total knee arthroplasty: risk of early revision compared to traditional bearings: an analysis of 62,177 primary cases. Acta Orthop Scand. 2013;84:145–52.

Long Term Outcome of Total Knee Arthroplasty. Condylar Constrained Prostheses

Konstantinos A. Bargiotas

Introduction

Constraint is a limitation of motion in a joint, which restricts one or more degrees of freedom in motion either due to an axis mechanism or to a conformity between two articulating surfaces [1]. In total knee arthroplasty (TKA) constraint is defined as the effect of the elements of the implant design which provides the stability needed when static and dynamic knee stabilisers are efficient [2]. The target for a pain free and well-functioning TKA is the achievement of a stable joint based on both adequate balance and function of the 'extrinsic' stability provided by the soft tissue envelope and the 'intrinsic' stability or constraint provided by the implant design. The balancing of these two elements and the avoidance of so-called kinematic conflict are the most challenging issues for surgical technique in TKA. With contemporary cruciate retaining or posterior stabilized TKAs restoration of normal knee kinematics depends on restoration of normal knee geometry and soft tissue balancing and thus requires as little implant constraint as possible [3]. When these principles cannot be met and the knee remains intra operatively unstable

or, during balancing, soft tissue structures fail, a more constrained implant should be used in order to prevent instability, pain and ultimately failure. Although controversy still exists concerning relative indications and the degree of constraint which is introduced in TKA, the use of the least constraint possible is generally advised [4, 5]. Constrained implants are commonly used in complex revision cases but they can also be utilized in difficult primary TKAs.

Constrained Knee Designs

Historically, the first implants allowed movement in a single axis, i.e. flexion-extension, as they were designed as hinges and therefore are referred to as first generation hinge implants. Such implants were relatively easy to use because the inherent stability of the hinge allowed for resection of all ligaments. Knee alignment was determined by the stems and there was no need for any restoration of basic knee biomechanics such as the curvature of the femoral condyles and the axis of original knee rotation. However, soon it became apparent that such designs produced unsatisfactory results, with unacceptable complication rates and very low long term survival rates [6, 7]. Later, a second degree of freedom in motion was introduced into hinged prostheses. The St. George knee was released in 1979, with rotation around a vertical axis being its

K.A. Bargiotas, MD, DSc
Orthopaedic Department,
University General Hospital of Larissa,
Mezourlo Region, Larissa 41110, Hellenic Republic
e-mail: kbargio@yahoo.gr

© Springer-Verlag London 2015
T. Karachalios (ed.), *Total Knee Arthroplasty: Long Term Outcomes*,
DOI 10.1007/978-1-4471-6660-3_18

characteristic design feature. Such implants are generally referred to as second generation or rotating hinge knees and their modern counterparts are in use today in cases where maximum degree of constraint is required.

During the same period the principle of knee joint resurfacing was introduced, aiming at restoration of normal knee kinematics based on reconstruction of normal knee shape and dimensions and balanced ligament function. The first example of this generation of implants is the total condylar TKA. Limited flexion, excessive femoral rollback and wear were the main problems of this type of implant [8, 9]. Initially the degree of conformity of the articulating surfaces was the only factor affecting stability. When the radii of curvature of both condyles are equal, pure rotation with no translation is expected between the femur and the polyethylene liner, provided that ligament balancing and joint line restoration is perfect. Later the degree of articulating surfaces conformity was reduced. The use of flat tibial components allows multiaxial, multiplanar mobility based entirely on the stability of the soft tissue envelope. Excessive femoral rollback, wear and aseptic loosening were also serious problems in these implant designs. In order to achieve an optimal balance between mobility and stability in both cruciate retaining and posterior stabilized implants a variety of implants have been manufactured. Several degrees of conformity between the femoral and tibial articulating surfaces and between medial and lateral knee compartments were utilized in order to provide adequate flexion and stability and to eliminate polyethylene wear. These implants are usually referred to as unconstrained knees.

Another way to increase constraint and to guide motion within certain limits is the addition of a polyethylene post articulating in a femoral intercondylar box, with a varying degree of conformity. These intercondylar stabilizing designs are sometimes referred to as guided motion TKAs and the degree of constraint escalates depending on the geometry and conformity of the post and cam mechanism. In semi-constrained posterior stabilized prostheses the polyethylene post is used to prevent posterior translation thus allowing varus/valgus displacement and rotation. From the original total condylar III TKA evolved the condylar contained (CCK) or varus valgus contained (VVC) TKAs which offer prevention of translation and stabilization in the sagittal plane. Via the introduction of a highly conforming polyethylene post, CCK designs provide protection against varus/valgus instability and limited or no rotation. Implants with minimal rotation of 2–5° are available from some manufacturers but, in general, unlike posterior stabilized or semi-constrained knees, CCKs are stabilized in two axes. In fully conforming post/cam mechanisms such as CCK, the wear rate of the polyethylene post has been reported to be high and with first generation liners fractures have also been reported [10] (Fig. 18.1). Improved methods of polyethylene liner molding and augmentation of the post by a screw or a metallic spike seem to have decreased the incidence of such fractures. Apart from type of design, surgical technique also plays a significant role. Gross rotational malposition and failure to reconstruct knee geometry increase rotational forces and wear of the post.

In a non- or semi-constrained design, forces generated in the knee joint during walking are counter balanced and absorbed by the soft tissue envelope in a way that resembles normal knee function. As the degree of constraint increases the amount of force absorbed by the implant rather than the soft tissues is increased and transmitted to the bone implant interface in the form of shear forces. Early loosening of constrained, first generation hinge implants was thus attributed to increased shear forces being transferred to the interface. Although condylar constrained devices of first and second generation are based on a totally different design philosophy, fears that increased shear forces will cause early loosening made the use of long stems mandatory. In recent years, concerns have been raised about the need for such stems. Their contribution to long term stability of the implant has been challenged and a number of drawbacks have been highlighted, such as the difficulty of removing these stems (especially cemented ones), the risk of diaphyseal fractures and increased cost. It seems reasonable,

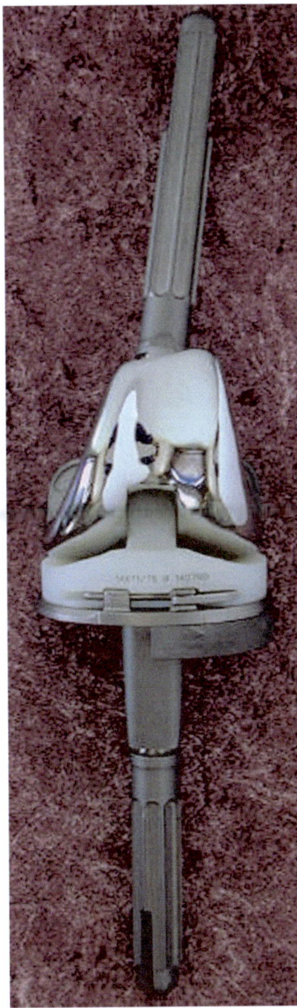

Fig. 18.1 Condylar Constrained Implant. A tall tibial post articulates in the intercondylar femoral box. 1.2° of valgus/varus and 2–3° of rotation are allowed in this particular implant. Most implants are fully constrained in both axes (Courtesy of BIOMET)

based on some latter reports, that CCK implants can be used either with very short stems or even without in cases with good bone quality. Controversy also exists concerning the use of cement for fixation of the stems. While femoral and tibial prostheses are cemented in almost all CCK TKAs, most contemporary knee systems offer a choice between cemented and uncemented stems. Traditional long cemented stems have proved extremely difficult to revise, especially in cases of infection where complete removal of the

cement is mandatory. Proponents of uncemented stems believe that these stems are easier to remove, although more technically demanding on implantation, and the likelihood of aseptic loosening appears to be lower [11].

Indications

When, in both primary and revision arthroplasty, ligaments are functional and varus-valgus alignment is adequate, a contemporary unconstrained or semi-constrained condylar prosthesis should be used. Whether a flexion – extension gap technique or a tensioning device is used, the algorithm of ligament releases which should be employed in order to create a well balanced knee in flexion and extension have been thoroughly described in the literature [3]. Limitations and failures of these techniques have also been reported and in such cases "intrinsic" implant constraint is necessary. In early revisions, 21–27 % of failures are due to instability [12, 13]. As mentioned above, it is generally accepted that as little as possible constraint should be used in any TKA. Constraint should in fact be proportional to the degree of ligament instability, escalating from a conventional cruciate retaining TKA when the posterior cruciate ligament and collaterals are intact to a rotating hinge device in cases of complete absence of ligaments. The decisive factor which dictates implant choice is not bone loss but the degree of ligamentous stability. There is no consensus regarding the amount of instability which indicates the use of CCK TKA. It has been suggested that 7–10 mm of persistent instability of the lateral and medial ligamentous complex should be used as an indication for conversion to a CCK [14]. In a recent study which included only primary TKAs, laxity greater than 5 mm was used as an indication for conversion from a posterior stabilized to a CCK implant [15] (Fig. 18.2). CCK implants are generally recommended when either medial or lateral collateral ligaments are absent or insufficient in order to balance both flexion and extension gaps [2, 16–18]. The posterior cruciate ligament, if present, should be sacrificed. CCK implants are not suitable for cases of excessive instability such as in the absence

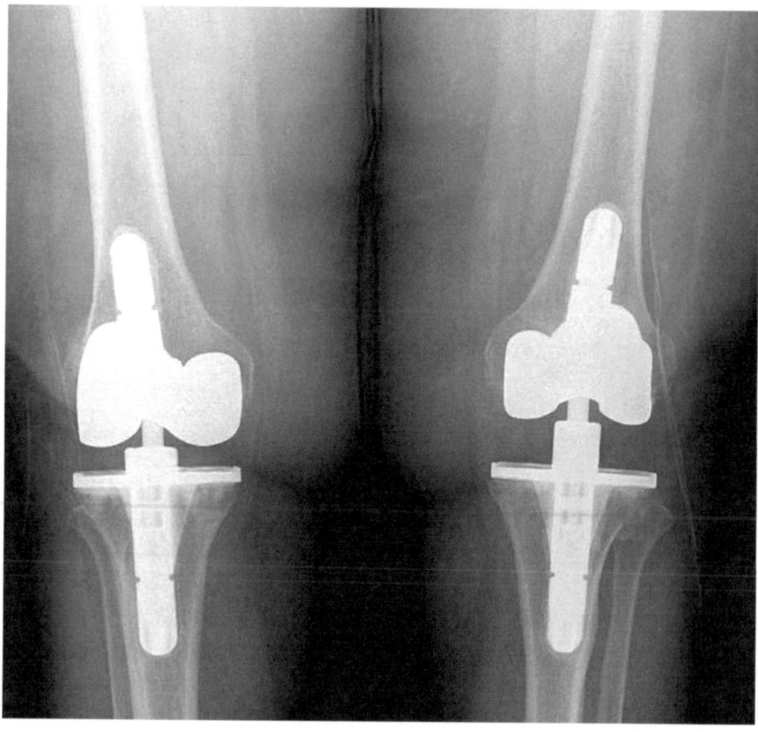

Fig. 18.2 Bilateral CCK implants in primary TKA at 10 years follow up with pristine radiologic appearance. Short cemented stems were used

of both collateral ligaments. In such cases, despite a tall post, dislocation may occur in deep flexion [19] and the use of rotating hinge devices is indicated. In primary cases, excessive varus or valgus deformity is considered to be an indication for a CCK prosthesis. Although the degree of deformity may not be clearly confirmed, deformities that exceed 25–30° usually need extensive soft tissue release and such procedures may end up in collateral ligament failure, significant alteration of the joint line and flexion-extension gap mismatch. In such cases the utilization of a CCK is considered an intra-operative decision and since soft tissue release tends to fail, especially in severely deformed valgus knees, CCK TKAs should be available on site. Moreover, in valgus knees with more than 17–20° of deformity, the peroneal nerve might be injured when extensive lateral release is utilized [8]. It appears that the use of a CCK has more predictable results compared to extensive soft tissue balancing in terms of pain, function and complication rates [20]. Controversy also exists concerning the use of a rotation hinge rather than a CCK. As mentioned above, McAuley et al. [21] highlighted the risk of CCK dislocation when the

soft tissue envelope presents gross instability rather than insufficient flexion and extension gap balance in both varus and valgus knees. In such conditions a rotating hinge or even a hinge implant should be considered, given that numerous dislocations have been reported even in rotating hinge TKAs [21]. Barrack [17, 18] has summarized three requirements for the use of a CCK TKA instead of a hinged implant; flexion-extension gap mismatch should be less than 10 mm, joint line restoration should be within 10 mm and the antero-posterior femoral diameter should be restorable. In cases where the collaterals are completely missing and/or Barrack's criteria cannot be met, a more constrained device such as a hinged or a rotating hinge prosthesis should be utilized in order to prevent dislocation and gross instability [2, 4] (Table 18.1). Although controversy exists over the use of CCK in excessive varus knees, in our experience CCK provides more predictable results in severely deformed knees (>30° of varus with extensive wear of the medial tibial condyle, large osteophytes and attenuation of the lateral collateral ligament) than a cruciate retaining or a posterior stabilized TKA. Especially in older,

Table 18.1 Knee balance and degree of constraint

Constrain	PCL	MCL	LCL	Flexion/extension gap	Joint line	Femoral diameter
CR	✓	✓	✓	Equalized	Normal	Normal
PS	–	✓	✓	Equalized	Normal	Normal
CCK	–	+/–	+/–	<10 mm	<10 mm	Normal or restored
Rotating Hinge	–	–	–	>10 mm	>10 mm	Not restored

CR cruciate retaining, *PS* posterior sacrifice, *PCL* posterior cruciate ligament, *MCL & LCL* medial & lateral collateral ligament (According to Lachiewicz et al. [26] and Barracks criteria [17, 18])

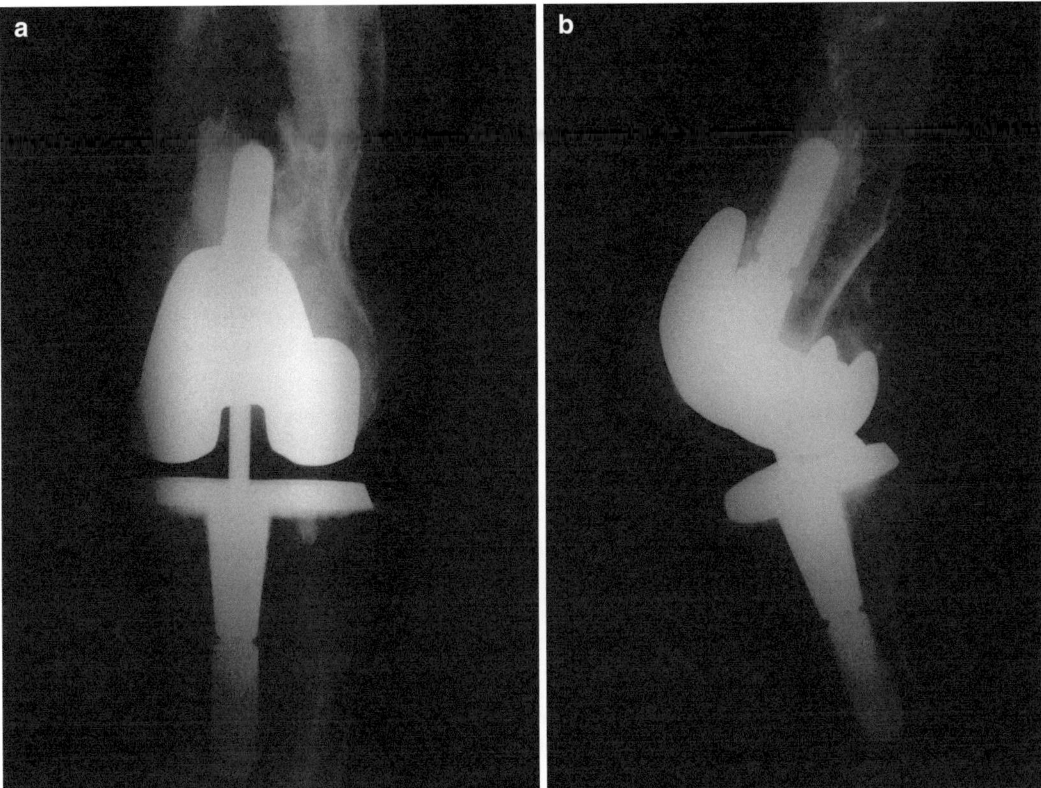

Fig. 18.3 (a) AP radiograph of a CCK prosthesis implanted on a severely deformed femur. Post traumatic cases impose unique problems and unpredictable modes of instability. Rotational stability of the femoral stem rely on the large intercondylar box and sclerotic condyle bone. (b) Lateral radiograph: A longer stem was impossible to be inserted in the femoral side

often overweight, patients the CCK prosthesis reduces the risk of instability and postoperative pain and provides stability which enhances early rehabilitation [22].

Patients with secondary arthritis due to severe intra-articular or extra-articular trauma, unusual coronal, and sagittal and rotational deformities present with unique patterns of bone defects and ligamentous instabilities which can lead to unpredictable intraoperative technical problems. In such knees the use of CCK or even a hinge TKA might be necessary (Fig. 18.3). Bone defects should not be considered an indication for constrained TKA. Provided that reconstruction of the femoral or tibial condyles with grafts and/or augments is feasible, the joint line is not severely displaced and collateral ligaments are stable both in flexion and extension, a stemmed posterior stabilized or even a cruciate retaining implant should be considered. As a general rule, a CCK TKA should be used in cases where residual instability in the coronal and/or sagittal plane is evident with trial components and when staged releases have failed to balance the knee. The choice of the degree of constraint is merely an intra-operative decision based on individualized parameters. The surgeon should be ready to adjust constraint in order to achieve stability with adequate range of motion. In cases where, despite releases, there is residual flexion or extension contracture one should move on to sacrificing contracted soft tissue elements even if they should be replaced by intrinsic implant constraint. It is the author's belief that from cruciate retaining to rotating hinge TKAs, all options should be considered especially in revision surgery and difficult primary knees with significant axis deviation and bone defects.

Surgical Considerations

In CCK motion is guided by the post/cam mechanism. The same mechanism practically restricts valgus or varus deviation of the anatomical axis of the knee to an angle built-in by the manufacturer. Additionally, if long uncemented stems are to be used the positioning of the femoral and tibial components are determined by the stems both in the coronal and sagittal planes. Regardless of the anatomy of the femoral and tibial condyles and possible bone loss, the implants have to be in perfect alignment with the anatomical axis of both the tibia and femur since the stems fill and match the intramedullary canal and firmly engage the cortices. As a consequence, depending on variations of femoral curvature (in the sagittal plane), there is a risk of either notching of the anterior femoral cortex or, more commonly, of anterior placement of the femoral component. While the former is of little significance since the distal locking stem protects from fractures, the latter when excessive can increase loads on the patella and decrease flexion. In this case undersizing of the femoral component or the use of a thinner

tibia insert or both might help to increase motion. On the tibial side the tibial tray might protrude medially or even laterally predisposing to residual pain (Fig. 18.4). Also, undersizing is not always possible or it may not solve the problem. Gross rotation of the tray is not recommended since mal-rotation may create very high loads on the post and the interface thus causing patella instability. Several manufactures offer off-set stems and/or adaptors that allow for two dimensional displacement of the tray or femoral stem in relation to the intramedullary stem. The need for detailed pre-operative planning is well documented in the literature and is obviously of paramount importance when dealing with complex cases and distorted anatomy. It is important that a full range of implants be available to the surgeon.

Finally, a surgeon must keep in mind that the amount of bone that needs to be excised between the condyles is often considerably more than the amount that is taken out with a PS prosthesis. The "box" is thus deeper and its "walls", i.e. the femoral condyles, thinner. If it is not cut in perfect alignment with the stem, it will then force the femoral insert during impaction against the condyle and fracture it, compromising stability. Extreme care should be taken during insertion of both trial and final components. When the box appears to be tight additional cuts should be made.

The Stem Debate

Experience with first generation Hinged prostheses, which suffered from early failure due to loosening, raised fears about the long term outcome of CCK knees. The use of long cemented stems is considered to be mandatory in all CCK prostheses regardless of bone quality and stock. However, data on the biomechanical effect of a stemmed component on bone implant interface are sparse. One group reported the biomechanical testing of CCK devices implanted with diaphyseal stems. They report a 20–60 % reduction of strain on the cancellous bone interface depending on bone quality. The authors concluded that in the use of CCK in cases with bone deficiencies or poor quality, stems should be used in order to reduce

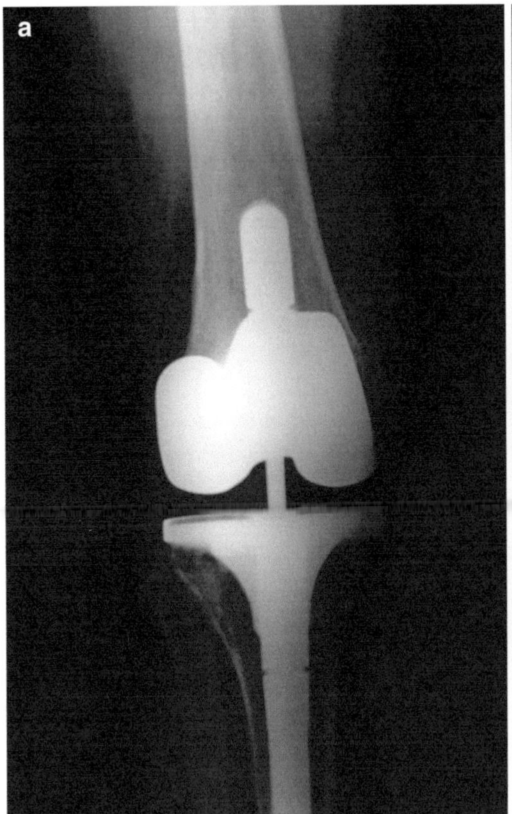
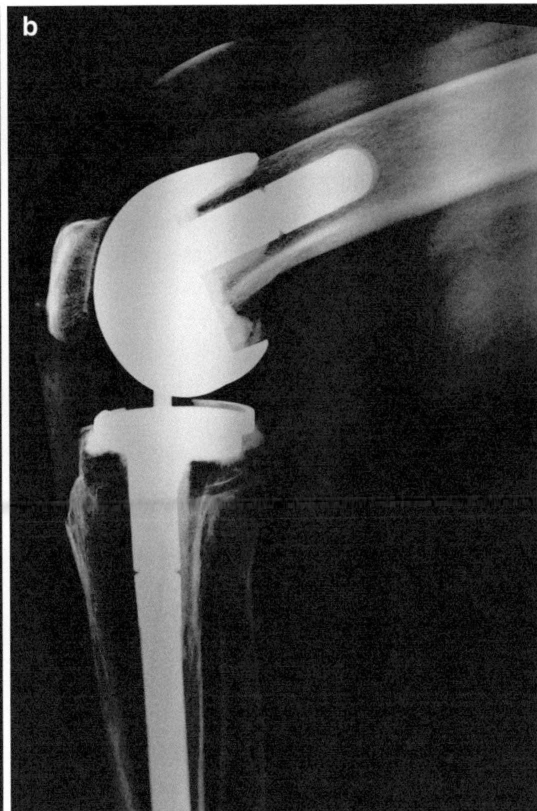

Fig. 18.4 AP (**a**) and Lateral (**b**) of a primary TKA in a valgus knee. Long fluted stem was used in tibia due to poor metaphyseal bone quality. (**a**) The tibial tray is hanging slightly lateral on AP. Long diaphyseal stabilized stems determine the final position of the tray. (**b**) They allow rotation but do not allow medio-lateral transposition but do not allow medio-lateral transposition

interface strain and to protect longevity [23, 24]. Today though, there is a growing body of clinical data suggesting that stems do not alter the clinical outcome of CCK prostheses in primary and revisions cases when there is adequate bone stock of relatively good quality. Sotereanos et al. [15] reported satisfactory results at 7 years of CCKs implanted in primary knees with small 30 mm cemented extensions which do not engage the diaphysis. In two other CCK studies, in which no stems were used, results were comparable to those of unconstrained implants [25, 26]. Most contemporary knee systems today offer cementless stems inserted into the diaphysis in a press-fit manner. These stems offer improved stability and are easier to remove if necessary. Today, however, their use is not mandatory in every CCK. An individualized approach should be followed based on bone stock and quality. In cases with poor metaphyseal bone, intra-operative fractures or large un-contained defects of the tibia, distal bearing stems should be used. On the femoral side, the large intercondylar box provides additional rotational stability when the condyles are dense and intact. In such an environment a long stem might not be necessary. In cases where condylar bone is missing the stem tends to be unstable in all three planes. A long diaphyseal press fit stem should then be utilized.

Outcome Data

There are a growing number of studies which report favorable results with the use of CCK knees. Despite initial fears, it seems that the use of

CCK TKAs has gradually become popular in both revision and difficult primary cases. Unfortunately, however, the majority of these reports are not without limitations. Very few are implant specific or studies designed to investigate a specific, implant related issue. Most are retrospective cohorts of CCK TKAs, and study populations are mixed. Primary and revision cases have been included in the same group and the results are not stratified accordingly. Furthermore, most studies include two generations of CCK or a variety of implants [27, 28]. Follow up is relatively short, since most of them do not exceed 10 years, and the number of patients is usually small. There is a need for improved studies especially related to controversial issues such as the need for stems and above all the indications for the use of such implants. These issues are still evolving and the limits are not clear at the moment.

Kim and Kim [29] have reported a 96 % survival rate of the components at 7.2 years in 114 revision cases. In another report of 57 revisions treated with either posterior stabilized or constrained type implants a 94 % survival rate at 40 months and 74 % at 99 months follow up was reported and almost all failures were attributed to extensor mechanism failure or residual instability of PS implants [30]. Haddad et al. [31] retrospectively analyzed causes and outcomes of 349 revision cases treated with PS, CCK or rotating hinge implants. Although follow up was relatively short (ranging from 12 to 60 months) the study failed to demonstrate significant differences between implant type with an overall survivorship of 90 % and a trend for less ROM for Rotating Hinge devices. Comparable results in mixed cohorts of primary and revision CCK cases with survivorship ranging from 92 to 96 % and no implant related complications compared to revision cohorts have been reported [27, 32].

In the largest cohort of CCK implants in primary TKAs, 192 knees were followed up to 10 years and no implant related failures were reported with radiolucent lines being also insignificant [33]. In a series of 55 CCK implants without diaphyseal stem extensions, no component loosening at six 6 years follow up was reported [26]. In a series of 44 primary CCK TKAs, in elderly patients with valgus knees, no prosthetic failures were reported over a longer period of time. Superior functional results and fewer complications such as peroneal nerve palsy and residual pain, in severe valgus knees (>17°), have been reported with the use of CCK implants when compared to extensive lateral releases [20, 26]. In a recent study, excellent results have also been reported with primary CCK implants when the main indication was residual instability of 5 mm or more with trial components. Other authors have reported a 97 % survival rate at 7 years in a relatively young cohort of patients, with functional results and radiolucencies being comparable to those of PS TKAs [15].

Conclusions

Based on the existing body of literature and with all its limitations in mind, it looks possible today that previous fears expressed over implant stability have not materialized. All clinical reports, to our knowledge, agree that implant failure rates for CCK do not differ when compared to PS or CR implants. Aseptic loosening and radiolucencies have not proved disastrous as predicted, and it seems that CCK has a role both in primary and revision surgery in cases where stability and normal kinematics are in doubt. As indications are still evolving and the degree of constraint needed needs to be determined intra-operatively, a full range of implant constraints should be available at any time. Above all, surgeons must be aware of the limitations of the implant they routinely use and ready to convert to a more suitable one when necessary.

References

1. Wülker N, Lüdemann M. Failure in constraint: "Too Much". In: Bellemans J, Ries MD, Victor J, editors. Total knee arthroplasty. Heidelberg: Springer Medizin Verlag; 2005. p. 69–72. Chapter 11.
2. Morgan H, Battista V, Leopold SS. Constraint in primary total knee arthroplasty. J Am Acad Orthop Surg. 2005;13:515–24.
3. Whiteside LA. Soft tissue balancing: the knee. J Arthroplasty. 2002;17(S1):23–72.

4. Gallagher JA, Bourne RB. Role of implant constraint in revision total knee replacement: striking the balance. Orthopedics. 2004;27:995–6.

5. Naudie DD, Rorabeck CH. Managing instability in total knee arthroplasty with constrained and linked implants. Instr Course Lect. 2004;53:207–15.

6. Hoikka V, Vankka E, Eskola A, Lindholm TS. Results and complications after arthroplasty with a totally constrained total knee prosthesis (GUEPAR). Ann Chir Gynaecol. 1989;78:94–6.

7. Hui FC, Fitzgerald RH. Hinged total knee arthroplasty. J Bone Joint Surg Am. 1980;62A:513–9.

8. Robinson RP. The early innovators of today's resurfacing condylar knees. J Arthroplasty. 2005;20:2–26.

9. Vince KG, Insall JN, Kelly MA. The total condylar prosthesis. 10- to 12-year results of a cemented knee replacement. J Bone Joint Surg (Br). 1989;71B:793–7.

10. Lombardi AV, Mallory TH, Fada RA, Adams JB, Kefauver CA. Fracture of the tibial spine of a total condylar III knee prosthesis secondary to malrotation of the femoral component. Am J Knee Surg. 2001;14:55–9.

11. Nakama GY, Peccin MS, Almeida GJ, Lira Neto Ode A, Queiroz AA, Navarro RD. Cemented, cementless or hybrid fixation options in total knee arthroplasty for osteoarthritis and other non-traumatic diseases. Cochrane Database Syst Rev. 2012;(10):CD006193.

12. Fehring TK, Odum S, Griffin WL, Mason JB, Nadaud M. Early failures in total knee arthroplasty. Clin Orthop. 2001;392:315–8.

13. Sharkey PF, Hozack WJ, Rothman RH, Shastri S, Jacoby SM. Why are total knee arthroplasties failing today? Clin Orthop. 2002;404:7–13.

14. Sculco TP. The role of constraint in total knee arthroplasty. J Arthroplasty. 2006;21(S4):54–6.

15. Maynard LM, Sauber TJ, Kostopoulos VK, Lavigne GS, Sewecke JJ, Sotereanos NG. Survival of primary condylar-constrained total knee arthroplasty at a minimum of 7 years. J Arthroplasty. 2014;29:1197–201.

16. Donaldson WF, Insall JN, Sculco TP, Ranawat CS. Total condylar III knee prosthesis. Long-term follow-up study. Clin Orthop. 1988;226:21–8.

17. Barrack RL. Rise of the rotating hinge in revision total knee arthroplasty. Orthopedics. 2002;25:1020–58.

18. Barrack RL. Evolution of the rotating hinge for complex knee arthroplasty. Clin Orthop. 2001;392:292–9.

19. McAuley JP, Engh GA. Constraint in total knee arthroplasty: when and what? J Arthroplasty. 2003;18(S1):51–4.

20. Easley ME, Insall JN, Scuderi GR, Bullek DD. Primary constrained condylar knee arthroplasty for the arthritic valgus knee. Clin Orthop. 2000;380:58–64.

21. Ward WG, Haight D, Ritchie P, Gordon S, Eckardt JJ. Dislocation of rotating hinge knee prostheses. A report of four cases. J Bone Joint Surg Am. 2005;87:1108–12.

22. Lampe F, Hille E. Failure in constraint: "Too Little". In: Bellemans J, Ries MD, Victor J, editors. Total knee arthroplasty. Heidelberg: Springer Medizin Verlag; 2005. p. 74–83. Chapter 12.

23. Rawlinson JL, Peters LE, Campbell DA, Windsor R, Wright TM, Bartel DL. Cancellous bone strains indicate efficacy of stem augments in constrained condylar knees. Clin Orthop. 2005;440:107–16.

24. Rawlinson JJ, Closkey RF, Davis N, Wright TM, Windsor R. Stemmed implants improve stability in augmented constrained condylar knees. Clin Orthop. 2008;466:2639–43.

25. Nam D, Umunna BP, Cross MB, Reinhardt KR, Duggal S, Cornell CN. Clinical results and failure mechanisms of a nonmodular constrained knee without stem extensions. HSS J. 2012;8:96–102.

26. Anderson JA, Baldini A, MacDonald JH, Pellicci PM, Sculco TP. Primary constrained condylar knee arthroplasty without stem extensions for the valgus knee. Clin Orthop. 2006;442:199–203.

27. Hartford JM, Goodman SB, Schurman DJ, Knoblick G. Complex primary and revision total knee arthroplasty using the condylar constrained prosthesis: an average 5-year follow-up. J Arthroplasty. 1998;13:380–7.

28. Lachiewicz PF, Soileau ES. Ten-year survival and clinical results of constrained components in primary total knee arthroplasty. J Arthroplasty. 2006;21:803–8.

29. Kim YH, Kim JS. Revision total knee arthroplasty with use of a constrained condylar knee prosthesis. J Bone Joint Surg Am. 2009;91A:1440–72.

30. Peters CL, Hennessey R, Barden RM, Galante JO, Rosenberg AG. Revision total knee arthroplasty with a cemented posterior-stabilized or constrained condylar prosthesis: a minimum 3-year and average 5-year follow-up study. J Arthroplasty. 1997;12:896–903.

31. Hossain F, Patel S, Haddad FS. Midterm assessment of causes and results of revision total knee arthroplasty. Clin Orthop. 2010;468:1221–8.

32. Hwang SC, Kong JY, Nam DC, Kim DH, Park HB, Jeong ST, Cho SH. Revision total knee arthroplasty with a cemented posterior stabilized, condylar constrained or fully constrained prosthesis: a minimum 2-year follow-up analysis. Clin Orthop. 2010;2:112–20.

33. Anderson JA, Baldini A, MacDonald JH, Tomek I, Pellicci PM, Sculco TP. Constrained condylar knee without stem extensions for difficult primary total knee arthroplasty. J Knee Surg. 2007;20:195–8.

Long Term Outcome of Total Knee Arthroplasty Rotating Hinge Designs

Demetrios Kafidas and Theofilos Karachalios

Introduction

At the dawn of knee arthroplasty (TKA), in the early 1950s of last century, prostheses were exclusively simple hinges, moving only on the sagittal plane and lacking any rotation. Pioneer prostheses were the Walldius (1951) and the Stanmore (1952) knees. Later, the Shiers (1954), Young (1963), St. Georg (1970) and Guepar prostheses (1970) were used [1–3]. All of these were first generation hinges (Figs. 19.1, 19.2, 19.3, and 19.4). Some hinges followed the low friction principle, like the Blauth prosthesis (Fig. 19.4) and other adopted low friction too but reminding more of a CCK design, like the Sheehan knee (Fig. 19.5) [1, 4]. Initially, failure rates were high and were attributed to excessive torsional and shearing forces acting on the bone cement interface. Aseptic loosening frequently occurred and structural failure of the components was occasionally appeared [2, 3, 5–11]. Wear particles, originating from the articulating

metallic surfaces, were often contributed to osteolysis process and subsequent loosening [6, 9]. In addition, infection and periprosthetic fractures were frequently seen, and when such an arthroplasty failed, revision or arthrodesis became very demanding procedures due to extensive bone resection during index surgery [8–10, 12, 13].

In early 1970s condylar TKA designs became increasingly popular due to their efficacy [14, 15]. Since then first generation of hinged prostheses became less attractive. In the late 1970s, the second generation hinged prostheses, the so called rotating hinge (RH) prostheses, were developed in order to facilitate reconstruction of certain more complex cases (difficult to address with condylar designs). Rotating hinges permitted motion both in the sagittal and the transverse plane (rotation), aiming at decreasing adverse high stresses on bone cement interface. Normal knee motion was better reproduced, since the so called home screw mechanism was feasible. Compared to first generation hinges, decreased loosening rates and improved gait pattern were achieved [2, 9, 16–18].

Condylar designs still remain the gold standard for a wide variety of cases, especially in primary TKA. However, certain indications are better met using constrained prostheses, and there is an ongoing controversy for the use of RHs or constrained condylar prostheses [19]. Defined indications and the choice of the

D. Kafidas, MD
Orthopaedic Department, University of Thessalia,
Larissa, Hellenic Republic

T. Karachalios, MD, DSc (✉)
Orthopaedic Department, Faculty of Medicine,
School of Health Sciences, University of Thessalia,
University General Hospital of Larissa,
Mezourlo region, 41110 Larissa, Hellenic Republic
e-mail: kar@med.uth.gr

© Springer-Verlag London 2015
T. Karachalios (ed.), *Total Knee Arthroplasty: Long Term Outcomes*,
DOI 10.1007/978-1-4471-6660-3_19

Fig. 19.1 The Stanmore prosthesis (lateral view in flexion and extension) – a simple metallic hinge

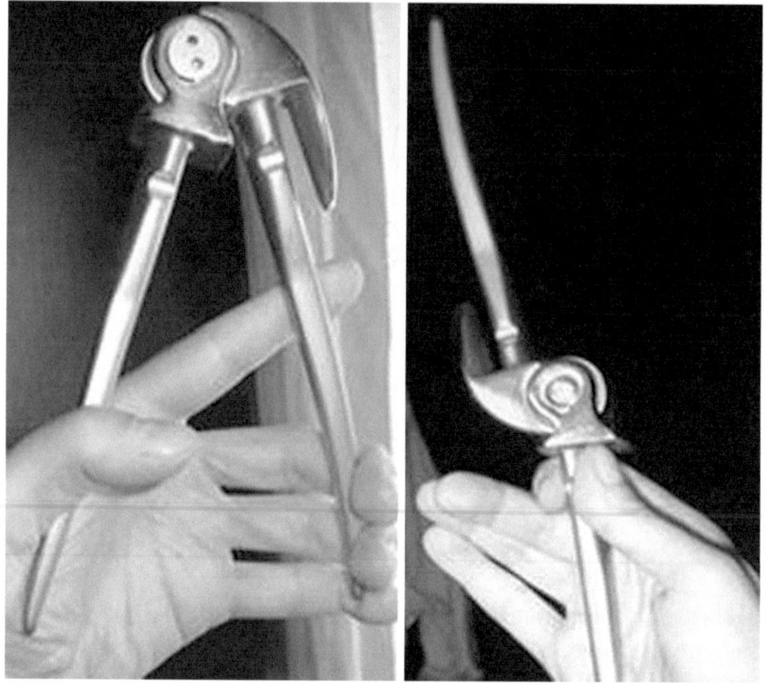

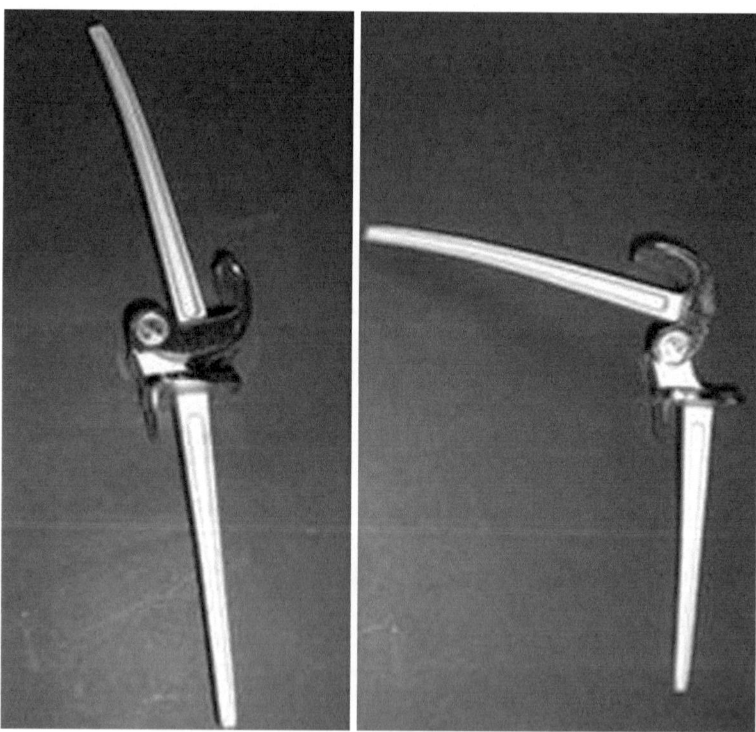

Fig. 19.2 The French GUEPAR prosthesis (lateral view in extension and flexion)

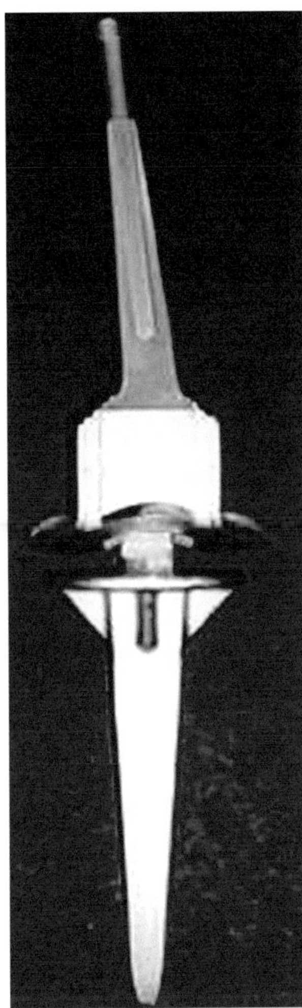

Fig. 19.3 St. Georg prosthesis (Waldemar Link GmbH, Hamburg, Germany). Anterior view. Classic hinge, precursor of the Endo-Modell prosthesis

appropriate type of RH TKA determines their outcome (in combination with other factors such as surgical technique, surgeon and patient related factors).

Types of Rotating Hinge Designs

Various designs of RH's have been used so far. Their main difference is the design of the articulating mechanism. A widely used RH is the Endo-Modell (Waldemar Link GmbH, Hamburg, Germany). Having been used from the mid 1980s, numerous clinical studies showed satisfactory results (Fig. 19.6) [20–24]. The hinge consists of a T-shaped mechanism which articulates with the femoral condyles, allowing flexion and extension. The early design allowed distraction between the femoral bush and the tibial stud, but subsequently, in order to avoid dislocations, an antiluxation mechanism was routinely used. The distal part of the hinge ends as a femoral bush, of which the interior cavity is covered by a polyethylene layer. Inside this hollow bush or cylinder a metallic tibial stud is articulating, rising from the tibial component and allowing rotation (Fig. 19.6a). Rotation, although depending on degree of flexion, does not exceed 20–30°, since at this point the femoral condyles approach and decelerate against the intercondylar eminence of the tibial tray under the tension provided by the soft tissue envelope, which consists of the remaining capsule, ligaments, muscles and tendons. This implant was initially designed for primary arthroplasty preserving the patellofemoral joint (Fig. 19.6c), while subsequently it was also available with a patellar flange and button (Fig. 19.6a, b) in order to facilitate revision arthroplasty and to address patellofemoral osteoarthritis, with or without patellar resurfacing. According to the manufacturer, bone resections are minimal, especially with the initial design which had no femoral flange, resembling resections of condylar prostheses (Fig. 19.6c). Thus, despite its long cemented stems, revision is considerably facilitated.

Compared to the Endo-Model implant, two other RH's, the Modular Segmental Kinematic Rotating Hinge (Howmedica, Rutherford, NJ) and the Noiles Prosthesis (Joint Medical Products, Stamford, CT) (Fig. 19.7) present a different design, since their axis is rotating inside the polyethylene tibial tray. Thus, rotation does not take place in the joint level but in a more wider and distal area, inside the tibial component. The Kinematic Rotating Hinge was designed exclusively for complex knee replacement, as after tumor resection or in complex knee revision with massive bone loss or ligamentous instability not amenable for a CCK arthroplasty [25, 26]. Initial designs had an all polyethylene tibial component while more recent designs have a metal-backed

Fig. 19.4 Blauth Prosthesis (Aesculap, Tuttlingen, Germany), simple hinge with low friction design (femoral condyles on polyethylene)

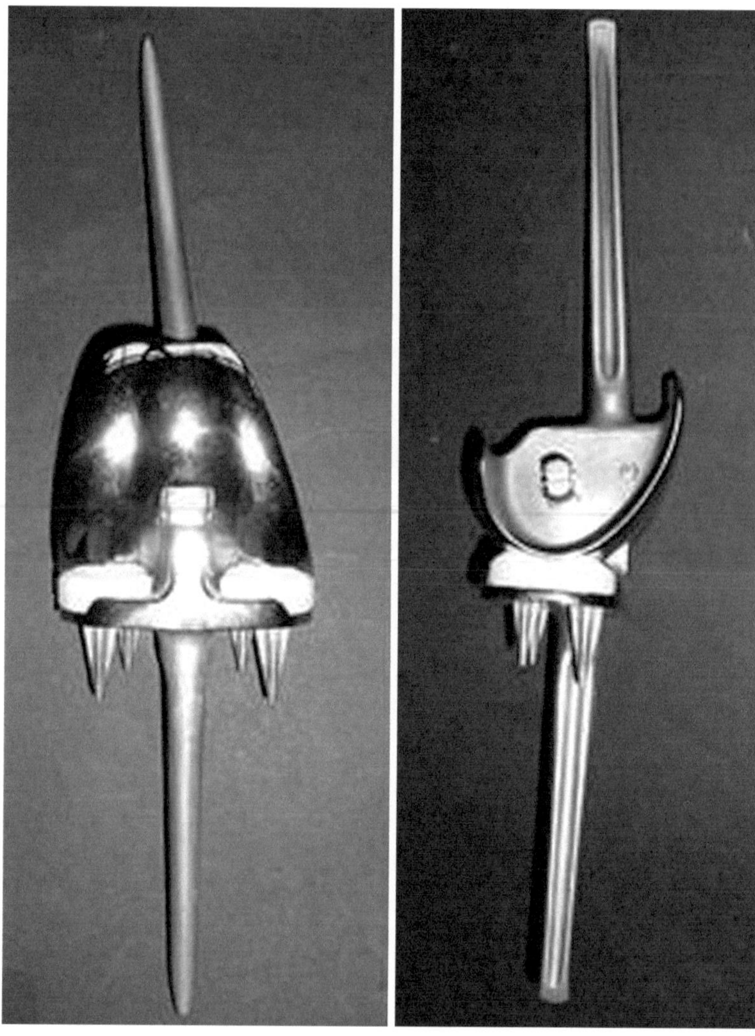

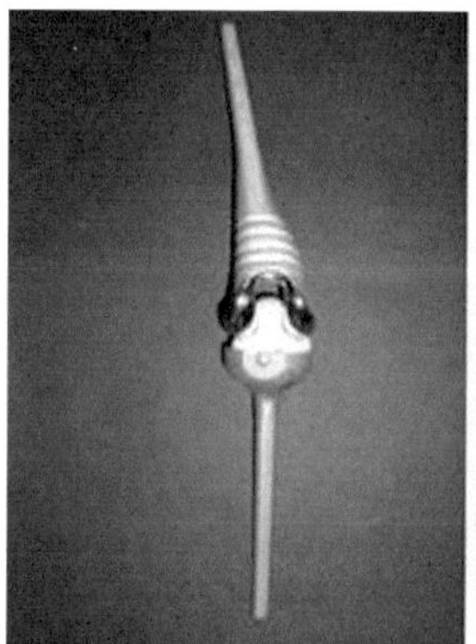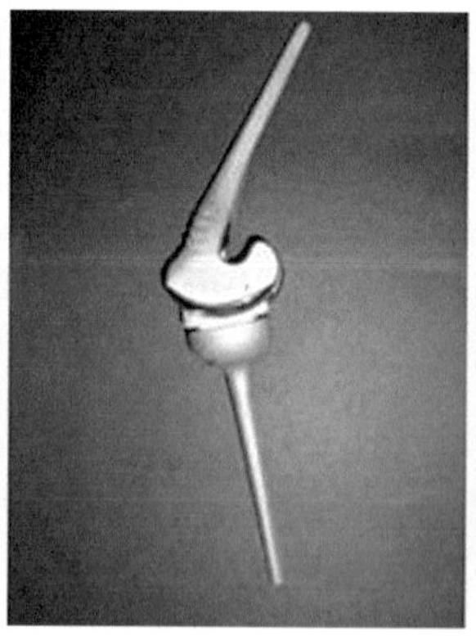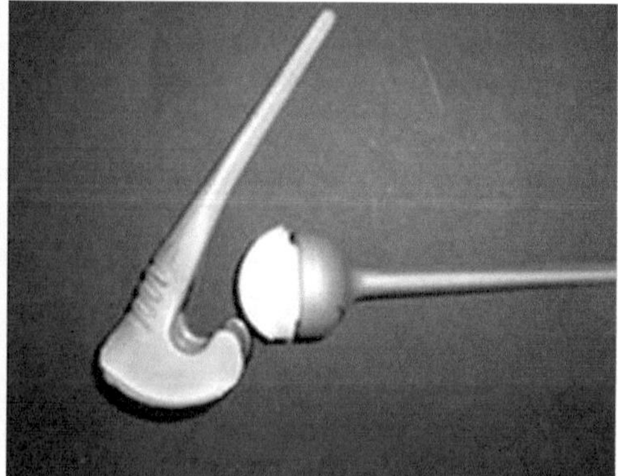

Fig. 19.5 Constrained condylar type design, the Sheehan prosthesis (1971). Anterior view, lateral view in slight flexion and demounted in lateral view. Low friction principle had been applied. Loosening, especially of the tibial component, was a constant concern

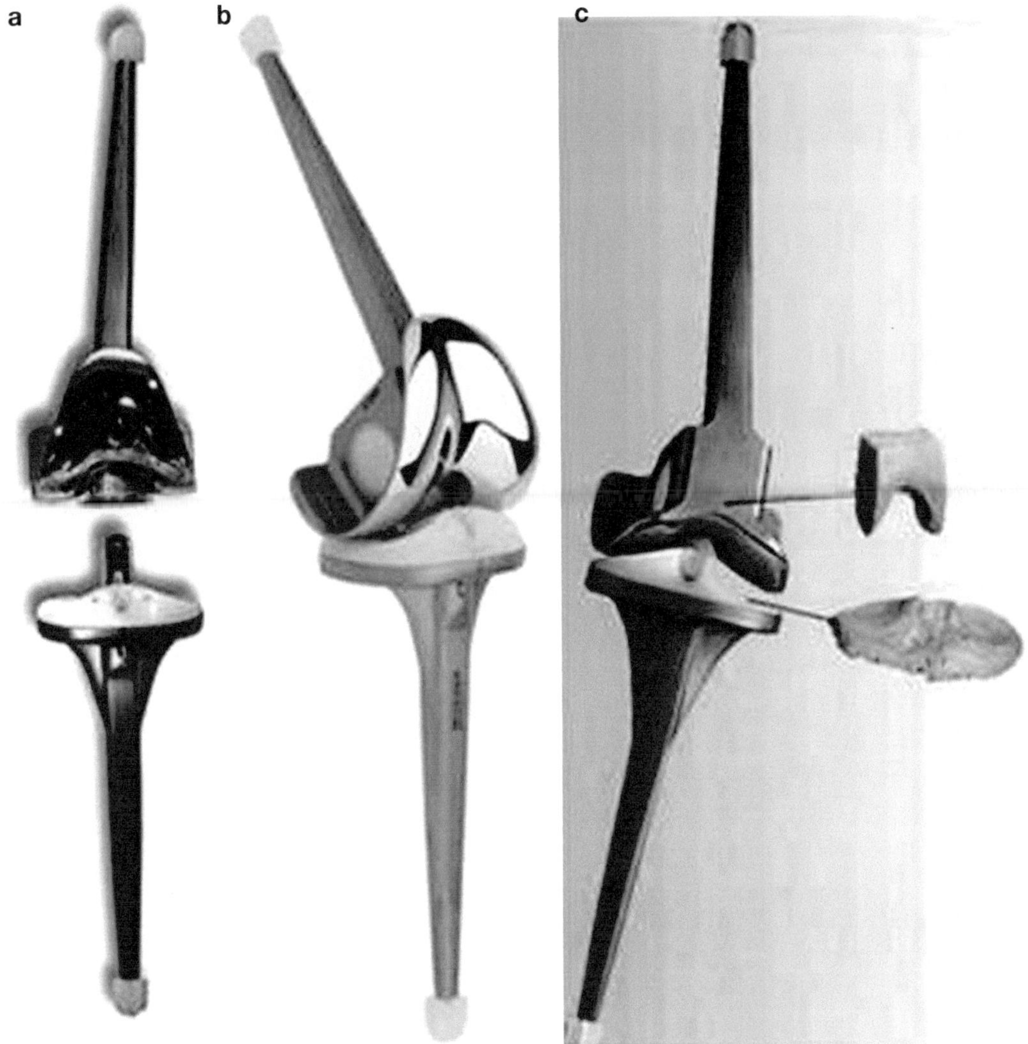

Fig. 19.6 The Endo-Modell prosthesis (Waldemar Link GmbH, Hamburg, Germany). The prosthesis disengaged (**a**), mounted in an oblique perspective (**b**) and almost from the front showing sparing bone resections (**c**). The former (**c**) is the initial design, preserving the patellofemoral articulation

tibial component. Only minor differences, compared to the Kinematic Hinge, were present in the Noiles prosthesis although the latter demanded more extensive bone resections, especially in the tibia due to its larger tibial component (Fig. 19.7). Another hinge design, evolving out of the Noiles prosthesis and also exclusively used for revision, has been introduced in the S-ROM Modular Knee (Johnson & Johnson Orthopaedics, Raynham, MA) (Fig. 19.8). The hinge mechanism consists of a femoral peg fixed inside the tibial polyethylene stem which rotates inside the metallic tibial component. Rotation takes place beneath the polyethylene tray, reminding somewhat of a rotating platform knee. Since designed for revision purposes, it is equipped with adequately long femoral and tibial stems. Available for complex knee arthroplasty, and especially salvage surgery, is also the Finn knee rotating hinge, being the centerpiece of the OSS prosthesis (orthopaedic salvage system). This is a highly modular implant, providing a

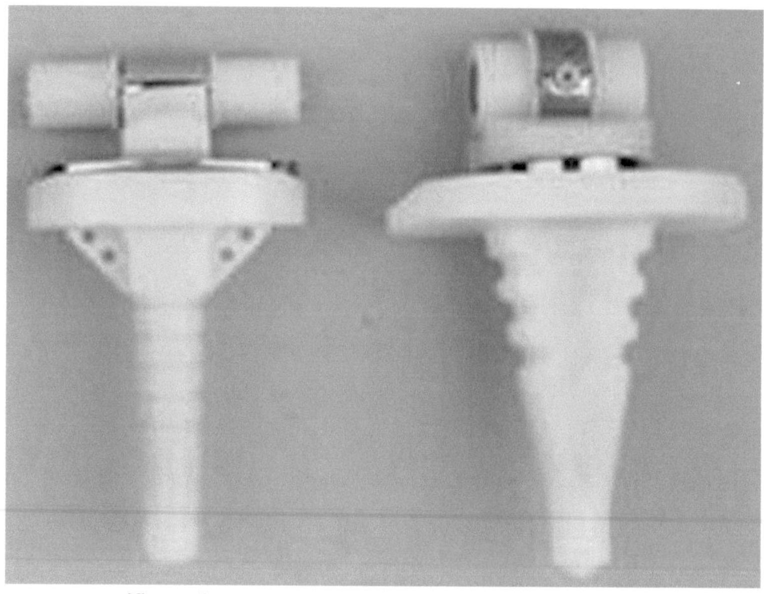

Fig. 19.7 Kinematic rotating and noiles hinge – classic rotating hinge designs with a femoral yoke mechanism and rotating tibial stem inside the tibial polyethylene

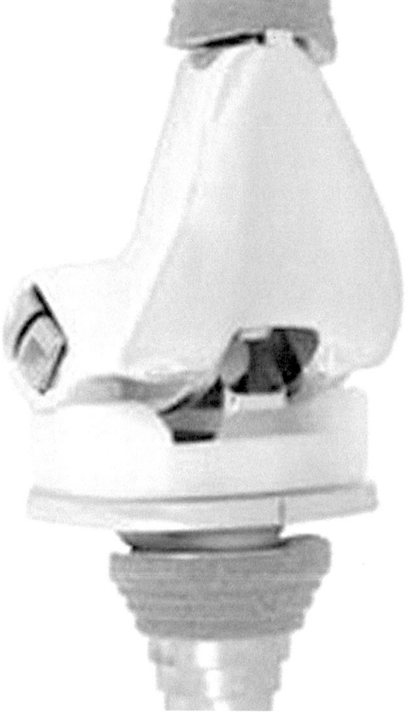

Fig. 19.8 S-ROM modular knee, consisting of a femoral hinge which is fixed inside the tibial tray which provides rotation within the tibial component, in a rotating platform manner

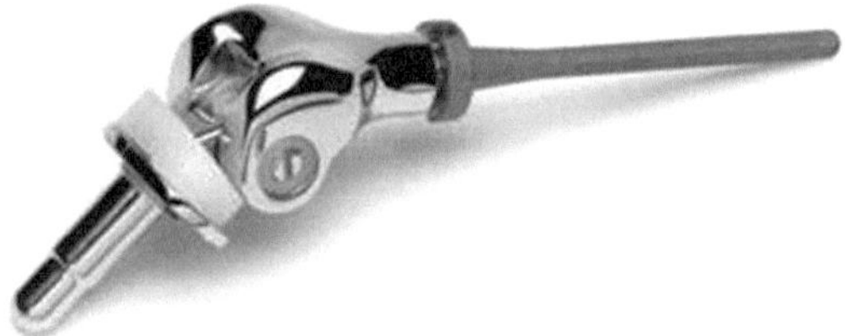

Fig. 19.9 The Finn rotating knee incorporated in one of the combinations of the OSS salvage systems. All these three prostheses are designated only for complex cases of knee arthroplasty

variety of components in order to address complex cases (Biomet, Warsaw, IN) (Fig. 19.9).

More recently (late 1990s), the Solution RT rotating hinge was introduced for primary and revision surgery (PLUS Endoprothetik AG, Switzerland, and since the year 2007 Smith & Nephew, Memphis, TN) in an attempt to reproduce normal kinematics, in terms of both home screw mechanism and femoral roll back (Fig. 19.10). If needed, femoral and tibial components are provided with modular stems, fixed with PMMA. The femoral rotation cone is articulated with the polyethylene liner inside a

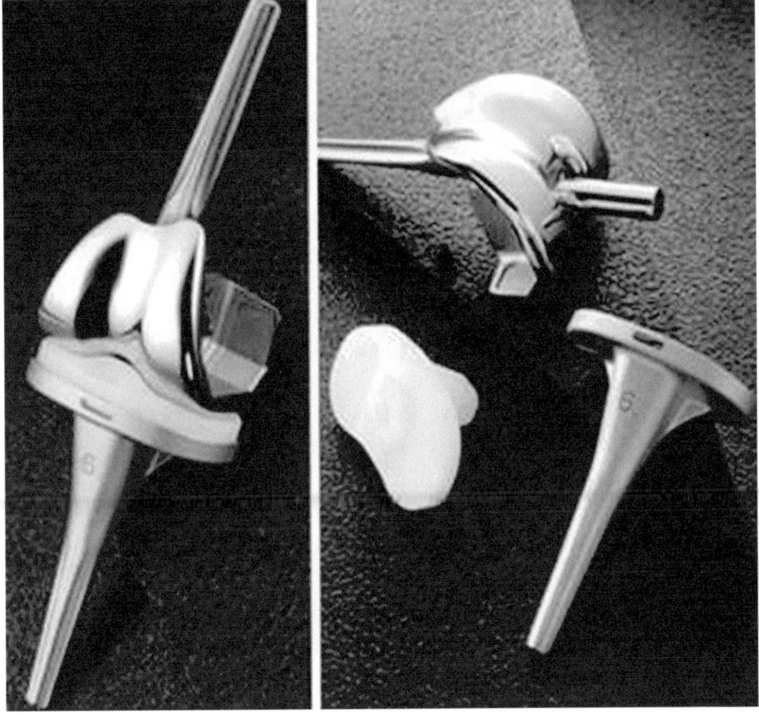

Fig. 19.10 The solution RT mounted and in components

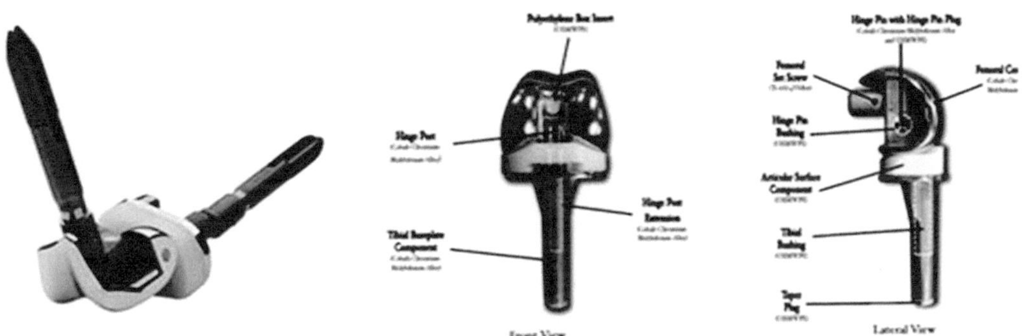

Fig. 19.11 (**a**) Legion HK, modern rotating hinge prosthesis in flexion and slight rotation, (**b**) The rotating hinge mechanism of the Zimmer NexGen rotating hinge

centrally placed bore permitting flexion, extension and rotation. Bone cuts are as sparing as with condylar prostheses except of the cuts for the femoral box. Although no specific patellar component is available, it is recommended, if needed, to use the patellar component of the respective condylar prosthesis. Recently, the same manufacturer (Smith & Nephew, Memphis, TN) introduced a similar RH implant, called Legion HK, aiming at the reproduction of normal knee kinematics (Fig. 19.11a). The same principles are present in the Zimmer NexGen Rotating Hinge prosthesis (Zimmer, Warsaw, IN). It seems that Solution RT, Legion HK and NexGen Rotating Hinge are rotating hinges of similar design and kinematics.

Indications

There are various types of RH's with different design and properties. When defining their indications one should interpret the literature based on different issues such as first generation implants, rotating or not rotating designs and on the fact that they are designated purely for revision or complex knee surgery. Skepticism regarding RH's is justified, since major complications are more difficult to be successfully managed during revision, compared to condylar implants, usually due to severe bone loss. In primary TKA, the indications for RH based on the degree of bone deformity and ligamentous instability is not clearly defined. Similarly, it is difficult to define indications for either constrained condylar (CCK) or RH implants when revision or complex knee surgery has to be performed. Several authors [2, 9, 27–29] use RH arthroplasties in revision and complex knee surgery only and propose strict indications such as (a) anteroposterior instability, especially if there is a very large flexion gap compared to the extension gap, (b) complete absence of the medial collateral ligament, (c) lateral rotational instability due to complete absence of any lateral stabilizing structures and (d) complete absence of any functional extensor mechanism resulting in a swing-through gait [27].

In North America, hinged implants were almost completely abandoned until the appearance of the RH's. In Central Europe, instead, hinged implants and especially RH's were extensively used, resulting in a respectable experience, even in primary RH arthroplasty. The indications for example for the primary Endo-Model TKA, as published by its developers, included gross deformity and instability, since deformity correction and balancing are easily achieved, while with condylar implants similar results can be achieved only by applying strict indications and performance of meticulous and precise surgical techniques [1]. Another indication for primary RH TKA is rheumatoid arthritis, since it can lead to progressive capsuloligamentous deficiency [1]. Condylar TKAs, in rheumatoid knees may develop late (after the 5th postoperative year) recurrence of malalignment without component loosening.

Clinical Outcome of RH's

When evaluating RH's, it is necessary to separate primary arthroplasty from complex knee surgery, either revision or salvage surgery. Moreover, RH implants proved more satisfactory than first generation hinged implants since complications, especially infection and loosening, were significantly reduced and walking pattern was improved [2, 9, 16–18, 30]. Therefore it seems inappropriate to restrict the use of RH TKA based on the memory of the poor results of fixed hinged implants. On the other hand, fixed hinge designs have been improved in the recent years. For example, Blauth TKA (Aesculap, Tuttlingen, Germany), a fixed hinge following the low friction principle, showed a 98 % survival rate at 10 years and 94 % at 20 years, though in low demand and senile patients [31]. Such high survival rates were also recorded in another study with the same implant. However, function seemed compromised, since average flexion was 95° only and half of the patients were able to stand up from a seated position with the support of their arms only, indicating limited knee flexion [32].

A literature search for RHs efficacy and clinical outcomes in cases with revision and complex knee surgery, no high quality studies (RCTs) were found. Most of them are relatively small cohort studies, retrospective and with a short follow-up. Therefore, no evidence based conclusions can be drawn.

The Noiles prosthesis, one of the early types of RH's (Fig. 19.8a), was evaluated in a small series of 18 complex TKAs. A 56 % failure rate was reported in terms of a HSS-score less than 60 points at 5 years follow up [2]. Major complications included femoral component subsidence, 5.1 mm on average, more pronounced in rheumatic patients (10 mm on average). Although such results seem disappointing, these cases were demanding salvage procedures. The Kinematic Rotating Hinge (Fig. 19.8a) was evaluated in a series of 38 knees (15 primaries and 23 revisions) available for follow up, out of 50 complex TKAs, with strict patients' selection criteria [9]. Clinical outcome in terms of pain, function and ROM was found improved at an average of 50 months follow up. A high complication rate was recorded including patellofemoral problems in 13 knees (34 %), deep infection in 8 knees (21 %), mechanical failure of the components in 8 knees (21 %) and loosening in 3 (7.9 %). Such high complication rates in mid term are not acceptable, but one has to keep in mind the severity of the cases. The authors stated that RH's should be reserved only for knees with complete absence of medial or lateral capsuloligamentous structures.

In contrast, satisfactory clinical outcomes have been reported with other RH's designs implanted as primary TKA with appropriate indications. Such an example is the Endo-Modell RH implant. In an initial retrospective report of 1,837 primary RHs (1,639 knees were available for follow up), a low aseptic loosening rate of 0.8 % and an infection rate of 1.9 % was documented at an average follow-up of 6.5 years [20]. In 1.8 % of the cases postoperative patellectomy or hemipatellectomy, due to severe patellofemoral pain, was performed, while mild patellofemoral pain was recorded in 12.6 % of them. Material failure, dislocations and instability occurred in 2 % of cases. Fifty-four per cent of the patients were pain free and 40 % reported mild pain only. Overall rate of patient satisfaction was 95 %, with 83 % of the patients reporting to be very satisfied and 12 % satisfied. Survival rate, with revision for any reason as the end point, was 94 % at 8 years follow up. In a similar retrospective, 7–8 years follow up study, of 230 primary TKAs using this implant, mainly for severe valgus or varus deformity, for rheumatoid arthritis and posttraumatic arthritis, complication rates were low (2.6 % for aseptic loosening, 0.4 % for malalignement, 2.6 % for infection, 0.4 % for nervous lesions and 1.7 % for patellofemoral complaints addressed by patellectomy) [21]. Authors showed these complication rates were found lower when compared to those recorded with the use of the fixed St. Georg hinge (with a follow up existing 20 years). It would be interesting to focus on the overall postoperative patellofemoral pain rate. Engelbrecht, one of the developers of this RH implant, suggested that when the femoral component is placed in

extension, condyles shift anteriorly increasing the forces in the patellofemoral joint and thus triggering equivalent symptoms [1]. Apart of surgeon related factors leading to patellofemoral symptoms, other implant related issues such as the trochlea design remain a matter of concern in hinged implants since the articulating mechanism restricts the depth of the trochlea. Infection rate is also high when compared to condylar implants mainly due to the bulky structure of the implant and the complexity of the surgery [31, 33]. In another study with 100 Endo-Modell primary TKAs, a 94 % survival rate at a mean follow up of 11 years was recorded leading to the conclusion that results were favorably comparable to condylar implants [24]. Early infection rate was 2 %, while patellofemoral maltracking was observed in 6 % of the procedures. Neither progressive radiolucent lines and migration, nor polyethylene wear were found. However, in another long term study with 98 primary RH TKAs the cumulative survival rate was 79.8 % at 10 years and 75.8 % at 15 years [34]. The authors suggested the use of RH arthroplasty in instability and revision cases only.

Satisfactory outcomes were reported when the Endo-Model RH implant was used in a series of 113 knees revised for loosening (47 %), periprosthetic fracture (24 %), infection (17 %) and instability or dislocation at a mean follow up of 2.1 years [22]. Despite difficulties encountered in such revision procedures, HSS scores were rated as good (51 %) or excellent (16 %) and seldom as fair (23 %) or poor (10 %). Satisfactory implantation and proper knee alignment was achieved in all cases due to the use of femoral and tibial stems. Deep infection occurred in 2 knees (2 %) which were originally revised for infection. Femoral aseptic loosening, secondary to allograft failure, was found in 6 (5 %) knees. Closed joint manipulation was performed in 5 (4 %) knees, while 2 femorotibial dislocations (2 %), 1 patellofemoral subluxation (1 %), 2 patellar fractures (2 %) and 2 screw disengagements were encountered. In a study with 53 revision arthroplasties using the same implant, improvement of clinical scores was seen at an average of 12.9 years follow up [35]. While early complications were easily addressed, late complications were significant. They mainly included mechanical failure of the hinge in 9 arthroplasties (17 %), with 6 cases needing re-revision while the other 3 were left unrevised due to the fact that they were asymptomatic and stable. Despite these complications, the authors concluded that rotating hinges are indicated in cases of revision TKA and when instability is present, since their results are not inferior to other less constrained revision implants.

The Solution RT RH TKA (Fig. 19.10) assigned both for primary and revision arthroplasty, mainly implanted in Europe, showed satisfactory outcomes and postoperative improvement of all clinical scores [36]. The clinical performance of the Kinematic Rotating Hinge (KRH) TKA (Fig. 19.7), used in complex surgery, was studied in a cohort of 58 patients who were available for final follow up at a mean of 6.3 years postoperatively [5]. Six knees underwent revision procedure for infection, while the majority due to bone loss, ligamentous deficiency, periprosthetic fractures and combinations of all of these. Clinical scores improved considerably in Category A patients (unilateral or bilateral TKAs with the other knee successfully replaced) and in Category C patients (multiple arthritic joint involvement medical infirmities), while in patients with a symptomatic contralateral knee (Category B) improvement was recorded but not in a statistically significant level. Range of movement was also improved significantly. Patients were satisfied in 68 % of cases, while no improvement or even worsening was reported in 6 % and 10 % of patients, respectively. A high complication rate was recorded, reaching the level of 49 %, while quite frequently (17 %) complications were two or even more. Reoperation was necessary in 19 (27 %) knees, while 9 (13 %) knees were revised due to aseptic loosening. Deep infection rate was high (10 knees- 14.5 %). Patellofemoral complications (13 %) and mechanical failure (10 %) were also quite frequent, the latter appearing as fractures of the tibial plastic sleeve of the original prosthetic design in four cases (Fig. 19.7), fractures of four tibial stems, a fracture of one femoral condyle and one case of fracture of the bushing and the axle. The authors concluded that these results were acceptable, since they were implanting the KRH in very challenging knee revisions and in their opinion the implantation of rotating hinges should be reserved for complex salvage knee surgery only. Compared to the initial short term study presented by Rand et al. [9], patellofemoral complications, implant loosening and fractures were found less frequently, due to the fact that surgical techniques had evolved, paying particular attention to the rotational placement of the components or to the intraoperative evaluation of patellar tracking, and to the KRH tibial component change of design from all polyethylene to metal backed.

In a retrospective short term study of revision TKA surgery, the S-ROM RH TKA clinical outcome was evaluated in 15 patients and compared to that of 87 patients who underwent revision using standard condylar revision implants at an average of 4.25 years of follow up [6]. Knees in the rotating hinge group presented more severe derangement and pathology and no revision for infection had been included in this study. Despite the fact that S-ROM implant was used in more complex cases, comparable clinical scores and ROM to those of the condylar group were observed and appropriate knee alignment was achieved in all cases of hinged revisions.

Walker and Mantkelow [19] compared revision TKA surgery using RHs in 14 knees and varus valgus constrained implants (VVC) in 12 knees. In the same study mechanical simulation of three VVC and two RH designs was also evaluated. It was found that hinged implants were more stable during simulation since the VVC's gradually developed at least 6° of varus deformity whereas the hinges showed no significant change [19]. This tendency could lead to progressive deformation of the plastic post, as it was found in one case in which the post was even metallically reinforced [37], or even to breakage of the post as in a case of a Total Condylar III prosthesis [38]. Signs of instability were also recorded clinically in the group of VVC's, affecting knee scores, both in the anteroposterior and the coronal plane [19]. Scores for ROM, pain and radiolucent lines were similar in both groups. RH's showed better function scores, though without statistical significance. Further, as it was evaluated by a questionnaire, correlation between operated and non-operated knee was stronger in the RH group, indicating a better clinical performance when compared to the VVC group. The authors proposed to reconsider the use of RH's due to the stability provided, to reproducible knee alignment, to the rotational element of motion and to a more reliable function.

Clinical Considerations

Total knee arthroplasty, primary or revision, should be mainly a soft tissue procedure regardless which type of implant is chosen. It seems that even rotating hinges, despite their intrinsic stability, are depending quite a lot on the soft tissue envelope which should be preserved as much as possible. In a cohort of 200 RH primary TKAs, no mechanical failures, as material breakage or dislocations, were initially encountered, while in the following years, due to more generous ligamentous detachments, mechanical complications increased up to the level of 1.7 % [20]. Based on this observation, surgeons became again more cautious, avoiding excessive ligamentous release and the rate fell again to 0.4 % and finally the authors suggested the preservation of any possible remaining capsule, ligaments and muscles [20]. Too generous soft tissue and collateral ligament releases can result in respective elongation of the collaterals, leading to knee recurvatum [39] along with coronal instability. In such a setting, apart of mechanical failure inappropriate stress transmission is also expected increasing the chances for component loosening, periprosthetic fractures and polyethylene wear.

Investigating the etiology of the relatively frequent patellofemoral complications after RH arthroplasty, apart from factors already mentioned such as incorrect sagittal placement of the femoral component, the relatively shallow trochlear groove due to the underlying hinge mechanism, other important factors emerge. Knees, requiring RH implants, often present with severely malfunctioning patellofemoral joint, since deformity affects both alignment and rotation predisposing to a more difficult reconstruction of anterior knee mechanics [41]. It is evident that previous surgery also affects the integrity of the patellofemoral articulation imposing additional difficulties. This correlation between severity of cases and patellar pain is evident when comparing results after primary and revision RH arthroplasty. So it is extremely important to apply all principles of current implantation techniques, like component orientation (in coronal, sagittal plane and rotation), soft tissue balancing, flexion and extension gap balancing, joint line preservation, intraoperative control and correction of patellar tracking, e.g. by lateral release or tibial tubercle transfer [42]. It is noted that in third generation RH's special attention has been paid in order to provide an adequately deep trochlear groove [40, 42]. In cohort studies of salvage knee surgery using RH's, infection rates were very high, between 14.5 and 17 %, due to the severity and complexity of these cases [5, 9, 22]. Infection is known to be more frequent in revision arthroplasty [43, 44], while any previous surgical procedure, like osteotomies, internal fixation etc., predisposes to infection [45, 46]. Another factor present in all RH designs is the bulk of the implant, offering greater surfaces and favoring microorganisms in the race for the surface [31, 33]. Infection rates in primary RH arthroplasty were recorded 1.9–2.6 % [20, 21].

Reported rates of periprosthetic fractures complicating RH arthroplasty vary. As for infection, periprosthetic fracture rates depend on severity and complexity of cases. Factors related are hinged design [7, 13], revision arthroplasty [47, 48], corticoid treatment [49–51] and neurologic disease [50].

In constrained knee implants, considerable forces and moments are directly transferred to the stems, challenging their fixation to the bone. In comparison to simple hinges loosening rates decreased significantly with rotating hinges [2, 9, 16–18]. The incidence of loosening for RH's in primary arthroplasty has been reported from 0.8 to 2.6 % in mid term retrospective studies [20, 21], while in complex knee arthroplasty it was 7.9–13 % [5, 9]. In the latter study revision was either necessary or scheduled in 2.9 % while the remaining cases were under close radiologic and clinical follow up [5].

Conclusions

The majority of primary TKAs are satisfactorily undertaken with contemporary condylar prostheses. In some cases of gross knee deformity as well as in revision knee arthroplasty rotating hinges are of value, due to their intrinsic stability and a more reproducible reconstruction of alignment. It is necessary, however, to implant such designs following strict indications, since if less constraint is required other options, like varus valgus constrained prostheses, should be preferred in order to provide better conditions in case of future revision surgery. Generally, gross knee instability with or without severe bone loss is an indication for RH TKA. Severe knee deformity could also be more reliably addressed with RH's. It may be preferable to use such implants in elderly patients. It is evident that results are also surgeon-related, since challenging cases, primary or revision, demand adequate training and experience.

Clinical experience, starting from the early 1980s, has led to sequential improvements of these implants such as trochlea design, bone sparing osteotomies, off-set stems, wedges etc. Improved surgical techniques have also contributed to better outcomes. It seems that in future, further evidence based improvements of the implants will provide better long term outcomes.

References

1. Engelbrecht E. Die Rotationsendoprothese des Kniegelenks. Berlin: Springer; 1984.
2. Shindell R, Neumann R, Connolly JF, Jardon OM. Evaluation of the noiles hinged knee prosthesis. A five-year study of seventeen knees. J Bone Joint Surg Am. 1986;68A:579–85.
3. Grimer RJ, Karpinski MRK, Edwards AN. The long-term results of Stanmore total knee replacement. J Bone Joint Surg Br. 1984;66B:55–62.
4. Bargar WL, Cracchiolo III A, Amstutz HC. Results with the constrained total knee prosthesis in treating severely disabled patients and patients with failed total knee replacements. J Bone Joint Surg Am. 1980;62A:497–511.
5. Springer BD, Hanssen AD, Sim FH, Lewallen DG. The kinematic hinge rotating prosthesis for complex knee arthroplasty. Clin Orthop. 2001;392:283–91.
6. Barrack RL. Evolution of the rotating hinge for complex total knee arthroplasty. Clin Orthop. 2001;392:292.
7. Jones RE. Management of complex revision problems with a modular total knee system. Orthopedics. 1996;19:802–4.
8. Karpinski MR, Grimer R. Hinged knee replacement in revision arthroplasty. Clin Orthop. 1987;220:185–91.
9. Rand JA, Chao EY, Stauffer RN. Kinematic rotating-hinge total knee arhtroplasty. J Bone Joint Surg Am. 1987;69A:489–97.
10. Knutson K, Lindstrand A, Lidgren L. Survival of knee arthroplasties. A nation-wide multicentre investigation of 8000 cases. J Bone Joint Surg Br. 1986;68B:795–803.
11. Hui FC, Fitzgerald Jr RH. Hinged total knee arthroplasty. J Bone Joint Surg Am. 1980;62A:513–9.
12. Windsor RE, Bono JV. Infected total knee replacements. J Am Acad Orthop Surg. 1994;2:44–53.
13. Chmell MJ, Moran MC, Scott RJ. Periarticular fractures after total knee arthroplasty: principles of management. J Am Acad Orthop Surg. 1996;4:109–16.
14. Insall JN, Hood RW, Flauwn LB, Sullivan DJ. The total condylar knee prosthesis in gonarthrosis. A five to nine-year follow-up of the first one hundred consecutive replacements. J Bone Joint Surg Am. 1983;65A:619–28.
15. Ranawat CS, Flynn WF, Saddler S, Hansraj KK, Maynard MJ. Long-term results of the total condylar knee arthroplasty: a 15-year survivorship study. Clin Orthop. 1993;286:94–102.
16. Engelbrecht E, Nieder E, Strickle E, Keller A. Intrakondyläre Kniegelegksendoprothese mit Rotationsmögligkeit. Endo Model Chir. 1981;52:368–75.
17. Walker PS, Emerson R, Potter T, Scott R, Thomas WH, Turner RH. The kinematic rotating hinge: biomechanics and clinical application. Orthop Clin North Am. 1982;13:187–99.
18. Shaw JA, Balcom WGRB. Total knee arthroplasty using the kinematic rotating hinge prosthesis. Orthopedics. 1989;12:647–54.
19. Walker PS, Mantkelow ARJ. Comparison between a constrained condylar and a rotating hinge in revision knee surgery. Knee. 2001;8:269–79.
20. Engelbrecht E, Nieder E, Klüber D. Ten to twenty years of knee arthroplasty at the Endo-Klinik: a report on long-term follow-up of the St. Georg hinge and the medium-term follow-up of the rotating knee Endo-Modell. In: Niwa S, Yoshino S, Kurosaka M, Shino K, Yamamoto S, editors. Reconstruction of the knee joint, vol. 186. Tokyo: Springer; 1997. p. 3–15.
21. Plutat J, Friesecke C, Klüber D. Scharnierendoprothese Endo-Modell – Modell mit Zukunft? Erfahrungen und Ergebnisse nach 20-jähriger Anwendung. Orthopade. 2000;29:56–8.

22. Lombardi Jr AV, Mallory TH, Eberle RW, Adams JB. Rotating hinge prosthesis in revision total knee arthroplasty: indications and results. Orthop Surg Surg Technol Int. 1997;VI:379–82.
23. Pradhan NR, Bale L, Kay P, Porter ML. Salvage revision total knee replacement using the Endo-Model rotating hinge prosthesis. Knee. 2004;11:469–73.
24. Petrou G, Petrou H, Tilkeridis C, Stavrakis T, Kapetsis T, Kremidas N, Gavras M. Medium-term results with a primary cemented rotating-hinge knee replacement. J Bone Joint Surg Br. 2004;86B:813–7.
25. Elia EA, Lotke PA. Results of revision total knee arthroplasty associated with significant bone loss. Clin Orthop. 1991;271:114–21.
26. Argenson JN, Aubaniac JM. Total knee arthroplasty in femorotibial instability. Orthopade. 2000;29(S1):45–7.
27. Cameron HU, Hu C, Vyamont D. Hinge total knee replacement revisited. Can J Surg. 1997;40:278–83.
28. Scuderi GC. Revision total knee arthroplasty. How much constraint is enough? Clin Orthop. 2001;392:300–5.
29. Dennis DA, Berry DJ, Engh G, Fehring T, Mac Donald SJ, Rosenberg AJ, Scuderi G. Revision total knee arthroplasty. J Am Acad Orthop Surg. 2008;16:442–54.
30. Attenborough CG. The Attenborough total knee replacement. J Bone Joint Surg Br. 1978;60B:320–6.
31. Böhm P, Holy T. Is there a future for hinged prostheses in primary knee arthroplasty? A 20-year survivorship analysis of the Blauth prostheses. J Bone Joint Surg Br. 1998;80B:302–9.
32. Steckel H, Klinger HM, Baums MH, Schutz W. Langzeiterfahrungen mit der Knietotalendoprothese nach Blauth – Stellenwert achsgeführter Kniegelenkendoprothesen. Z Orthop. 2005;143:30–5.
33. Inglis AE, Walker PS. Revision of failed knee replacements using fixed-axis hinges. J Bone Joint Surg Br. 1991;73B:757–61.
34. Bistolfi A, Lustig S, Rosso F, Dalmasso P, Crova M, Massazza G. Results with 98 Endo-Modell rotating hinge prostheses for primary knee arthroplasty. Orthopedics. 2013;36:746–52.
35. Bistolfi A, Rosso F, Crova M, Massazza G. Endomodell rotating-hinge total knee for revision total knee arthroplasty. Orthopedics. 2013;36:1299–306.
36. Malzer U. RT-PLUS/RT-PLUS modular. Modulare revisions endoprothetik des Kniegelenks. Berlin: Springer; 2011.
37. Robie BH, Daellenbach KK, Bolanos A, Wright TM. Retrieval analysis of constrained condylar tibial components. Trans Orthop Res Soc. 1997;22:644–6.
38. McPherson EJ, Vince KG. Breakage of a total condylar III knee prosthesis. A case report. J Arthroplasty. 1993;8:561–3.
39. Krackow KA, Weiss APC. Recurvatum deformity complicating performance of total knee arthroplasty. A brief note. J Bone Joint Surg Am. 1990;72A:268–71.
40. Westrich GH, Mollano AV, Sculco TP. Rotating hinge total knee arthroplasty in severely affected knees. Clin Orthop. 2000;379:195–208.
41. Eckhoff DG. Effect of limb malrotation on malalignment and osteoarthritis. Orthop Clin North Am. 1994;25:405–14.
42. Parker DA, Dunbar MJ, Rorabeck CH. Extensor mechanism failure associated with total knee arthroplasty: prevention and management. J Am Acad Orthop Surg. 2003;11:238–47.
43. Hanssen A, et al. Instructional course lectures AAOS: evaluation and treatment of infection at the site of total hip or knee arthroplasty. J Bone Joint Surg Am. 1998;80A:910–22.
44. Peersman G, Laskin R, Davis J, Peterson M. Infection in total knee replacement: a retrospective review of 6489 total knee replacements. Clin Orthop. 2001;392:15–23.
45. Wilson MG, Kelley K, Thornhill TS. Infection as a complication of total knee-replacement arthroplasty. Risk factors and treatment in sixty-seven cases. J Bone Joint Surg Am. 1990;72A:878–83.
46. Wymenga AB, van Horn JR, Theeuwes A, Muytjens HL, Sloof TJ. Perioperative factors associated with septic arthritis after arthroplasty. Prospective multicenter study of 362 knee and 2,651 hip operations. Acta Orthop Scand. 1992;63:665–71.
47. Merkel KD, Johnson EW. Supracondylar fracture of the femur after total knee arthroplasty. J Bone Joint Surg Am. 1986;68A:29–43.
48. Cain PR, Rubash HE, Wissinger HA, et al. Periprosthetic femoral fractures following total knee arthroplasty. Clin Orthop. 1986;208:205–14.
49. Aaron RK, Scott R. Supracondylar fracture of the femur after total knee arthroplasty. Clin Orthop. 1987;219:136–9.
50. Boggoch E, Hastings D, Gross A, et al. Supracondylar fracture of the femur adjacent to resurfacing and Macintosh arthroplasties of the knee in patients with rheumatoid arthritis. Clin Orthop. 1980;229:213–20.
51. Figgie MP, Goldberg VM, Figgie III HE, et al. The results of treatment of supracondylar fracture above total knee arthroplasty. J Arthroplasty. 1990;5:267–76.

Clinical Outcome of Total Knee Megaprosthesis Replacement for Bone Tumors

20

Vasileios A. Kontogeorgakos

Introduction

Amputation used to be the most common treatment for malignant bone tumors. However, tremendous advances in medical therapy and surgical reconstruction techniques and materials over the last three decades have allowed for limb salvage in the majority of patients.

The most common malignant bone tumors are chondrosarcoma, osteosarcoma and Ewing's sarcoma [1]. Chondrosarcoma is a bone malignancy of adulthood, resistant to chemotherapy and radiotherapy; thus wide excision with negative margins is the suggested treatment option [1]. Osteosarcoma and Ewing's sarcoma mainly develop in children and young adults [1]. These pathologies frequently develop around the knee joint, as the distal femur and proximal tibia growth plate demonstrate a high growth rate [2, 3]. Both of these sarcomas are considered chemosensitive and most of the suggested treatment protocols include neoadjuvant chemotherapy followed by tumor wide resection and post operative

chemotherapy based on the degree of tumor necrosis induced by chemotherapy [1].

Marcove was one of the pioneers of limb salvage for tumors around knee in the 1970s [4]. At that time, custom-made prostheses were used. After biopsy and tissue diagnosis of malignancy, 4–6 weeks were required for prosthesis manufacture and Rosen introduced the concept of preoperative chemotherapy in the waiting period [5].

Currently, for patients at skeletal maturity and with a primary malignant bone tumor around the knee, limb salvage is indicated when resection to negative margins can be achieved and remaining soft tissues are adequate for wound closure and function. Contamination of the knee synovial fluid with malignant cells, either from intra-articular extension of a malignant tumor or an intra-articular hematoma caused by a pathologic fracture or incorrect intra-articular biopsy, may be an indication for amputation. In such cases an alternative to above knee amputation is a Van Ness rotationplasty or an extra-articular knee resection [6–8]. For patients who have not reached skeletal maturity, limb salvage and reconstruction with an adult type mega-prosthesis can be performed when limb length discrepancy is anticipated to be less than 3 cm [3]. As distal femur or proximal tibia oncological resection sacrifices collateral ligaments, a degree of constraint is required in total knee mega-prosthesis. Initially tumor megaprostheses were cemented, custom made, with fixed hinge mechanisms. The

V.A. Kontogeorgakos, MD, DSc
Department of Orthopaedic Surgery,
ATTIKON University General Hospital,
Athens, Hellenic Republic, Greece

Medical School, University of Athens,
Athens, Hellenic Republic, Greece
e-mail: vaskonto@gmail.com

© Springer-Verlag London 2015
T. Karachalios (ed.), *Total Knee Arthroplasty: Long Term Outcomes*,
DOI 10.1007/978-1-4471-6660-3_20

principal mode of failure was the high rate of aseptic loosening [9].

In 1982, the Kotz Modular Femur Tibia Reconstruction (KMFTR) System was introduced. The KMFTR prosthesis used uncemented stems and a fixed hinge system. The next step in the evolution of knee megaprostheses was the rotating hinge mechanisms that compensated for ligamentous instability but allowed for knee rotation, resulting in better functional outcome and lower loosening rates [10–12]. Several studies have documented comparative oncological outcomes between limb salvage and amputation and limb salvage offers better functional outcome [13, 14]. Bernthal et al. evaluated 24 patients (7 proximal femoral replacements, 9 distal femoral replacements, and 8 proximal tibia replacements) in a gait laboratory at a mean of 13.2 years after their reconstruction [15]. Median O_2 consumption and walking speed among the endoprosthesis groups was not different from the control patients. Patients with proximal tibia replacements had reduced knee extension and flexion strength compared with patients in other reconstruction groups. All groups had an efficient gait and were active at home and in the community at a mean of 13.2 years after surgery.

Although endoprosthetic reconstruction for bone tumor defects allows for a functional limb, an increased number of complications are encountered. Unwin et al. in 1993 classified failure of tumor endoprosthesis as biological (infection), biomechanical (loosening and fracture) or mechanical (prosthesis breakage and servicing procedures such as change of bushings) [16]. A multicenter study in 2010 followed 2,174 skeletally mature patients who received a large endoprosthesis for tumor resection. Five modes of failure were identified and classified: soft-tissue failures (Type 1), aseptic loosening (Type 2), structural failures (Type 3), infection (Type 4), and tumor progression (Type 5). The relative incidences are significantly different and dependent on anatomic location [17].

There is debate over the most appropriate method for fixation of the medullary stems: cemented vs uncemented. Obviously, cemented stems offer the advantage of immediate stability

of the prostheses which allows for full weight bearing after soft tissue healing. Uncemented prostheses need protected weight bearing until osseointegration is achieved. However, patients with malignant bone tumors frequently receive prolonged chemotherapy regimens, develop quadriceps muscle atrophy after biopsy and protected weight bearing and may have limited life expectancy. On the other hand, first generation cemented megaprostheses had a high revision rate due to aseptic loosening with bone loss. Compress implants are newer designs which use a spring-loaded component that exerts continuous high compression forces, inducing bone hypertrophy at the bone–prosthesis interface [18, 19]. The functional results as well as the complications encountered for knee mega-prosthesis reconstructions are not the same for distal femur and proximal tibia bone resections. Indeed, endoprosthetic survival seems to be better for tumors of the distal femur compared to the distal tibia [9, 20].

Distal Femur Endoprostheses

Proximal tumors can be resected with an anterolateral or more commonly an anteromedial approach that facilitates major vessel identification and protection (Fig. 20.1). Malignant bone tumor can invade the cortex and extend to soft tissue (extra-compartmental tumors T2, on the Enneking classification system) [21]. However, popliteal vessels and nerves are infrequently involved by the tumor. In such a case, after the vessels are dissected out, an envelope of quadriceps musculature covering the soft tissue extension should be excised with the distal femur. The rectus femoris muscle is rarely infiltrated by tumor extension and thus can be spared for retention of the extension mechanism. Remaining musculature can be rearranged to cover the prosthesis and enhance rotational stability and strength of knee extension [22]. The length of bone resection is an important factor for aseptic loosening of the prosthesis as resection of more than 40 % of the distal femur has a negative influence on prosthetic survival [9, 23].

Cemented Fixation

Unwin et al. in 1996, reviewed 1,001 Stanmore cemented custom made prostheses with fixed hinge mechanisms, inserted before 1992 as a primary replacement for bone tumor [9]. The probability of avoiding aseptic loosening for 10 years was reported as 93.8 % for the proximal femur, 67.4 % for the distal femur and 58 % for proximal tibia replacements. The amputation rate due to complications for the entire group was 8.6 %. Myers et al. in 2007, reported on 335 patients who underwent distal femoral replacement [24]. A total of 192 patients remained alive with a mean follow-up of 12 years. All prostheses were custom made. One hundred and sixty two patients had a fixed-hinge design and 173 a rotating-hinge of which 143 had a hydroxyapatite (HA) collar. Only 15 prostheses were uncemented. Patellar resurfacing was not routinely performed. Early failure was usually due to infection or breakage of the prosthesis whereas late failure was more likely to be due to aseptic loosening. If aseptic loosening was taken as the endpoint, the rotating-hinge

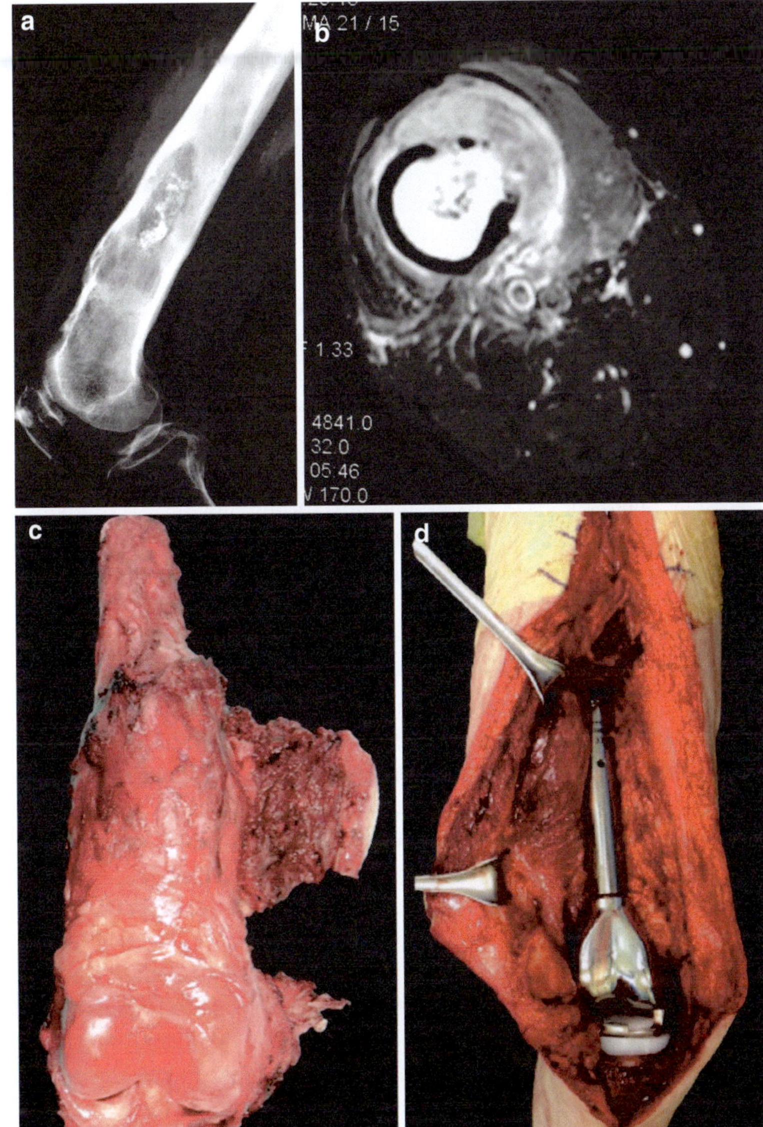

Fig. 20.1 A 70 years old male presented with progressive knee- distal femur pain over 3 months. (**a**) X-ray reveals a predominantly lytic lesion with intra-lesional calcifications of the distal metaphysis- diaphysis of the femur. (**b**) MRI axial T2 FS image reveals cortex erosion and soft tissue extension. Closed biopsy was consistent with high grade chondrosarcoma. (**c**) The patient underwent wide tumor resection. Distal femur specimen. (**d**) Cemented rotating hinge prosthesis was inserted. (**e, f**) X-rays 3 months post operatively

Fig. 20.1 (continued)

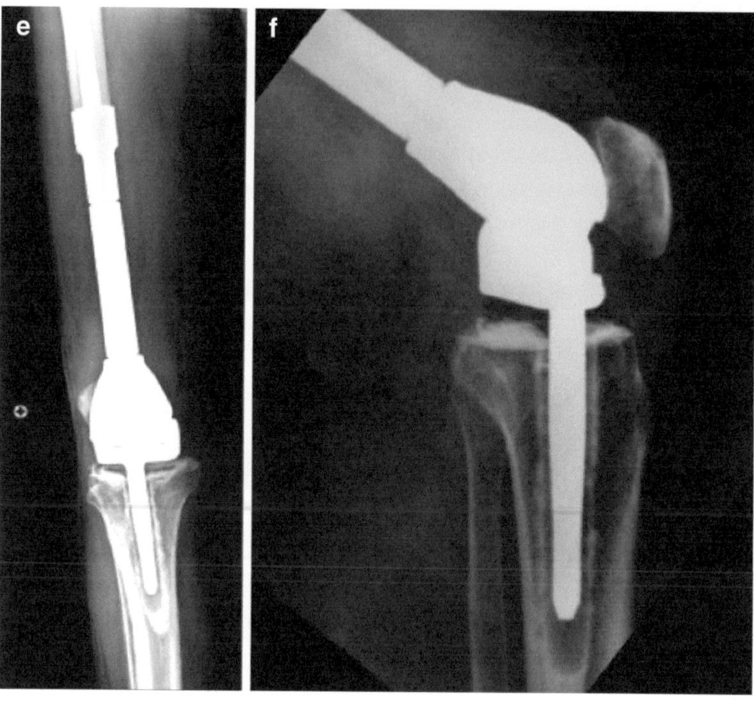

design with an HA collar was least likely to fail. The risk of revision for aseptic loosening of a fixed-hinge was 35 % at 10 years compared with 24 % for a rotating-hinge without an HA collar and 0 % for a rotating-hinge with an HA collar. Rebushing of the primary endoprosthesis was needed in 55 prostheses (45 fixed-hinge, 10 rotating-hinge). The overall infection rate was 9.6 %. Amputation was performed in 6 % for local recurrence and in 4.5 % of patients due to infection. Schwartz et al. in 2009, compared 85 modular distal femoral implants to 101 custom-casted designs [12]. All prostheses were cemented with a rotating hinge mechanism. The modular components had a greater 15-year survivorship than the custom-designed implants: 93.7 % versus 51.7 %, respectively. 9.7 % of the patients ultimately required amputation. The authors conclude that long-term survivors should expect at least one or more revision procedures in their lifetime. Bergin et al. in 2012, published the results of 104 distal femoral reconstructions [25]. They focused their analysis on the impact of the bone/stem ratio on aseptic loosening rate. All patients received a cemented modular prosthesis. Survival for 104 stems from aseptic loosening was 94.6 % at 10

and 15 years and 86.5 % at 20 years. The bone/stem ratio independently predicted aseptic failure. Patients with stable implants had larger stem sizes and lower bone/stem ratios than those with loose implants (14.5 mm versus 10.7 mm and 2.02 versus 2.81, respectively). The largest cause of failure in this study was infection (11.7 %) while 5.8 % of the implants were revised because of stem fracture.

Uncemented Fixation

Batta et al. has reported a high rate of aseptic loosening for custom-made uncemented, distal femoral endoprosthetic replacements [26]. Nine out of 69 implants (13 %) had to be revised due to aseptic loosening. All aseptically loose implants were diagnosed within the first 5 years. Capanna et al. in 1993, reports the results of 95 modular uncemented KMFTR tumor prostheses for distal femoral resections [27]. The femoral stem had two lateral flanges at right angles to each other, each with three holes to allow the passage of a total of six screws through the stem and cortex. Clinical results were excellent or good in 75 %.

Local recurrence of the tumors developed in five patients. The polyethylene bushes failed in 42 % of cases at an average of 64 months postoperatively, causing varus-valgus instability or locking, usually painless. The infection rate was 5 % for primary cases and was correlated to the extent of quadriceps excision. Bone remodeling around the femoral stem was evaluated on X-rays using the Rizzoli system. According to this system, in grade A there is no change, Grade B there is cortical sclerosis, Grade C there is cortical cancellation, Grade D there is distal sclerosis and proximal atrophy and in Grade E there is proximal osteolysis. In their series Grade D remodeling occurred in 47 % of the prostheses fixed with six screws and in only 11 % with three screws. Stem breakage occurred in 6 % and was associated with the use of narrow stems and extensive quadriceps excision. Most of the fractures occurred though the proximal screw hole. Lan et al. used dual-energy X-ray absorptiometry (DEXA) to evaluate the extent of periprosthetic bone remodelling around the KMFTR prosthesis for distal femoral reconstruction [28]. Bone loss around the KMFTR prosthesis was maximal at the distal end of the femur and progressively decreased towards the proximal end of the stem. Ten patients with implants fixed by screws were found to have a mean loss of bone mineral density (BMD) of 42 % in the most distal part of the femur, while the 13 without screw fixation had a mean loss of 11 %. Mittermayer et al. in 2002, reported on 251 uncemented reconstructions with the KMFTR system or the Howmedica Modular Reconstruction System (HMRS) [29]. Aseptic loosening rate at 10 years was 4 % for proximal femur, 24 % for distal femur replacements and 15 % for proximal tibia. The first radiological signs of aseptic loosening were always seen at the most proximal or distal part of the anchorage stem at a mean of 12 months after the first implantation. Griffin et al. in 2005, examined the risk factors associated with prosthetic failure for the KMFTR uncemented tumor prosthesis of 74 distal femoral [30]. For the distal femoral prosthesis the aseptic loosening rate was very low (2.7 %), the infection rate was 6.8 %, tumor local recurrence was 6.8 %, and the stem fracture rate 5.4 %.

All stem fractures occurred through components with six holes for transverse screw fixation produced before 1994. No fractures occurred through newer components with only three holes.

Proximal Tibia Replacements

For proximal tibia resections the common surgical approach is the anterior with proximal medial femoral extension, allowing for popliteal space exploration, identification of the popliteal neurovascular bundle, the trifurcation of the popliteal artery, arterial branches to gastrocnemius heads and common peroneal nerve (Fig. 20.2).

The reported results for proximal tibia replacement megaprostheses are frequently inferior to the distal femur. Two inherent characteristics of proximal tibia resection surgery are considered to be the principal causes for this outcome: defective attachment of the patellar tendon and the lack of available soft tissue. The attachment of the patellar tendon should be resected at least a few millimeters from the tibial tubercle in cases of malignancy, in order to achieve a clear oncological margin, thus resulting in a shortened tendon stump. In order to restore the continuity of the extensor mechanism, augmentation of the stump with synthetic or biological material is frequently necessary. This is the weak point for this step of reconstruction as reliable and effective long-term attachment of the tendon to the implanted prosthesis is not always successful. We frequently observe a gradual proximal migration of the patella on a lateral X-ray and a clinical lag of active, but full passive knee extension. Colangeli et al. in 2007, performed gait analysis of knee megaprostheses for proximal tibia tumors [31]. Functional performance during gait was abnormal in moss cases, consistent with weakness of the extensor apparatus and knee extension lag. Knee stability was supported by the intrinsic prosthesis biomechanics. The inadequacy of surrounding soft tissue for tension free coverage of the prosthesis (especially the metaphyseal part of the prosthesis) is the other major issue. Frequently, the proximal tibia has to be resected en block with the proximal fibula and an envelope of soft tissue for safe negative tumor margins. An important step in the evolution of limb sparing surgery for proximal tibia tumors was the concept of a local rotational flap of gastrocnemius head for prostheses coverage and anchorage of the patellar tendon [32, 33]. More recently the use of the Trevira attachment tube has been introduced to enhance joint capsule stability and tendon attachment [34]. The tube is directly attached to the tibial prosthesis with non-absorbable sutures. Fibroblasts migrate into the tube's mesh, so that attachment of soft tissue takes place. In Hardes et al.'s series most of the patients were able to actively extend their knee [35].

Cemented Fixation

Myers et al. in 2007, reported on 194 patients who underwent a cemented proximal tibial replacement, with 95 having a fixed hinge design and 99 a rotating-hinge with a hydroxyapatite collar [10]. The median age of the patients was 21.5 years. At a mean follow-up of 14.7 years, 115 patients remained alive. Rebushing of the primary endoprosthesis was needed in 36 patients (20 fixed-hinge, 16 rotating-hinge). The risk of revision for aseptic loosening in the fixed-hinge knees was 46 % at 10 years. This was reduced to 3 % in the rotating-hinge knee with a hydroxyapatite (HA) collar. Amputations were carried out in 17.5 % of patients either for local tumor recurrence or

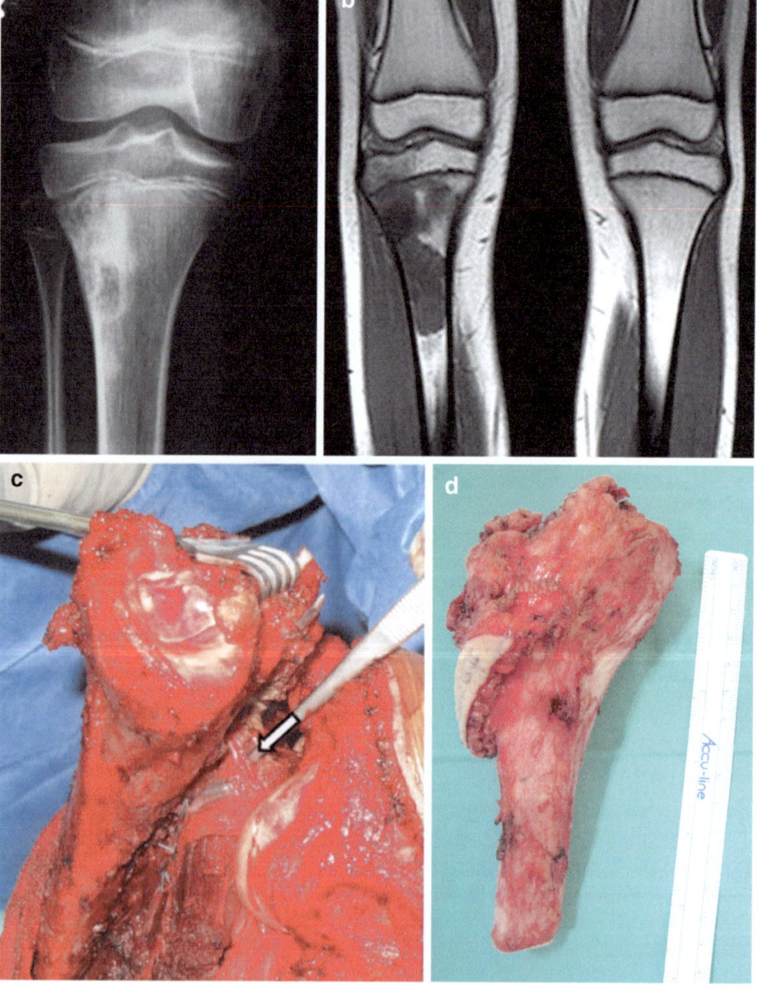

Fig. 20.2 A 12 years old female had right vague proximal tibia pain for a month. (**a**) anterior posterior x-ray reveals mixed sclerotic and lytic areas at the metaphyseal area. (**b**) MRI T1 coronal image shows a low to iso-intense signal to muscle lesion of the metaphysis extending to proximal tibial epiphysis. Biopsy of the lesion diagnosed osteosarcoma. The patient followed neo-adjuvant chemotherapy (**c**) Intraoperative view. Popliteal artery is dissected and the branch of the anterior tibial artery (*arrow*) is identified and ligated. (**d**) The proximal 14 cm of the tibia with proximal fibula 5 cm was resected en block. (**e**) A cemented modular hinge rotating prosthesis is inserted 1 cm longer. (**f**) The patellar tendon is sutured with heavy sutures over the porous coated anterior surface of the prosthesis. The medial gastrocnemius head is dissected and ready to rotate over the prosthesis and tendon attachment. (**g**) Lateral x-ray 6 months post operatively. The patient had 10° extension lag

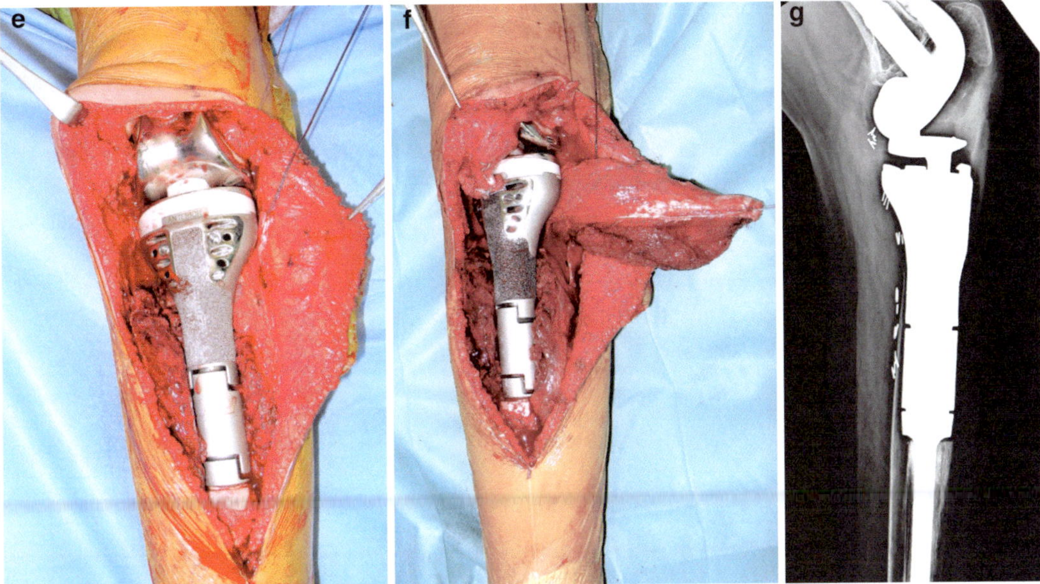

Fig. 20.2 (continued)

infection. Before gastrocnemius flaps were used the risk of amputation at 10 years following surgery was 28 %. Since the introduction of flaps, this has fallen to 14 %. Schawrtz et al. in 2010, retrospectively reviewed 52 cemented proximal tibial endoprosthetic reconstructions [12]. All prostheses had rotating hinge mechanisms; in 98 % this was the Kinematic rotating-hinge mechanism. Post-operatively all patients had their knee immobilized for a month. The failure of the rotating-hinge mechanism necessitating replacement of the bushings, axle, tibial bearing, or polyethylene was 23.1 % at a mean of 8.9 years postoperatively. Delayed wound healing or minor postoperative wound dehiscence was observed in 13.5 % of patients. The incidence of deep infection and local recurrence rate was 5.8 % and 5.8 % respectively while amputation had to be performed in 9.6 % of the patients. The use of an extramedullary porous ingrowth surface was associated with a lower incidence of aseptic loosening [12, 36]. The 29 modular implants demonstrated a trend toward improved survival compared to the 23 custom-designed components, with a 15-year survivorship of 88 % versus 63 %. The final mean postoperative Musculoskeletal Tumor Society score at was 82 % of normal function [12].

Uncemented Fixation

Griffin et al. in 2005, examined the risk factors associated with prosthetic failure for the KMFTR uncemented tumor prosthesis in 25 proximal tibial implants [30]. For the proximal tibia prosthesis the aseptic loosening rate was 0 %, the infection rate 20 % and stem fracture rate 8 %. Flint et al. in 2006, reported on 44 uncemented proximal tibia reconstructions [37]. Although they had no case with aseptic loosening, 24 % of the prosthesis failed either due to infection, local tumor recurrence, stem fracture, rotational instability or vascular compromise. In 16 % of the patients amputation was carried out. The mean knee extension lag was 6° and the MSTS score was 75 %. Mavrogenis et al. in 2013, reviewed 225 patients with proximal tibial tumors treated with proximal tibial resection from 1985 to 2010 [38]. The prostheses used in this series were KMFTR, HMRS and the rotating hinge Global Modular Reconstruction System (GMRS). Fixation of the prosthesis was cementless in 209 and cemented in 16 patients. The overall survival of patients with sarcomas was 62 % at 10 years, while survival of megaprosthetic reconstructions was 78 % at 10 years, without any difference between fixed and rotating hinge megaprostheses. The overall complication rate was 25 %. The most common complications were infection (12 %), aseptic loosening (6 %), and extensor mechanism rupture (3 %). Infection rate was almost double in patients who had been administered chemotherapy. The mean extension lag from full active extension was 12°. MSTS function was significantly better in multivariate analysis for rotating compared to fixed hinge megaprostheses.

Infection

Infection is a frequent complication of knee megaprosthesis reconstruction ranging from 3.6 % to 37.5 %, and it is a leading cause for amputation [12, 39–44] (Fig. 20.3). Body image is significantly worse for patients undergoing late amputation after failed limb salvage [45]. Hardes et al. in 2006, reported on 30 patients with an infection associated with a tumor endoprosthesis [46]. Limb salvage related to the complication infection was achieved in 63.3 %. The mean number of revision operations per patient was 2.6. No patient receiving chemotherapy with a poor soft tissue condition had limb salvage surgery. A poor soft tissue condition was a significant risk factor for failed limb salvage. Jeys and Grimer, in 2009, stated that the risk of infection is life-long although infection most frequently occurs within 12 months from the last surgical procedure [43]. The most common pathogenic organism is coagulase-negative Staphylococcus and the most effective treatment for deep infection is two-stage revision [43, 47]. Previous radiotherapy increases the infection rate [47]. Flint et al. in 2007, reported on 11 patients who underwent removal of the prosthesis for infection [48]. They concluded that two-stage revision of uncemented tumor endoprostheses with retention of a well-ingrown stem could be associated with successful eradication of infection. Racano et al. in 2013, conducted a systematic review of the literature for clinical studies that reported infection rates in adults with primary bony malignancies of the lower extremity treated with surgery and endoprosthetic reconstruction [49]. This review

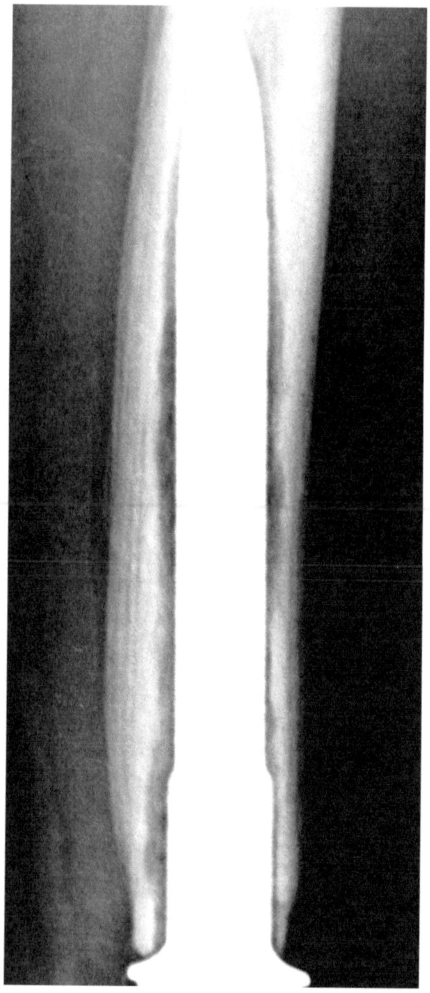

Fig. 20.3 X-ray of a distal femur uncemented stem with deep infection. Multiple solid periosteal reactions and intramedullary radiolucencies around stem

yielded 48 studies reporting on a total of 4,838 patients. The overall pooled weighted infection rate for lower-extremity LSS with endoprosthetic reconstruction was approximately 10 % with the most common causative organism reported to be Gram-positive bacteria in the majority of cases. The pooled weighted infection rate was 13 % after short-term postoperative antibiotics and 8 % after long-term postoperative antibiotics. Silver is well known for its anti-microbial properties. Silver coated megaprostheses are currently under investigation regarding their effect on incidence of deep infection and possible side effects [50, 51]. An in-vivo study in a rabbit model concludes that the silver coated Mutars megaprosthesis resulted in reduced infection rates without toxicological side effects [52]. Hardes et al. demonstrated a lower infection rate and less aggressive treatment of infection in patients treated with silver coated megaprostheses compared to titanium prostheses [53]. Shirai et al. in 2014, performed a clinical trial of iodine-coated megaprostheses to evaluate their safety and antibacterial effect [54]. Abnormalities of thyroid gland function were not detected. The authors conclude that the iodine-supported titanium megaprostheses were highly effective and showed promise in the prevention and treatment of infections in large bone defects.

Advances in chemotherapy have substantially increased the overall survival of patients for most of the primary bone malignant tumors. Limb salvage is currently the rule for most patients as it is associated with improved function without compromising oncological outcome [13, 14]. Massive allograft transplantation around the knee used to be an attractive treatment option. However, over the last decade massive allografts have gone out of favour because of prolonged time to union and a high number of complications: namely infection, nonunion and allograft fracture [55, 56].

Length of bone resection seems to be related with prosthesis longevity for both proximal tibia and distal femur resections [9]. The first designs of custom made cemented prostheses for tumors around the knee were characterized by a high rate of aseptic loosening. The original uncemented KMFTR prostheses with two flanges and six screw holes had a high rate of fatigue stem fractures because of increased stress shielding and stress resorption of bone under the flanges of the prosthesis. Thus the prosthesis has been modified from six to three screw holes. The rotating hinge mechanism is a significant development as it reduces rotational stress around the stem. Rotating hinge mechanisms seem to improve knee function and reduce aseptic loosening and stem breakage rates. However, metal ion cobalt (Co) and chromium (Cr) release is significantly higher in patients with megaprostheses compared to a standard rotating-hinge knee device [57]. Nowadays, the use of a fixed hinge mechanism should be considered in cases with large soft tissue resections and total femur replacements as

fixed mechanisms facilitate closed reduction in case of dislocation of the hip replacement. The use of a hydroxyapatite collar seems to reduce osteolysis from polyethylene particles as bone formation around the HA collar seals the medullary path for wear debri migration. Currently the use of modular replacement systems with rotating hinge mechanisms, either with cemented or uncemented stems, for reconstruction of bone and joint defects is not only limited for reconstruction after tumor surgery but is also extended for difficult post-traumatic or cases of infection. Patients close to skeletal maturity and older can be treated with available modular adult type endoprostheses. Modular prostheses offer the advantage of immediate availability. Additionally, the surgeon can adjust the length of bone resection based on the principles of oncological surgery and intra-operatively construct and implant the prosthesis. Although modularity of implanted endoprosthesis raises concerns about increased aseptic loosening, newer prostheses have shown very good survival rates compared to older custom designs [12]. Custom made prosthesis manufacturing should be reserved for unusual tumor location, large bone defects, skeletal immaturity and difficult revision cases.

Infection is still a major problem for megaprosthesis reconstruction. The incidence is much higher compared to conventional prosthesis. Development of deep infection with poor soft tissue quality frequently results in amputation. The use of a gastrocnemius rotation flap for coverage of the proximal tibia prosthesis seems to reduce the infection rate and increase the function of the extensor apparatus. Use of silver coated or iodine-supported prostheses may also help to reduce infection rates.

Conclusion

The overall complication rate for megaprostheses reconstruction for the distal femur and proximal tibia is relatively high but limb salvage is feasible in the vast majority of patients. The overall oncological and functional outcome with newer prostheses is satisfactory, although long-term survivors will probably undergo prosthesis revision in their lifetime.

References

1. National comprehensive cancer network. Bone cancer. J Natl Compr Canc Netw. 2013;11:688–723.
2. Simon MA, Springfield D, editors. Surgery for bone and soft-tissue tumors. Philadelphia: Lippincott-Raven; 1998. Chap 24a.
3. Abudu A, Grimer R, Tillman R, Carter S. The use of prostheses in skeletally immature patients. Orthop Clin North Am. 2006;37:75–84.
4. Marcove RC. En bloc resection of osteogenic sarcoma. Can J Surg. 1977;20:521–8.
5. Rosen G, Marcove RC, Caparros B, Nirenberg A, Kosloff C, Huvos AG. Primary osteogenic sarcoma: the rationale for preoperative chemotherapy and delayed surgery. Cancer. 1979;43:2163–77.
6. Hillmann A, Hoffmann C, Gosheger G, Krakau H, Winkelmann W. Malignant tumor of the distal part of the femur or the proximal part of the tibia: endoprosthetic replacement or rotationplasty: functional outcome and quality-of-life measurements. J Bone Joint Surg Am. 1999;81A:462–8.
7. Capanna R, Scoccianti G, Campanacci DA, Beltrami G, De Biase P. Surgical technique: extraarticular knee resection with prosthesis-proximal tibia-extensor apparatus allograft for tumors invading the knee. Clin Orthop. 2011;469:2905–14.
8. Hardes J, Henrichs MP, Gosheger G, Gebert C, Höll S, Dieckmann R, Hauschild G, Streitbürger A. Endoprosthetic replacement after extra-articular resection of bone and soft-tissue tumours around the knee. Bone Joint J. 2013;95:1425–31.
9. Unwin PS, Cannon SR, Grimer RJ, Kemp HB, Sneath RS, Walker PS. Aseptic loosening in cemented custom-made prosthetic replacements for bone tumours of the lower limb. J Bone Joint Surg Br. 1996;78B:5–13.
10. Myers GJ, Abudu AT, Carter SR, Tillman RM, Grimer RJ. The long-term results of endoprosthetic replacement of the proximal tibia for bone tumours. J Bone Joint Surg Br. 2007;89:1632–7.
11. Malo M, Davis AM, Wunder J, Masri BA, Bell RS, Isler MH, Turcotte RE. Functional evaluation in distal femoral endoprosthetic replacement for bone sarcoma. Clin Orthop. 2001;389:173–80.
12. Schwartz AJ, Kabo JM, Eilber FC, Eilber FR, Eckardt JJ. Cemented endoprosthetic reconstruction of the proximal tibia: how long do they last? Clin Orthop. 2010;468:2875–84.
13. Simon MA, Aschiliman MA, Thomas N, Mankin HJ. Limb-salvage treatment versus amputation for osteosarcoma of the distal end of the femur. J Bone Joint Surg Am. 1986;68A:1331–7.
14. Rougraff BT, Simon MA, Kneisl JS, Greenberg DB, Mankin HJ. Limb salvage compared with amputation for osteosarcomamof the distal end of the femur: a long-term oncological, functional, and quality-of-life study. J Bone Joint Surg Am. 1994;76A:649–56.
15. Bernthal NM, Greenberg M, Heberer K, Eckardt JJ, Fowler EG. What are the functional outcomes of endoprosthetic reconstructions after tumor resection? Clin Orthop. 2014.
16. Unwin PS, Cobb JP, Walker PS. Distal femoral arthroplasty using custom made prostheses: the first 218 cases. J Arthroplasty. 1993;8:259–68.
17. Henderson ER, Groundland JS, Pala E, Dennis JA, Wooten R, Cheong D, Windhager R, Kotz RI, Mercuri M, Funovics PT, Hornicek FJ, Temple HT, Ruggieri P, Letson GD. Failure mode classification for tumor endoprostheses: retrospective review of five institutions and a literature review. J Bone Joint Surg Am. 2011;93A:418–29.
18. Kramer MJ, Tanner BJ, Horvai AE, O'Donnell RJ. Compressive osseointegration promotes viable bone at the endoprosthetic interface: retrieval study of compress implants. Int Orthop. 2008;32:567–71.
19. Bini SA, Johnston JO, Martin DL. Compliant prestress fixation in tumor prostheses: interface retrieval data. Orthopedics. 2000;23:707–11.
20. Torbert JT, Fox EJ, Hosalkar HS, Ogilvie CM, Lackman RD. Endoprosthetic reconstructions: results of long-term followup of 139 patients. Clin Orthop. 2005;438:51–9.
21. Enneking WF, Spanier SS, Goodman MA. A system for the surgical staging of musculoskeletal sarcoma. Clin Orthop. 1980;153:106–20.
22. Malawer M. Distal femoral resection with endoprosthetic reconstruction. In: Malawer MM, Sugarbaker PH, editors. Musculoskeletal cancer surgery, Chapter 30. Dordrecht, The Netherlands: Kluwer Academic Publishers; p. 459.
23. Kawai A, Lin PP, Boland PJ, Athanasian EA, Healey JH. Relationship between magnitude of resection, complication, and prosthetic survival after prosthetic knee reconstructions for distal femoral tumors. J Surg Oncol. 1999;70:109–15.
24. Myers GJ, Abudu AT, Carter SR, Tillman RM, Grimer RJ. Endoprosthetic replacement of the distal femur for bone tumours: long-term results. J Bone Joint Surg Br. 2007;89:521–6.
25. Bergin PF, Noveau JB, Jelinek JS, Henshaw RM. Aseptic loosening rates in distal femoral endoprostheses: does stem size matter? Clin Orthop. 2012;470:743–50.
26. Batta V, Coathup MJ, Parratt MT, Pollock RC, Aston WJ, Cannon SR, Skinner JA, Briggs TW, Blunn GW. Uncemented, custom-made, hydroxyapatite-coated collared distal femoral endoprostheses: up to 18 years follow-up. Bone Joint J. 2014;96:263–9.
27. Capanna R, Morris HG, Campanacci D, Del Ben M, Campanacci M. Modular uncemented prosthetic reconstruction after resection of tumours of the distal femur. J Bone Joint Surg Br. 1994;76B:178–86.
28. Lan F, Wunder JS, Griffin AM, Davis AM, Bell RS, White LM, Ichise M, Cole W. Periprosthetic bone remodelling around a prosthesis for distal femoral tumours. Measurement by dual-energy X-ray absorptiometry (DEXA). J Bone Joint Surg Br. 2000;82B:120–5.
29. Mittermayer F, Windhager R, Dominkus M, Krepler P, Schwameis E, Sluga M, Kotz R, Strasser G. Revision of the Kotz type of tumour endoprosthesis for the lower limb. J Bone Joint Surg Br. 2002;84B:401–6.

30. Griffin AM, Parsons JA, Davis AM, Bell RS, Wunder JS. Uncemented tumor endoprostheses at the knee: root causes of failure. Clin Orthop. 2005;438:71–9.

31. Colangeli M, Donati D, Benedetti MG, Catani F, Gozzi E, Montanari E, Giannini S. Total knee replacement versus osteochondral allograft in proximal tibia bone tumours. Int Orthop. 2007;31:823–9.

32. Dubousset J, Missenard G, Kalifa C. Management of osteogenic sarcoma in children and adolescents. Clin Orthop. 1991;270:52–9.

33. Malawer MM, Price WM. Gastrocnemius transposition flap in conjunction with limbsparing surgery for primary sarcomas around the knee. Plast Reconstr Surg. 1984;73:741–9.

34. Gosheger G, Hillmann A, Lindner N, Rödl R, Hoffmann C, Bürger H, Winkelmann W. Soft tissue reconstruction of megaprostheses using a trevira tube. Clin Orthop. 2001;393:264–71.

35. Hardes J, Ahrens H, Nottrott M, Dieckmann R, Gosheger G, Henrichs MP, Streitbürger A. Attachment tube for soft tissue reconstruction after implantation of a mega-endoprosthesis. Oper Orthop Traumatol. 2012;24:227–34.

36. Ward WG, Johnson KS, Dorey FJ, Eckardt JJ. Extramedullary porous coating to prevent diaphyseal osteolysis and radiolucent lines around proximal tibial replacements. J Bone Joint Surg Am. 1993;75A:976–87.

37. Flint MN, Griffin AM, Bell RS, Ferguson PC, Wunder JS. Aseptic loosening is uncommon with uncemented proximal tibia tumor prostheses. Clin Orthop. 2006;450:52–9.

38. Mavrogenis AF, Pala E, Angelini A, Ferraro A, Ruggieri P. Proximal tibial resections and reconstructions: clinical outcome of 225 patients. J Surg Oncol. 2013;107:335–42.

39. Bickels J, Wittig JC, Kollender Y, Henshaw RM, Kellar-Graney KL, Meller I, Malawer MM. Distal femur resection with endoprosthetic reconstruction: a long-term follow up study. Clin Orthop. 2002;400:225–35.

40. Horowitz SM, Lane JM, Otis JC, Healey JH. Prosthetic arthroplasty of the knee after resection of a sarcoma in the proximal end of the tibia: a report of sixteen cases. J Bone Joint Surg Am. 1991;73A:286–93.

41. Malawer MM, Chou LB. Prosthetic survival and clinical results with use of large-segment replacements in the treatment of high-grade bone sarcomas. J Bone Joint Surg Am. 1995;77A:1154–65.

42. Wu CC, Henshaw RM, Pritsch T, Squires MH, Malawer MM. Implant design and resection length affect cemented endoprosthesis survival in proximal tibial reconstruction. J Arthroplasty. 2008;23:886–93.

43. Jeys L, Grimer R. The long-term risks of infection and amputation with limb salvage surgery using endoprostheses. Recent Results Cancer Res. 2009;179:75–84.

44. Morii T, Morioka H, Ueda T, Araki N, Hashimoto N, Kawai A, Mochizuki K, Ichimura S. Deep infection in tumor endoprosthesis around the knee: a multi-institutional study by the Japanese musculoskeletal oncology group. BMC Musculoskelet Disord. 2013;14:51.

45. Robert RS, Ottaviani G, Huh WW, Palla S, Jaffe N. Psychosocial and functional outcomes in long-term survivors of osteosarcoma: a comparison of limb-salvage surgery and amputation. Pediatr Blood Cancer. 2010;54:990–9.

46. Hardes J, Gebert C, Schwappach A, Ahrens H, Streitburger A, Winkelmann W, Gosheger G. Characteristics and outcome of infections associated with tumor endoprostheses. Arch Orthop Trauma Surg. 2006;126:289–96.

47. Grimer RJ, Belthur M, Chandrasekar C, Carter SR, Tillman RM. Two-stage revision for infected endoprostheses used in tumor surgery. Clin Orthop. 2002;395:193–203.

48. Flint MN, Griffin AM, Bell RS, Wunder JS, Ferguson PC. Two-stage revision of infected uncemented lower extremity tumor endoprostheses. J Arthroplasty. 2007;22:859–65.

49. Racano A, Pazionis T, Farrokhyar F, Deheshi B, Ghert M. High infection rate outcomes in long-bone tumor surgery with endoprosthetic reconstruction in adults: a systematic review. Clin Orthop. 2013;47:2017–27.

50. Hussmann B, Johann I, Kauther MD, Landgraeber S, Jäger M, Lendemans S. Measurement of the silver ion concentration in wound fluids after implantation of silver-coated megaprostheses: correlation with the clinical outcome. Biomed Res Int. 2013;2013:763096.

51. Glehr M, Leithner A, Friesenbichler J, Goessler W, Avian A, Andreou D, Maurer-Ertl W, Windhager R, Tunn PU. Argyria following the use of silver-coated megaprostheses: no association between the development of local argyria and elevated silver levels. Bone Joint J. 2013;95:988–92.

52. Gosheger G, Hardes J, Ahrens H, Streitburger A, Buerger H, Erren M, Gunsel A, Kemper FH, Winkelmann W, Von Eiff C. Silver-coated megaendoprostheses in a rabbit model – an analysis of the infection rate and toxicological side effects. Biomaterials. 2004;25:5547–56.

53. Hardes J, von Eiff C, Streitbuerger A, Balke M, Budny T, Henrichs MP, Hauschild G, Ahrens H. Reduction of periprosthetic infection with silver-coated megaprostheses in patients with bone sarcoma. J Surg Oncol. 2010;101:389–95.

54. Shirai T, Tsuchiya H, Nishida H, Yamamoto N, Watanabe K, Nakase J, Terauchi R, Arai Y, Fujiwara H, Kubo T. Antimicrobial megaprostheses supported with iodine. J Biomater. 2014.

55. Gebhardt MC, Flugstad DI, Springfield DS, Mankin HJ. The use of bone allografts for limb salvage in high-grade extremity osteosarcoma. Clin Orthop. 1991;270:181–96.

56. Brigman BE, Hornicek FJ, Gebhardt MC, Mankin HJ. Allografts about the knee in young patients with high-grade sarcoma. Clin Orthop. 2004;421:232–9.

57. Friesenbichler J, Maurer-Ertl W, Sadoghi P, Lovse T, Windhager R, Leithner A. Serum metal ion levels after rotating-hinge knee arthroplasty: comparison between a standard device and a megaprosthesis. Int Orthop. 2012;36:539–44.

Long Term Outcome of Total Knee Arthroplasty. The Effect of Patella Resurfacing

Elias Palaiochorlidis and Theofilos Karachalios

Introduction

Resurfacing of the patella remains the most controversial issue in Total Knee Arthroplasty (TKA). After more than 20 years of debate, the question of whether or not to resurface the patella primary TKA remains controversial. Patellar complications during primary TKA have emerged as a major cause of failure [1] (Figs. 21.1 and 21.2). Placement of the patellar component is usually more difficult than placement of any other component in TKA and it is often the first component to fail. There are no specialized jigs available to help the surgeon perform a precise patella cut, even in Computer Assisted Orthopaedic Surgery (CAOS). Despite manufacturers' efforts, there is no commercially available "perfect" jig [2].

E. Palaiochorlidis, MD, DSc
Orthopaedic Department, Center of Biomedical Sciences (CERETETH), University of Thessalia, Larissa, Hellenic Republic

T. Karachalios, MD, DSc (✉)
Orthopaedic Department, Center of Biomedical Sciences (CERETETH), University of Thessalia, Larissa, Hellenic Republic

Orthopaedic Department, Faculty of Medicine, School of Health Sciences, Center of Biomedical Sciences (CERETETH), University of Thessalia, University General Hospital of Larissa, Mezourlo region, Larissa 41110, Hellenic Republic
e-mail: kar@med.uth.gr

In this review we present the effect of patella resurfacing or non-resurfacing on the long term outcome of TKA based on a critical evaluation of existing of quality studies.

History

It is important to focus on the history of resurfacing in order to reveal why controversies have arisen, and then focus on current knowledge

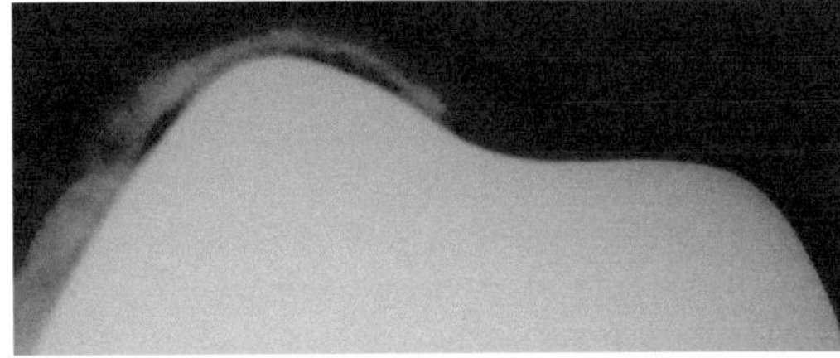

Fig. 21.1 Painful patellofemoral joint in TKA. Radiological appearance at 5 years follow up

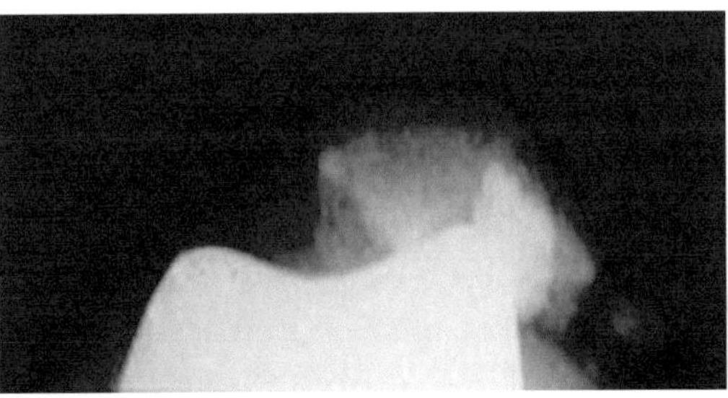

Fig. 21.2 Radiological appearance of a loose patella implant and patella fracture at 6 years follow up

© Springer-Verlag London 2015
T. Karachalios (ed.), *Total Knee Arthroplasty: Long Term Outcomes*,
DOI 10.1007/978-1-4471-6660-3_21

related to this issue. It has been demonstrated, right from the beginning, that extensor mechanism dysfunction is the most common reason for revision after TKA [3, 4]. However, the first generation of TKAs did not routinely offer patellar surfacing. Isolated patellofemoral joint replacement has existed since the 1950s, when McKeever reported a series of 40 patients with patellar resurfacing using a Vitallium implant screwed into the patella [5]. In the 1970s, Blazina and Lubinus introduced femoral groove components combined with patella resurfacing [6, 7]. Initial results and complication rates were disappointing, leading to high TKA revision rates [8]. As time passed and first generation TKA survival rates improved, patellofemoral problems became more apparent [9]. The development of second generation TKA and the publication of satisfactory mid-term results regenerated scientific interest in the patellofemoral compartment of TKA. When retropatellar resurfacing became available, better outcomes in terms of improvement of function and pain relief were obtained.

Subsequently the following questions were raised: (a) Should the patella always be resurfaced? (b) What is the role of implant design? (c) Are the problems related to technical error during implant placement (wrong size, malalignment, femoral or tibial component malrotation etc.) preventable?

Anatomical Issues

According to Dennis [10], the load sustained by the patellofemoral joint varies from 0.5 to 1 times body weight during normal walking, 3–4 times body weight during stair climbing and 8 times body weight during knee flexion. This entire load is distributed on a narrow contact surface, the patellofemoral joint. When resurfacing the patella, the contact surface becomes even narrower leading to a load increase per area unit. Patella resurfacing decreases the contact surface more than non-resurfacing [11]. Singerman [12] demonstrated that patellofemoral contact forces are similar to normal without patella resurfacing in TKA, while Matsuda [13] declared that contact stress changes per area

unit are affected by femoral component design, especially during knee flexion greater than 60°. It is important to note that some femoral component designs cause a patella inclination of more than 10° during knee flexion [14]. Evaluation of contact stress in metal backed patella implants with a mobile polyethylene insert showed both decreased and increased values [11, 15]. A literature search has shown that the developing contact stress per area unit is greater than the failure limit of the polyethylene insert [11]. It should be expected that higher wear rates and component failure would appear. Clinically, however, this did not happen often for several reasons (e.g., soft tissue adaptation, pseudomeniscus formation etc.). Recently, two important anatomical issues have appeared: anatomical alignment and the morphology of the distal femoral patella groove [16, 17].

Issues of Surgical Technique

Errors in surgical technique are the most common reason for patellofemoral joint complications. Thus surgery aims at correct alignment and balance of the extensor mechanism, and a surgeon must decide whether to replace the patellar or not [3, 18]. The surgical approach should be such as to avoid knee tightening and patella malalignment. Patellofemoral ligament resection is required [19]. Release of the patellofemoral ligament as described by Krackow [19] helps to laterally retract the patella which enhances exposure, thus improving patellar tracking and avoiding excessive soft tissue tightness. Principles of efficient patella resurfacing include (Fig. 21.3): (a) *restoration of normal patellar thickness*, which requires correct measurement, avoidance of over or under resection of the patella (a 1–2 mm decrease in patella thickness is perhaps allowed) (Fig. 21.4) [20]. (b) *Creation of symmetrical patellar facets*. Asymmetric inadvertent resurfacing occurs in 10–15 % of cases, even in the hands of experienced surgeons, which leads to increased patella inclination and instability [21]. (c) *Preservation of intact patella vascularization by* protecting the fat pad, the superior lateral artery of the knee during patellar release and

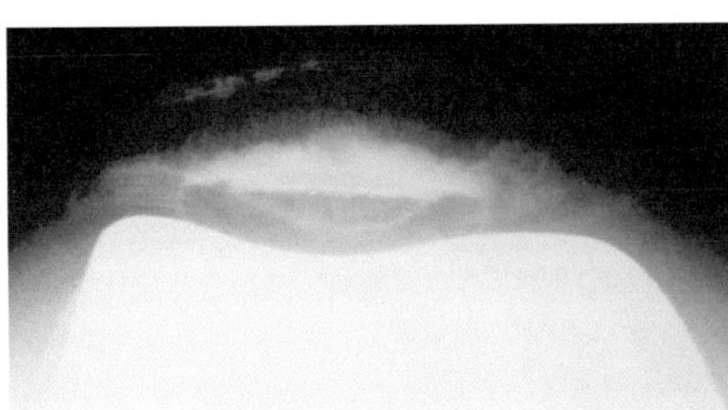

Fig. 21.3 Radiological appearance of satisfactory patella resurfacing at 12 years follow up

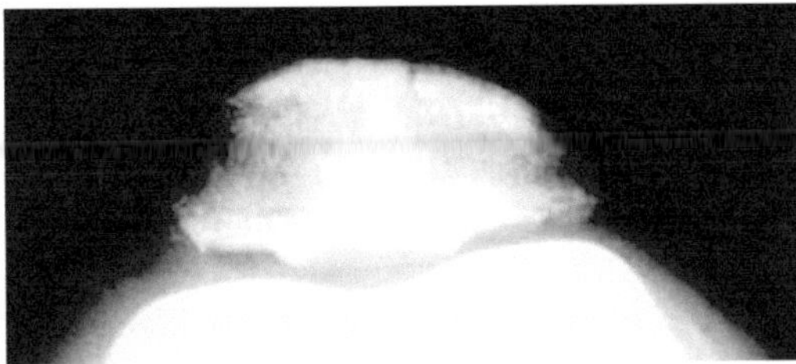

Fig. 21.4 Radiological appearance of a thick patella with overstuffing of the patellofemoral joint

intraosseous vascularization avoiding implants with one big central peg which may lead to patellar fracture (using implants with three pegs instead), (d) *Patellar tracking restoration* with lateral release or tibial tubercle displacement. Patellar tracking is better assessed when the tourniquet is released, before the soft tissues are sutured and by avoiding the stabilizing effect of the thumb when examining the knee during full range of movement, (e) *Optimal femoral, tibial and patellar component orientation.* Optimal femoral component placement is determined by 3° of external rotation, slight lateral displacement, neutral alignment in the sagittal plane and no anterior displacement [22]. Optimal tibial component placement is determined by slight lateral displacement in the frontal plane and rotationally centered in the medial aspect of the tibial tubercle. Finally, optimal patellar placement is determined by slight medial displacement of an implant of correct size and in neutral vertical alignment. Partial bursectomy using cautery, followed by some degree of denervation, is also recommended and (f) *Avoiding Soft tissue impingement.* Optimal patella implant design should meet the following criteria: (a) It should

be symmetrical (oval central dome) or anatomical, (b) it should have three pegs instead of one big central one due to the risk of fracture and osteonecrosis, (c) it should not be metal-backed.

When intraoperative evaluation reveals patellar malalignment (Fig. 21.5) and instability, malpositioning of the TKA implant should be excluded. If this is not the case, lateral patellar retinacular ligament release should be performed, to try to preserve the superior lateral geniculate artery and vastus lateralis tendon. If maltracking persists, medial imbrication should be performed [3]. Alternatively, tibial tuberosity transfer should be considered. It is a safe technique which requires the transferal of a large spiky bone fragment facing distally [23, 24].

Surgical technique is probably more important than certain design features of the femoral and tibial components in minimizing the incidence of patellofemoral complications. A persistent problem with surgical technique is the variability of component alignment which is seen using the currently available alignment guides [4]. Eckhoff et al. [17] compared four different methods of determining tibial component rotation, for instance, and found a range of 20° from 2° internal rotation to 19° external rotation. A similar study has evaluated the alignment and rotation of the femoral component. Olcott and Scott [22] evaluated four commonly used methods of determining component rotation and found that flexion gap asymmetry occurred in 10–30 % of patients depending on the anatomical landmarks used to determine femoral component rotation [22].

Component Design

Early femoral component designs were not anatomical and were characterized by a shallow flat trochlear groove which resulted in a relatively high incidence of patellar subluxation and dislocation. The priority in early cruciate retaining components was minimal bone resection which resulted in the acceptance of a shallow groove [4]. Contemporary designs are anatomical and have incorporated a separate inter condylar bone cut in order to allow resection of adequate depth

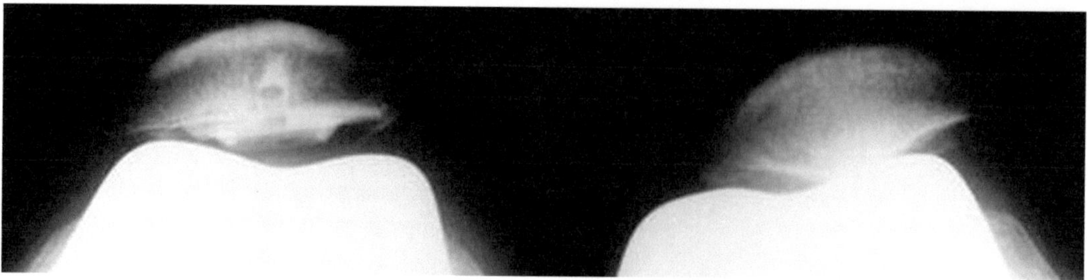

Fig. 21.5 Radiological appearance of patella tilt and instability in bilateral TKA (*right* nonresurfaced and *left* resurfaced)

and replication of a normal anatomical trochlear groove [25]. Another design feature is the distal extent of the trochlear groove. Earlier designs did not provide support for the patellar component other than two small areas of point contact beyond 90° of flexion. By extending the metal surface of the trochlea farther distally, higher contact areas and lower contact stresses can be maintained beyond 90° of flexion [4]. This feature has been incorporated into some recent designs. There is evidence that this design feature is particularly advantageous when the patellar is left unresurfaced [13].

Replace or Not. The Decision
(Figs. 21.6 and 21.7)

Some authors suggest routine resurfacing of the patella due to large numbers of cases with residual anterior knee pain, increased rates of both secondary patellar replacements (revision) and other reoperations in TKAs without patellar

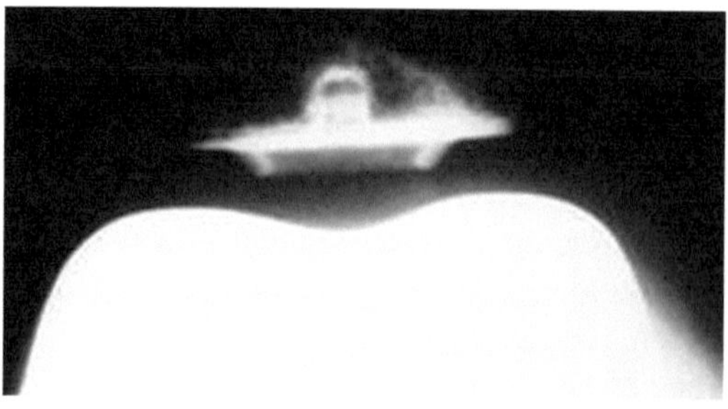

Fig. 21.6 Satisfactory radiological appearance of a resurfaced patella in an asymptomatic TKA at 16 years follow up

resurfacing [26–28]. Others find no reason to support routine patellar resurfacing [29–31]. They suggest that patella complications are found more often in a resurfaced group than in a group without resurfacing [29–31]. A selective decision based on factors such as patella thickness, the presence of preoperative anterior knee pain, the severity of degenerative changes in the patella or rheumatoid arthritis and the experience of the surgeon has also been suggested [32–34].

The native patella is more physiological and anatomical when compared with a resurfaced patella. Problems associated with patellar tilt and over stuffing of the patellofemoral joint are minimized when the native patella is not replaced. The most widely used argument against patellar resurfacing is the higher complication rate reported with patellar resurfacing. It is true that fractures, dislocations, extensor disruption and osteonecrosis have been reported without patellar resurfacing, but their incidence increases significantly and new complications appear with the increasing practice of patellar resurfacing [35–37]. New complications related to patellar resurfacing include component wear, dissociation, loosening, and patellar clunk syndrome [38, 39].

Arnold et al. [40] conclude that using a blood supply preserving approach and a biomechanically sound TKA without patellar replacement achieves excellent long term results. They also showed that the patellofemoral joint is an important problem after TKA [40]. Ogon et al. [31] have concluded that patellar complications were more often found in the resurfaced group than in the group without resurfacing. The results indicate no overall advantage of patella resurfacing

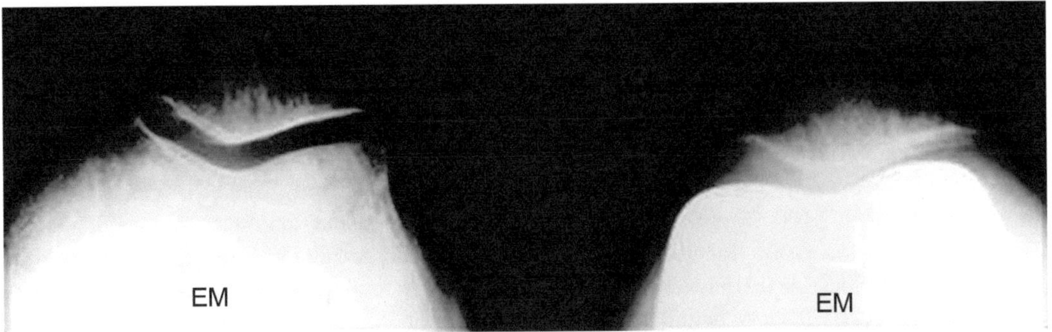

Fig. 21.7 Satisfactory radiological appearance of a nonresurfaced in an asymptomatic TKA at 14 years follow up

compared with patella retention in the long run [41]. Barrack [41] has noted that every study to date supports the idea that kinematics are more abnormal when the patella is resurfaced than when it is retained. He also suggests that patello-femoral contact areas are higher and contact stresses are lower in the native patella compared with the resurfaced patella in TKA. Virtually every clinical study of bilateral knee arthroplasty in which one patella has been resurfaced and the other has not showed either equivalent results or a preference for the unresurfaced side. Laboratory and clinical data indicate that not resurfacing the patella is a viable if not a preferable option in most TKA patients [41]. Feller [42] reports that stair climbing ability was significantly better in the patellar retention group. Although there were no complications related to patellar resurfacing, in the mid-term no significant benefit was found from resurfacing the patella during TKA for osteoarthritis, unless it was severely deformed [42]. Proponents of patellar resurfacing argue that the native patella is more physiological and ana-tomical in the normal knee, but once the mechan-ics and surfaces of the joint are altered with arthroplasty, these advantages are lost. Patellar kinematics have been shown to be more variable after arthroplasty when compared with normal knees [43, 44]. With time, the prolonged effects of cartilage to metal contact become detrimental [36, 45]. High patellofemoral loads are also thought to contribute to cartilage deterioration over time [46]. This has been confirmed in vivo, based on numerous reports documenting significant carti-lage erosion at the time of secondary resurfacing,

despite the fact that healthy appearing cartilage was found at index TKA [47, 48]. In vitro and in vivo evidence of deterioration over time pro-vides a compelling argument in favor of patellar resurfacing.

Revision rates due to patella resurfacing have been reported as high as 50 %, with an overall complication rate ranging from 5 % to 55 % in all TKAs [49, 50]. Poor results have been attrib-uted to inferior prosthetic designs and surgical technique. Metal backed patella designs, which showed increased wear, loosening, and polyeth-ylene dissociation, have provided the majority of undesirable data related to prosthetic design [51, 52]. This issue has improved with the use of all polyethylene, three pegged patella compo-nents [53]. Asymmetric patellar resection, patel-lofemoral joint overstuffing and excessive patella resection have also contributed to high complication rates. Surgical techniques for patella resection which emphasize patellar resection reproducing equal facet thickness, native patellar height and tracking and respect-ing vascular supply have produced complication rates from 0 % to 4 % [42, 54].

Various quality studies concerning patella resurfacing (including randomised controlled tri-als (RCTs), prospective studies, meta-analyses and systematic reviews) have been published but no final conclusion has yet been drawn. It has to be stressed that early studies were performed using non-anatomic and non-patella friendly femoral components which is, in our opinion, a serious negative confounding factor. Several investigators have reported superior results in patients having patellar resurfacing. Ranawat [55], in a 5–10 year follow up of 100 TKAs with patellar resurfacing, reports good to excellent results in the majority of patients with only a 2 % complication rate. Rand [56] evaluated 50 TKAs and showed an average Hospital for Special Surgery score of 92, 100 % good or excellent results, and no evidence of fracture, loosening, subluxation, or dislocation in mid-terms. Levitsky et al. [57] reports on 79 TKAs without resurfacing and on 13 bilateral TKAs with unilateral resurfacing. Of the 13 bilateral TKAs with unilateral resurfacing patient preference was 46 % equivocal, 46 % favoring resurfacing, and 7.7 % favoring non-resurfacing. Abraham et al. [58] evaluated 100 Variable Axis TKAs with 5–9 years follow up. Fifty three knees were non-resurfaced and 47 knees were resurfaced. No difference in pain or function was detected, but a statistically significant difference was observed in resting pain in the non-resurfaced knees. Overall, this study showed a trend to greater anterior knee pain in the non-resurfaced group. Picetti reports on 100 Total Condylar TKAs without patella resurfacing. An average follow up of 4.5 years 71 % good or excellent results were recorded. Forty percent of patients reported abnormal stair climbing and 29 % experienced patellofemoral pain. However, there was no control group and Total Condylar knee arthroplasty used had radically different design features than current designs. Boyd et al. [59] has shown that secondary resurfacing produced inferior results in their study of 891 Duopatellar TKAs at an average follow up of 6.5 years. Four hundred and ninety five patellae were not resurfaced and 396 were resurfaced. There was a 12 % complication rate in the non-resurfaced group compared to a 4 % complication rate in the primary resurfaced group. Ten percent of the patients who did not have resurfacing experienced postoperative patellofemoral pain compared to less than 1 % of the patients who had resurfacing. Most importantly, 10 % of patients who had secondary resurfacing for patellofemoral pain continued to have pain after secondary resurfacing and had a higher rate of skin slough, infection, and decreased ROM. However, this study included patients with inflammatory arthritis. When the analysis was restricted to patients with osteoarthritis, the complication rate was comparable between the two groups with 6 % of knees without resurfacing experiencing complications compared to 4 % among patients who had resurfacing. Again, this was an older design component that does not meet current design standards. Superior functional results have been reported with patella resurfacing. Schroeder-Boersch et al. [60] compared 20 resurfaced knees with 20 unresurfaced knees at a minimum of 2 years follow up. Better functional results were observed in the resurfaced knees, leading the authors to conclude that regular resurfacing is indicated in patients with OA. Twenty two patients with advanced patellofemoral disease who had bilateral TKAs were investigated by Enis et al. [61]. In all patients, the right side was treated with patellar resurfacing, whereas the left patella was not resurfaced. The resurfaced knees had superior isokinetic measurements, less patellofemoral pain, and were preferred by patients.

Results in the inflammatory arthropathy population have been consistently in favor of routine patellar resurfacing. Shoji [62] first reported on a population of 35 patients with RA who had bilateral TKAs with one side being resurfaced and the other side not. At an average follow up of 2.7 years, there was no difference in terms of pain, function, motion, or muscle power. Later, Kajino [63] evaluated the same group of patients 6 years after surgery. An increase in pain while standing, ascending or descending stairs, and patellofemoral tenderness in patients without patellar resurfacing was reported. Patients also presented radiographic erosive changes on the articular surface of the patella in previously unresurfaced patellas. Keblish et al. [34, 64] report no difference in clinical results between the two sides. Enis et al. [61] studied cases of bilateral TKA with and without patellar resurfacing using the Townley Knee (DePuy) and found that patients had a preference for the resurfaced side.

Barrack et al. [65] report the results of an RCT study using the Miller-Galante II total knee replacement which found no difference in knee score or patient satisfaction; however, 10 % of patients without resurfacing subsequently underwent resurfacing. Among the patients who had bilateral knee replacements with one side resurfaced and the other side not resurfaced, the knee scores were equivalent and patients expressed no preference for one side over the other. A minimum 5 year follow-up report of this same group of patients continued to show no significant difference between the groups [72]. The incidence of anterior knee pain increased in both groups, but more in the patients who had had resurfacing [53]. Bourne et al. [66] conducted a similar RCT study using the AMK TKA. Fifty patellas were resurfaced and 50 were not. At 2 years follow up less pain and greater flexion was recorded in patients without resurfacing. There were no differences reported in function, stair climbing, or extension torque. Four percent of the patients without resurfacing, however, required patellar resurfacing due to anterior knee pain. Later, Burnett and Bourne [47] report on these same 100 patients at 8–10 years follow up. At 4 years, pain was equal in the two groups and subjective pain questionnaires at final follow-up of 8–10 years showed that patients who had had resurfacing had less anterior knee pain with stair climbing and walking and overall higher patient satisfaction scores. A progression of cartilage degeneration during secondary resurfacing for pain was also observed.

Wood et al. [54] and Barrack et al. [65] have reported a higher rate of postoperative anterior knee pain in patients who did not have patellar resurfacing at the time of their index TKA. Wood et al. report on 228 Miller-Galante II TKAs with an average follow-up of 4 years [54]. Reoperation rates for patellofemoral problems were at the same level (12 % in the non-resurfaced and 10 % in the resurfaced group). There was a lower incidence of postoperative knee pain and better results for stair descent in the patients who had had resurfacing. The only statistically significant predictor of postoperative knee pain in this study was the absence of patellar resurfacing. Barrack et al. report on 118 TKAs (58 resurfaced and 60 not resurfaced). There was a higher incidence of postoperative anterior knee pain and reoperation rates in the non-resurfaced group at 30 months

follow up [65]. Selective resurfacing was evaluated in a RCT of Kinemax TKAs based on intraoperative patella cartilage and osteophyte criteria [67]. A slight superiority of the resurfaced compared to the non- resurfaced and selective resurface groups was reported in terms of the Bristol Knee Score at 5–10 years follow up.

Current Trends

There is a consensus to perform patella resurfacing in cases of primary patellofemoral arthritis in older patients when a severely deformed patella is present and does not track normally. Patella resurfacing should also be performed and in cases of inflammatory arthritis.

Patellar resurfacing should be avoided when the patella is small and osteopenic. In such cases resurfacing places the patella at high risk of patellar fracture or component loosening. Many surgeons tend to avoid resurfacing in young, active patients who have normal or near normal appearing articular cartilage. Recently, computer-assisted decision analysis has been applied to resurfacing of the patella in TKA [3]. This is a technique based on probability theory and Bayesian logic which uses computer software and meta-analysis of the available literature. Using this methodology, not resurfacing the patella becomes the procedure of choice if the probability of postoperative anterior knee pain with unresurfaced patellae decreases below 14 %, if the probability of having pain with a resurfaced patella increases above 8 %, or if patellar implant failure decreases below 80 % in a patient in a state of otherwise excellent health. Several studies have reported an incidence of postoperative anterior knee pain below 14 % with unresurfaced patellae and an incidence of anterior knee pain above 8 % with resurfaced patellae [59, 68, 69]. Surgeons can use these guidelines and, based on their experience, should determine whether patellar resurfacing is indicated in their patients.

If the patella is not resurfaced, it is important to choose a femoral component which is compatible with the native patella. Design features that seem to be favorable include a deep congruent trochlear groove that extends distally to maintain contact beyond 90° of flexion. Using such an implant, Kulkarni et al. [70] has reported excellent results with or without patellar resurfacing. The incidence of anterior knee pain was 7 % in the resurfaced group compared to 10 % in the non-resurfaced group. Moreover, only one patient in each group had pain severe enough to require medication. This indicates that at least with some designs, patellar resurfacing may not be necessary. If the patella is not resurfaced, patients should be informed that subsequent resurfacing may be necessary. If the patella is resurfaced routinely, it is incumbent on the surgeon to maintain a very low complication rate because several series without patellar resurfacing have achieved success in more than 90 % of patients [53]. The final decision on whether to resurface the patella rests with the surgeon, based on his level of training, experience, and intraoperative judgment of the status of patellofemoral articulation.

In evaluating the causes of patellofemoral problems in TKA a clearer understanding of the optimal technique and design of knee arthroplasty has emerged. It has become clear that the patella is vitally important in the overall success or failure of TKA. The occurrence of patellar complications, such as maltracking or anterior knee pain usually indicate an underlying problem in surgical technique, component design, or both. This explains why isolated patellar resurfacing is associated with a high rate of complications and persistent symptoms, why resurfacing a previously nonresurfaced symptomatic patella is associated with persistent or recurrent symptoms, and why even doing patellectomy after patellar fragmentation can fail to relieve symptoms. Conversely, normal patellar tracking and absence of any peripatellar symptoms is a strong indication of a successful arthroplasty procedure [70, 71]. In the process of understanding and minimizing patellofemoral symptoms and complications after TKA, we have gained a better understanding of optimal surgical techniques and implant design.

Churchill et al. [72] have suggested that in increasing femoral roll back in flexion, a reduction of the patellofemoral contact load is observed. In their study, posterior cruciate ligament substituting TKA produced the greatest and the most reproducible roll back. Moving the tibial post posteriorly further increased roll back, and increased roll back correlated with reduced patellar load. Quadriceps loads were reduced by increasing the roll back but to a smaller degree [72]. Harwin et al. [73] has stated that satisfactory patella resurfacing can be performed with minimal complications if the following technical considerations are met: 5–7° of valgus alignment; medial placement of the patellar component, taking care not to increase either the AP diameter of the knee or the thickness of the patella; avoiding internal rotation either in the tibia or in the femur and correct soft tissue balance. If anything goes wrong, patellofemoral complication is the usual outcome [74]. Pollo et al. [74] have evaluated kinematic and kinetic variables in the knee joint and no significant differences were found in the biomechanics of walking, stair climbing or chair rising in patients with or without a resurfaced patella. In other words, they did not find any advantage of patella resurfacing. Reuben [75] has proposed that TKA systems should include instrumentation that allows precise restoration of overall patellar thickness while maintaining a bony patellar thickness of at least 15 mm in order to produce the best results. They also conclude that patellar complications following total knee arthroplasty have begun to emerge as a major cause of failure. Stiehl et al. [76] suggest that kinematic abnormalities of the prosthetic patellofemoral joint may reduce effective extensor movement after TKA.

The majority of recent publications favour nonresurfacing of the patella in terms of anterior knee pain, functional outcome and patient satisfaction. Newer designs are compatible with the native patella and a satisfactory remodelling of the native patella can take place in nonresurfaced TKAs. It is presumed that the majority of future TKAs will be of the patella nonresurfacing type provided better implant prosthetic designs are available [77].

Several randomised trials have provided inconclusive evidence regarding this problem due to small sample sizes. Systematic reviews and meta-analyses have been performed in an attempt to clarify the issue. A meta-analysis by Parvizi et al. [78] included 14 RCTs and quasi-RCTs and demonstrated that the rate of anterior knee pain and patient satisfaction significantly favoured patellar resurfacing. They also observe no significant difference regarding reoperation rates between patella resurfaced and nonresurfaced groups. Nizard et al. [79] performed another meta-analysis pooled 12 RCTs and quasi-RCTs and reports that anterior knee pain and reoperation rates were in favour of resurfacing. Forster et al. [80] published a systematic review including three RCTs and reported that the overall rate of reoperation for a patellofemoral problem was 0.7 % in the resurfaced group and 12 % in the nonresurfaced group. Study data on clinical knee scores and anterior knee pain could not be analysed together as there was a significant heterogeneity. A meta-analysis presented by Pakos et al. [81], which included ten RCTs, shows that the RR of revision favoured patellar resurfacing and the RR of anterior knee pain also favoured patellar resurfacing in five trials. The standard mean differences calculated for the knee scores were not significantly different between the compared arms with substantial heterogeneity. In a recent systematic review, Li et al. [1] found that the relative risk of reoperation was significantly lower for the patellar resurfacing group than for the nonresurfacing group. The overall incidence of postoperative anterior knee pain in the 1,421 TKAs included was 12.9 % in the patellar resurfacing group and 24.1 % in the nonresurfacing group. The existing evidence indicates that patellar resurfacing can reduce the risk of reoperation with no improvement in postoperative knee function or patient satisfaction over TKA without patellar resurfacing. Whether it can decrease the incidence of anterior knee pain remains uncertain.

Systematic reviews and meta-analyses are affected not only by the quality of RCTs but also by the methodology whereby RCTs are selected for inclusion [82]. Because the included RCTs and methods used in each meta- analysis were different, the results of the above systematic reviews and meta-analyses are inconsistent. We have to stress again that an in depth evaluation of existing RCTs reveals that the majority used old non-anatomic femoral implants with primitive femoral grooves.

Indelli et al. [83] has suggested that newer femoral designs with softer edges and a deep, long femoral groove allow for a correct reproducibility of the patellofemoral conformity. In their study, the incidence of extensor mechanism complications appeared to be more related to poor surgical technique than to implant design. No revisions were performed in this case series. Average knee flexion at follow-up was 115°. Two major patello-femoral complications (6.6 %) were registered at final follow up. Radiological evaluation (Merchant's view) of the first painful knee showed a medial tilt of the replaced patella with a medial bony impingement. This complication was related to insufficient patellar bone removal, leaving the patella with an excessive cross section. Radiological evaluation of the second painful knee showed an asymmetric patellar bone cut, whereby the proximal pole of the patella had a diameter of 13.2 mm with respect to 9.8 mm in the distal pole, favouring patellar tilting and proximal soft tissue entrapment.

Obviously, there is a need or further research into this issue. In order to observe adverse events over the long term, patients' age should be taken into consideration when enrolling eligible participants. Further research should describe randomisation methods and the concealment of allocation of patients in more detail, at least use blinded outcome assessors and report whether intention to treat analysis is used. Reporting that conforms to the Consolidated Standards of Reporting Trials (CONSORT) is necessary [84]. Future trials should also perform cost-effectiveness analyses.

With the components, instrumentation, and techniques currently available, patellofemoral complications should no longer be the most common reason for TKA revision, or even a particularly common reason for reoperation. The patella should be resurfaced when the indications are s outlined above. For the remaining patients, who constitute the majority, this decision must be individualized on the basis of a surgeon's training and experience and an intraoperative assessment of the patellofemoral articulation.

References

1. Li S, Chen Y, Su W, Zhao J, He S, Luo X. Systematic review of patellar resurfacing in total knee arthroplasty. Int Orthop. 2011;35:305–16.
2. Gopinathan P. Patellar resurfacing vs non-resurfacing during primary total knee arthroplasty-a review of literature. Orthopaedics. 2004;1(2):e1.
3. Rand JA. The patellofemoral joint in total knee arthroplasty. J Bone Joint Surg Am. 1994;76A:612–20.
4. Barrack RL, Burak C. Patella in total knee arthroplasty. Clin Orthop. 2001;389:62–73.
5. McKeever DC. The classic: patellar prosthesis (1955). Clin Orthop. 2005;440:13–21.
6. Blazina ME, Fox JM, Del Pizzo W, Broukhim B, Ivey FM. Patellofemoral replacement 1979. Clin Orthop. 2005;436:3–6.
7. Lubinus HH. Patella glide bearing total replacement. Orthopaedics. 1979;2:119–27.
8. Crachiollo A, Benson M, Finerman M. A prospective comparative analysis of the first generation knee replacement. Polycentric vs. geometric knee arthroplasty. Clin Othop. 1979;145:37–46.
9. Laskin R. The patella need not to be resurfaced during total knee replacement. In: Controversies in total knee replacement. Oxford/New York: Oxford University Press; 2001. p. 187.
10. Dennis DA. Patellofemoral complications in total knee arthroplasty. A literature review. Am J Knee Surg. 1992;5:156–66.
11. Matsuda S, Ishinisi T, White SE, Whiteside LA. Patellofemoral joint after knee arthroplasty. Effect on contact area and contact stress. J Arthroplasty. 1997;12:790–7.
12. Singerman R, Gabriel SM, Kennendy JW. Patellar contact forces with and without patellar resurfacing in total knee arthroplasty. J Arthroplasty. 1999;14:603–9.
13. Matsuda S, Ishinisi T, Whiteside LA. Contact stresses with an unresurfaced patella in total knee arthroplasty: the effect of femoral component design. Orthopedics. 2000;23:213–28.
14. McLean CA, Laxer E, Casey J, Ahmet AM. The effect of femoral component designs on the contact and tracking characteristics of the unresurfaced patella in TKA. Orthop Trans. 1994;18:616.
15. Buechel FF, Pappas MJ, Makris G. Evaluation of contact stress in metal backed patellar replacements. Clin Orthop. 1991;273:190–7.
16. Feinstein WK, Noble PC, Kamaric E, Tullos HS. Anatomic alignment of the patellar groove. Clin Orthop. 1996;331:64–73.
17. Eckhoff DG, Burke BJ, Dwyer TF, Pring ME, Spitzer VM, VanGerwen DP. Sulcus morphology of the distal femur. Clin Orthop. 1996;331:23–8.
18. Scuderi GR, Insall NJ, Scott WN. Patellofemoral pain after total knee arthroplasty. J Am Acad Orthop Surg. 1994;2:239–46.
19. Krachow KA. Surgical procedure. In: Klein EA, editor. The technique of total knee arthroplasty. St Louis: CV Mosby; 1990. p. 168–237.
20. Hsu JC, Luo AP, Rand JA. Influence of patellar thickness on patellar tracking and patellofemoral contact characteristics after total knee arthroplasty. J Arthroplasty. 1996;11:69–80.
21. Pagnano MW, Trousdale RT. Inadvertent asymmetric resurfacing of the patella in total knee arthroplasty. Orthop Trans 1998–99;22:19.
22. Olcott CW, Scott RD. Femoral component rotation during total knee arthroplasty. Clin Orthop. 1999;367:3942.
23. Kirk P, Rorabeck CH, Bourne RB, Burkart B, Nott L. Management of recurrent dislocation of the patella following total knee arthroplasty. J Arthroplasty. 1992;7:229–33.
24. Whiteside LA. Distal realignment of the patellar tendon to correct abnormal patellar tracking. Clin Orthop. 1997;344:284–9.
25. Petersilge WJ, Oishi CS, Kaufman KR, Irby SE, Colwell Jr CW. The effect of trochlear design on patellofemoral shear and compressive forces in total knee arthroplasty. Clin Orthop. 1994;309:124–30.
26. Levai JP, McLeod CH, Freeman MA. Why not resurface the patella? J Bone Joint Surg (Br). 1983;65B:448–51.
27. Waters TS, Bentley G. Patellar resurfacing in total knee arthroplasty. A prospective, randomized study. J Bone Joint Surg Am. 2003;85A:212–7.
28. Tabutin J, Banon F, Catonne Y, Grobost J, Tessier JL, Tillie B. Should we resurface the patella in total knee replacement? Experience with the Nex Gen prosthesis. Knee Surg Sports Traumatol Arthrosc. 2005;13:5348.
29. Oh IS, Kim MK, You DS, Kang SB, Lee KH. Total knee arthroplasty without patellar resurfacing. Int Orthop. 2006;30:415–9.
30. Hasegawa M, Ohashi T. Long term clinical results and radiographic changes in the nonresurfaced patella after total knee arthroplasty: 78 knees followed for mean 12 years. Acta Orthop Scand. 2002;73:539–45.
31. Ogon M, Hartig F, Bach C, Nogler M, Steingruber I, Biedermann R. Patella resurfacing: no benefit for the long term outcome of total knee arthroplasty. A 10- to 16.3-year follow-up. Arch Orthop Trauma Surg. 2002;122:229–34.
32. Picetti GD, McGann WA, Welch RB. The patellofemoral joint after total knee arthroplasty without patellar resurfacing. J Bone Joint Surg Am. 1990;72A:1379–82.
33. Kim BS, Reitman RD, Schai PA, Scott RD. Selective patellar nonresurfacing in total knee arthroplasty. 10 year results. Clin Othop. 1999;367:81–8.
34. Keblish PA, Varma AK, Greenwald AS. Patellar resurfacing or retention in total knee arthroplasty.

A prospective study of patients with bilateral replacements. J Bone Joint Surg (Br). 1994;76B:930–7.

35. Clayton ML, Thirupathi R. Patellar complications after total condylar arthroplasty. Clin Orthop. 1982;170:152–7.

36. Gomes LS, Bechtold JE, Gustilo RB. Patellar prosthesis positioning in total knee arthroplasty: a roentgenographic study. Clin Orthop. 1988;236:72–81.

37. Healy WL, Wasilewski SA, Takei R, Oberlander M. Patellofemoral complications following total knee arthroplasty: correlation with implant design and patient risk factors. J Arthroplasty. 1995;10:197–201.

38. Burnett RS, Boone JL, Rosenzweig SD, Steger-May K, Barrack RL. Patellar resurfacing compared with nonresurfacing in total knee arthroplasty. A concise follow-up of a randomized trial. J Bone Joint Surg Am. 2009;91A:256–67.

39. Beight JL, Yao B, Hozack WJ, Hearn SL, Booth Jr RE. The patellar "clunk" syndrome after posterior stabilized arthroplasty. Clin Orthop. 1994;299:139–42.

40. Arnold MP, Friedrich NF, Widmer H, Muller W. Patellar substitution in total knee prosthesis – is it important? Orthopade. 1998;27:637–41.

41. Barrack RL. Orthopaedic crossfire – all patellae should be resurfaced during primary total knee arthroplasty: in opposition. J Arthroplasty. 2003;3(S1):35–8.

42. Feller JA, Bartlett RJ, Lang DM. Patellar resurfacing versus retention in total knee arthroplasty. J Bone Joint Surg (Br). 1996;78B:226–8.

43. Komistek RD, Dennis DA, Mabe A, Walker S. An In vivo determination of patellofemoral contact positions. J Clin Biomech. 2000;15:29–36.

44. Stiehl JB, Komistek RD, Dennis DA, Keblish PA. Kinematics of the patellofemoral joint in total knee arthroplasty. J Arthroplasty. 2001;16:707–14.

45. Forster H, Fisher J. The influence of continuous sliding and subsequent surface wear on the friction of articular cartilage. Proc Inst Mech Eng. 1999;213:329–45.

46. Reilly TR, Martens M. Experimental analysis of the quadriceps muscle force and patellofemoral joint reaction force for various activities. Acta Orthop Scand. 1972;43:126–37.

47. Burnett RS, Bourne RB. Indications for patellar resurfacing in total knee arthroplasty. J Bone Joint Surg Am. 2003;85A:728–45.

48. Barrack RL, Bertot AJ, Wolfe MW, Waldman DA, Milicic M, Myers L. Patellar resurfacing in total knee arthroplasty: a prospective, randomized, double blind study with five to seven years of follow-up. J Bone Joint Surg Am. 1997;79A:1121–31.

49. Brick GW, Scott RD. The patellofemoral component of total knee arthroplasty. Clin Orthop. 1988;231:163–78.

50. Dennis DA. Patellofemoral complications in total knee arthroplasty. In: Kesser JR, editor. Orthopaedic knowledge update 5. Home study syllabus. Rosemont: American Academy of Orthopaedic Surgeons; 1995. p. 283–9.

51. Stulberg SD, Stulberg BN, Hamati Y, Tsao A. Failure mechanisms of metal-backed patellar components. Clin Orthop. 1988;236:88–105.

52. Wasilewski SA, Frankel U. Fracture of polyethylene of patellar component in total knee arthroplasty, diagnosed by arthroscopy. J Arthroplasty. 1989;4(S1):19–22.

53. Barrack RL, Wolfe MW. Patellar resurfacing in total knee arthroplasty. J Am Acad Orthop Surg. 2000;8:75–82.

54. Wood DJ, Smith AJ, Collopy D, White B, Brankov B, Bulsara MK. Patellar resurfacing in total knee arthroplasty: a prospective, randomized trial. J Bone Joint Surg Am. 2002;84A:187–93.

55. Ranawat CS. The patellofemoral joint in total condylar knee arthroplasty: pros and cons based on five to ten year follow-up observations. Clin Orthop. 1986;205:93–9.

56. Rand JA. Patellar resurfacing in total knee arthroplasty. Clin Orthop. 1990;260:110–7.

57. Levitsky KA, Harris WJ, McManus J, Scott RD. Total knee arthroplasty without patellar resurfacing: clinical outcomes and long-term follow-up evaluation. Clin Orthop. 1993;286:116–21.

58. Abraham W, Buchanan JR, Daubert H, Greer III RB, Keefer J. Should the patella be resurfaced in total knee arthroplasty? Efficacy of patellar resurfacing. Clin Orthop. 1988;236:128–34.

59. Boyd Jr AD, Ewald FC, Thomas WH, Poss R, Sledge CB. Long-term complications after total knee arthroplasty with or without resurfacing of the patella. J Bone Joint Surg Am. 1993;75A:674–81.

60. Schroeder-Boersch H, Scheller G, Fischer J, Jani L. Advantages of patellar resurfacing in total knee arthroplasty: two year results of a prospective, randomized study. Arch Orthop Trauma Surg. 1998;117:73–8.

61. Enis JE, Gardner R, Robledo MA, Latta L, Smith R. Comparison of patellar resurfacing versus nonresurfacing in bilateral total knee arthroplasty. Clin Orthop. 1990;260:38–42.

62. Shoji H, Yoshino S, Kajino A. Patellar replacement in bilateral total knee arthroplasty: a study of patients who had rheumatoid arthritis and no gross deformity of the patella. J Bone Joint Surg Am. 1989;71A:853–6.

63. Kajino A, Yoshino S, Kameyama S, Kohda M, Nagashima S. Comparison of the results of bilateral total knee arthroplasty with and without patellar replacement for rheumatoid arthritis: a follow-up note. J Bone Joint Surg Am. 1997;79A:570–4.

64. Keblish T, Ogata K, Hara M. Comparison of cemented and cementless fixation resurfaced and unresurfaced patella on the press fit condylar type total knee arthroplasty. Proceedings of AAOS 66th annual meeting of the AAOS 1999.

65. Barrack RL, Wolfe MW, Waldman DA, Milicic M, Bertot AJ, Myers L. Resurfacing of the patella in total knee arthroplasty: a prospective, randomized, double blind study. J Bone Joint Surg Am. 2001;83A:1376–81.

66. Bourne RB, Roraback CH, Vaz M, Kramer J, Hardie R, Robertson D. Resurfacing vs not resurfacing the patella during total knee arthroplasty. Clin Orthop. 1995;321:156–61.
67. Newman JH, Ackroyd CE, Shah NA, Karachalios T. Should the patella be resurfaced during total knee replacement. Knee. 2000;7:17–23.
68. Insall JN, Ranawat CS, Aglietti P, Shine P. A comparison of four models of total knee replacement prostheses. J Bone Joint Surg Am. 1976;58A:754–65.
69. Insall JN, Tria AJ, Aglietti P. Resurfacing of the patella. J Bone Joint Surg Am. 1980;62A:933–6.
70. Kulkarni SK, Freema MAR, Poal-Manresa JC, Ascencio JI, Rodriguez JJ. The patellofemoral joint in total knee arthroplasty. Is the design of the trochlea the critical factor. J Artrhoplasty. 2000;15:424–9.
71. Bery DJ, Rand JA. Isolated patellar component revision of total knee arthroplasty. Clin Orthop. 1993;286:110–5.
72. Churchill DL, Incavo SJ, Johnson CC, Beynnon BD. The Influence of femoral rollback on patellofemoral contact loads in total knee arthroplasty. J Arthroplasty. 2001;16:909–18.
73. Harwin SF, Stein AJ, Stern RE. Patellofemoral resurfacing at total knee arthroplasty. Contemp Orthop. 1994;29:265–71.
74. Pollo FE, Jackson RW, Koeter S, Ansari S, Motley GS, Rathjen KW. Walking, chair rising and stair climbing after total knee arthroplasty: patellar resurfacing versus non-resurfacing. Am J Knee Surg. 2000;13:103–8.
75. Reuben JD, McDonald CL, Woodard PL, Hennington LJ. Effect of patella thickness on patella strain following total knee arthroplasty. J Arthroplasty. 1991;6:251–8.
76. Stiehl JB, Komistek RD, Dennis DA, Keblish PA. Kinematics of the patellofemoral joint in total knee arthroplasty. J Arthroplasty. 2001;16:706–14.
77. Barrack RL, Wolfe MW, Waldman DA. Patellar resurfacing in total knee arthroplasty. Proceedings of the 67th annual meeting of the AAOS, 2000.
78. Parvizi J, Rapuri VR, Saleh KJ, Kuskowski MA, Sharkey PF, Mont MA. Failure to resurface the patella during total knee arthroplasty may result in more knee pain and secondary surgery. Clin Orthop. 2005;438:191–6.
79. Nizard RS, Biau D, Porcher R, Ravaud P, Bizot P, Hannouche D, Sedel L. A meta-analysis of patellar replacement in total knee arthroplasty. Clin Orthop. 2005;432:196–203.
80. Forster MC. Patellar resurfacing in total knee arthroplasty for osteoarthritis: a systematic review. Knee. 2004;11:427–30.
81. Pakos EE, Ntzani EE, Trikalinos TA. Patellar resurfacing in total knee arthroplasty. A meta-analysis. J Bone Joint Surg Am. 2005;87A:1438–45.
82. Chen K, Guodong Li, Dong Fu, Chaoqun Y, Qiang Zhang, Zhengdong Cai. Patellar resurfacing versus nonresurfacing in total knee arthroplasty: a meta-analysis of randomised controlled trials. Int Orthop. 2013;37:1075–83.
83. Indelli PF, Marcucci M, Cariello D, Paolo P, Innocenti M. Contemporary femoral designs in total knee arthroplasty: effects on the patello-femoral congruence. Int Orthop. 2012;36:1167–73.
84. Moher D, Schulz KF, Altman DC. The CONSORT statement: revised recommendations for improving the quality of reports of parallel-group randomised trials. Lancet. 2001;357:1191–4.

Infected Total Knee Arthroplasty. Basic Science, Management and Outcome

Theofilos Karachalios and George Komnos

Introduction

Numbers of primary elective total knee arthroplasties (TKAs) are steadily increasing and so is the number of revisions. The most common complications after primary TKA are pneumonia, pulmonary embolism and wound or periprosthetic joint infection [1] (Fig. 22.1). Surgical site infection (SSI) is one of the most serious complications of TKA and may be the most common cause of early failure and revision [2, 3]. In Britain, it is estimated that 25 % of TKA revisions are due to infection [4]. The rate of periprosthetic infection varies across different studies. An average rate of 1 % is reported, although there are studies which present higher rates in primary (0.5–2 %) and revision surgery (2–5 %) [3]. Lower rates (0.31 %) are also reported from specialized centers with ultraclean operating theatres [5–7]. Infection after TKA leads to an increased risk of patient morbidity and mortality and to a higher cost for treatment. It is estimated that the annual cost of periprosthetic joint infection revisions exceeds $566 million in the United States and is growing [8]. The average cost of in hospital care is estimated to be double in SSI compared to non SSI patients [5]. The higher cost is related to extended hospital stays, frequent readmissions, prolonged use of antibiotics and higher postoperative rehabilitation periods.

There are well recognized risk factors which increase the risk for TKA infection such as rheumatoid arthritis, hemophilia, diabetes, obesity, hypertension, steroid therapy, poor general health, history of previous surgical procedures and wound related complications [9, 10]. Risk factors for perioperative SSI include male gender, liver disease, cancer, electrolyte disorders, congestive heart failure and pulmonary circulatory disease [5, 11]. As far as the pathogen is concerned, periprosthetic infections with MRSA are associated with higher rates of re-infection [12]. Approximately 72 % of pathogens seem to be Gram positive, 7 % Gram negative and 0,6 % fungal, while in around 21 % of the cases no organism has been identified.

T. Karachalios, MD, DSc (✉)
Orthopaedic Department, Center of Biomedical Sciences (CERETETH), University of Thessalia, Larissa, Hellenic Republic

Orthopaedic Department, Faculty of Medicine, School of Health Sciences, Center of Biomedical Sciences (CERETETH), University of Thessalia, University General Hospital of Larissa, Mezourlo region, Larissa 41110, Hellenic Republic
e-mail: kar@med.uth.gr

G. Komnos, MD
Orthopaedic Department, Center of Biomedical Sciences (CERETETH), University of Thessalia, Larissa, Hellenic Republic

Orthopaedic Department, General Hospital of Karditsa, Karditsa, Hellenic Republic

© Springer-Verlag London 2015
T. Karachalios (ed.), *Total Knee Arthroplasty: Long Term Outcomes*,
DOI 10.1007/978-1-4471-6660-3_22

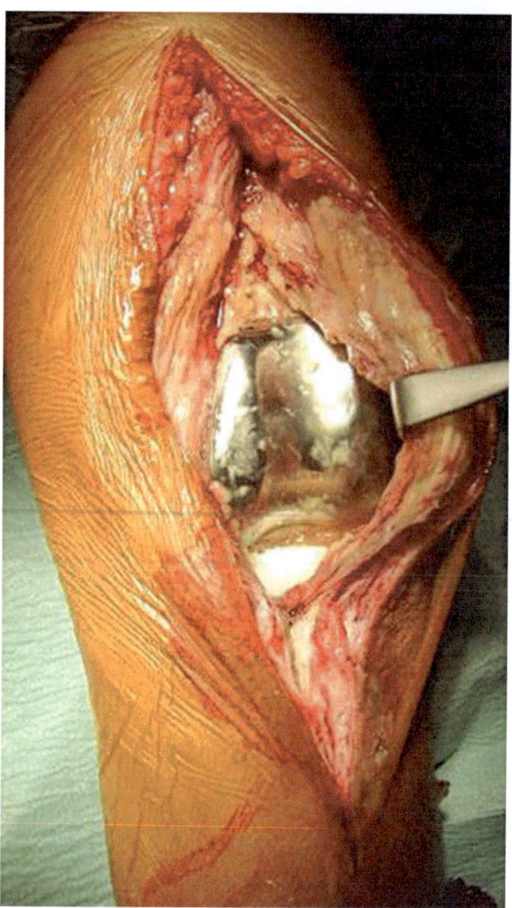

Fig. 22.1 Intraoperative view showing an infected TKA with biofilm formation

Diagnosis of an infected knee remains a challenge for orthopaedic surgeons. Swelling, tenderness and pain in an operated knee raises the suspicion for infection. Diagnosis depends on the clinical picture, plain radiographs, bone scans, serologic tests, routine blood work (ESR, CRP, interleukin-6 and glucose levels), knee aspiration and synovial fluid examination, intraoperative cultures and histology [3, 13–18]. Molecular diagnostic tests are now available for clinical use. Classification systems have been developed in order to aid the management of decision making. These systems were initially based on the time of appearance and duration of symptoms and signs (stage I – infections occurring within 6 weeks of implantation, stage II – infections being delayed chronic presentations, stage III – late infections occurring in a previously well-functioning joint and stage IV – an unexpected positive culture result in aseptic revision surgery) but it later became apparent that factors such as pathogen, patient (comorbidities, immunosuppression, medication) and the quality of local tissue are also important and determine outcome [19] (Fig. 22.2). Extensor mechanism and knee soft tissue envelope problems require a low threshold for early plastic surgery intervention.

Due to the heterogeneous nature of the disease, surgeons face several management challenges related to the numerous species of bacteria with variable antibiotic sensitivity, to abnormal bone and soft tissue environments, patients with comorbidities etc. (Fig. 22.3). Theoretically optimal treatment management is difficult to apply to all patients, and high quality comparative clinical data is lacking. Moreover, published data focus on control of infection (with a variable infection free time period), providing limited information about functional recovery, mechanical complications and aseptic loosening. Recently, an attempt has been made to draw diagnostic and treatment guidelines (consensus agreement) [20]. There is growing evidence that we are now dealing with a "different enemy". Staphylococcus aureus (MRSA), enterococcus (VRE), gram negatives (pseudomonas) or polymicrobial infections are all exhibiting more aggressive biological behavior. In the past a low percentage of pathogens were developing biofilm approximately 3 weeks after surgery [21, 22]. Now 80–90 % of the pathogens develop biofilm as early as 1–10 days [21, 22]. We therefore believe that the acute infection stage, published management strategies and literature data including interpretation of old series should be reconsidered.

Management Strategies

Treatment options vary. Prevention remains the key for the overall control of infection. Therapy depends on many factors such as the chronicity of the infection, stability of the components, medical status of the patient and is determined by surgeon experience and facilities [10, 17] (Fig. 22.3). Sometimes an infectious disease consultant is

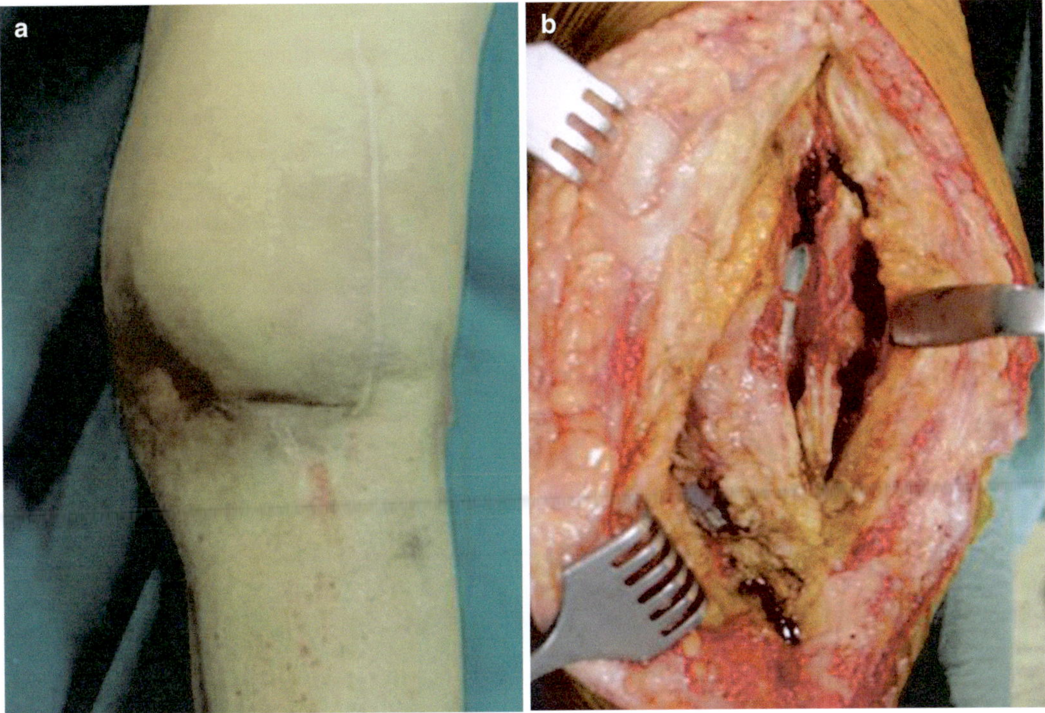

Fig. 22.2 (**a**) Preoperative appearance of compromised knee soft tissue envelop, (**b**) following wide infected tissue debridement extensor mechanism defects are found

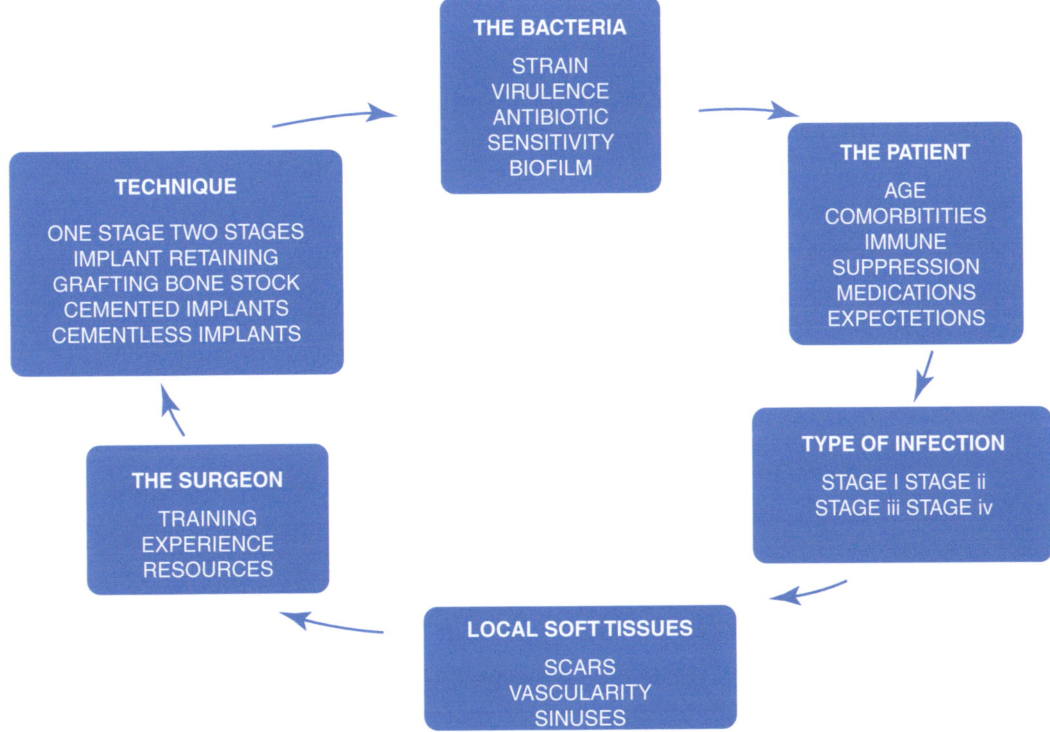

Fig. 22.3 Infected total knee arthroplasty management strategies. Factors influencing mid and long term outcome

also involved in the treatment care plan and advises about the best antibiotic and home care [18]. There are simple procedures like irrigation, implant retention after debridement and polyethylene exchange, and antibiotic suppression, or complex ones like one stage exchange technique, two stage exchange technique, arthrodesis, resection arthroplasty and amputation. The gold standard for infection control is still the two stage revision procedure [13, 15, 16, 23].

Debridement and retention of the implants is not widely accepted. It is the least invasive method; however, it requires careful patient selection. Debridement with component retention can be used with varying degrees of success (approximately 80 % clinical efficacy), especially in the acute postoperative period with only one attempt permitted [10, 24]. It is usually used in healthy patients with acute onset of symptoms and it results in better knee function [13] (Fig. 22.4). Arthroscopic debridement and retention of implants may also be used in acutely infected TKAs. This method is not widely used and therefore little is known about its role and success rate in the management of joint infection. Published data show 62.5 % success rate in a small sample of 16 acute infections followed up for 2 years [25].

The one stage exchange procedure is well established for infected THA with long term results at the level of 10 years. However, it is not widely supported and approved in the literature.

Nevertheless, it seems that single stage revision has its role in the management of TKA infections and its use is gaining popularity. It can be used in certain patients where the causative pathogen is known, no sinuses are present, the patient is not immunocompromised and there is no radiological evidence of component loosening or osteitis [4]. It has some advantages like less surgical procedures and therefore lower costs and lower hospitalization. One stage might provide better knee function but infection control remains unclear [26]. Goksan and Freeman published their results in 1992 with a success rate of 90.9 % at an average of 10 years [27]. Similar results were published in 2004 by Buechel et al. [28] who treated 22 infected knees with one stage exchange revision arthroplasty. Their results showed an infection free rate of 90 % with knee scores of 79,5 on average at 10 years follow up. In 47 patients treated with one stage exchange, 41 (87 %) were infection free at 3 years follow-up [26]. However, knee function was not improved when compared to that of historical control patients having two stage exchange. Parkinson et al. [11] presented "two in one technique" in 2008. It is similar to the two stage technique except that the time interval between the two procedures is minutes instead of 4–6 weeks, but this technique has an unconfirmed clinical outcome. There are studies showing that one stage exchange is not associated with higher rates of infection recurrence and failure (Table 22.1). They show survival rates of 87 % on

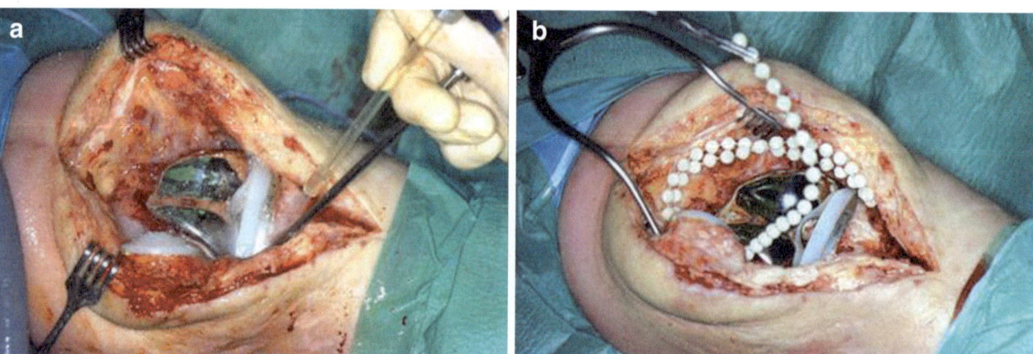

Fig. 22.4 Implant salvage in a TKA with early postoperative infection. (**a**) Wide infected tissue debridement, (**b**) temporary implantation of antibiotic loaded beads

Table 22.1 Clinical outcome studies with one stage exchange procedure

Study	Strategy	Number of patients	Mean follow up	Infection free survival rate (%)	Mean knee society function score (points)
Bauer et al. [30]	1 stage	30	52 months	67	62.5
Buechel et al. [28]	1 stage	22	10.2 years	90.9	
Göksan and Freeman [27]	1 stage	19	4.6 years	89	
Lu et al. [31]	1 stage	8	20 months	100	
Scott et al. [32]	1 stage	10		70	
VonFoerster et al. [29]	1 stage	104	5–15 years	73	

Table 22.2 Clinical outcome studies with two stage exchange procedure

Study	Year published	Number of infection free patients (%)	Mean follow up (months)
Insall et al. [49]	1983	10/11 (91)	34
Wilde and Ruth [50]	1988	9/10 (90)	33
Booth and Lotke [51]	1989	24/25 (96)	25
Teeny et al. [52]	1990	10/10 (100)	42.5
Wilson et al. [53]	1990	16/20 (80)	34
Masri et al. [54]	1994	22/24 (92)	26
Goldman et al. [42]	1996	58/64 (91)	90
Hirakawa et al. [55]	1998	41/55 (75)	62
Fehring et al. [56]	2000	51/55 (93)	36
Durbhakula et al. [57]	2004	22/24 (92)	33
Haleem et al. [43]	2004	87/96 (91)	86
Cuckler [33]	2005	43/44 (98)	62
Hoffman et al. [58]	2005	44/50 (88)	30
Bauer et al. [30]	2006	52/77 (67)	52
Hart and Jones [59]	2006	42/48 (88)	48.5
Kurd et al. [60]	2010	70/96 (73)	34.5
Westrich et al. [35]	2010	66/72 (90.7)	52
Sherrell et al. [34]	2011	55/83 (66)	50
Mahmud et al. [38]	2012	220/236 (93)	48

average at the level of 3 years follow up. Many authors believe that one stage revision produces reproducible high quality results and will soon achieve the same widespread acceptance in the knee as it does in infected hip arthroplasty. However, despite the low infection relapse rates published, the high failure rate of 27 % reported by Von Foerster et al. [29] in a large series of 118 infected knees suggest that further research is needed.

Two stage revision remains the gold standard for the management of infected TKA [3, 10, 11, 14, 24, 36, 37, 39]. It is reported to have higher infection free rates (Table 22.2). The method was first presented by Insall et al. in 1983 [39]. It involves prosthesis removal followed by delayed reimplantation. There is an interval of 4–6 weeks between the two procedures during which the patient is given antibiotic therapy. Tissue cultures taken during the first surgery can identify the infecting pathogen and define antibiotic treatment. When infection persists despite antibiotic therapy, the first stage of the procedure is repeated [40, 61]. Articulating or static spacers are used. Systematic infection, presence of sinus track, compromised soft tissues and unknown or antibiotic-resistant pathogens are also indications for the two stage procedure. A relative contraindication is acute infection caused by a known pathogen that can be managed with synovectomy and antibiotic therapy or the one stage procedure [41]. Disadvantages, compared to one stage procedure, are impaired mobility, joint stiffness and pain, higher cost of treatment and longer hospital stay [11]. Goldman et al. [42] found an infection free rate of 91 % at 10 years in a survey of 64 two stage procedures without the use of antibiotic loaded cement. A review of 253 two stage revision procedures in 2012 showed an overall infection free survival rate of 85 % at 5 years and 78 % at 10 years [38]. Haleem et al. [43] published a 77 % survival rate at 10 years for revision for any reason as an end point in a series of 96 two stage revision TKAs. Bauer et al. [30] published a multicenter retrospective study comparing one and two stage revisions for infection and found no difference between the two techniques in eradicating infection. As far as functional knee outcome is concerned, the one stage procedure showed better outcome. In a study from the Netherlands, which included 15 patients with mean follow up of 25 months, an attempt was made to compare the two stage procedure to debridement without implant removal. The infection free rate of the staged procedure was 100 % and only 37 % with the salvage procedure at a minimum 5 years follow up [44]. In another study with 20 infected TKAs, who were treated with the two stage procedure, no need for revision was recorded at an average of 6 years follow up [41]. In a recent systematic review with a large number of incidents (204 knees with one stage procedure and 1,421 with two stage) the infection free survival rate was 89.8 % for the two stage and 81.9 % for the one stage procedure at a mean follow up of 44 months [45]. Two stage reimplantation is still effective for treating contemporary pathogens, many of which are multi-antibiotic resistant (MAR). In a series of 75 infected TKAs, the infection free rates were similar to both MAR (91.2 %) and non MAR (91.3 %) infections at 2 years follow up [35].

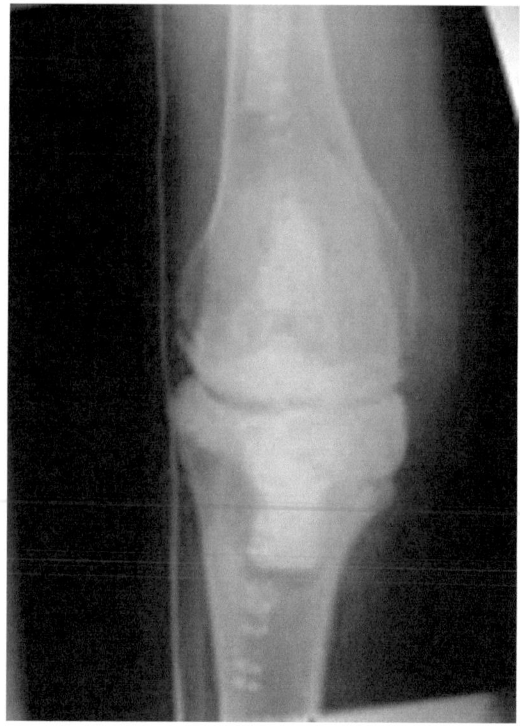

Fig. 22.5 Postoperative radiological AP view of a custom made antibiotic static spacer

Limited data is available concerning antibiotic loaded spacers used in two stage revisions. The standard of care includes implantation of an antibiotic loaded cement spacer to eradicate any organisms prior to reimplantation of the prosthesis. The traditional spacers used are static cement blocks inserted into the joint space (Fig. 22.5). More recent spacers include endoskeleton type, static cement spacers and articulating spacers (Fig. 22.6). Articulating spacers can be constructed intraoperatively or from commercial components. Their use is becoming increasingly popular. In a review published in 2014 which included 962 TKAs treated with articulating spacers and 707 TKAs with static ones, an infection relapse rate of 9.7 % in the static and 7.9 % in the articulating group was found at an average 4 years follow up [40]. However, the reoperation rate for additional complications was higher in the articulating spacer group. In another study, greater range of motion was observed in patients

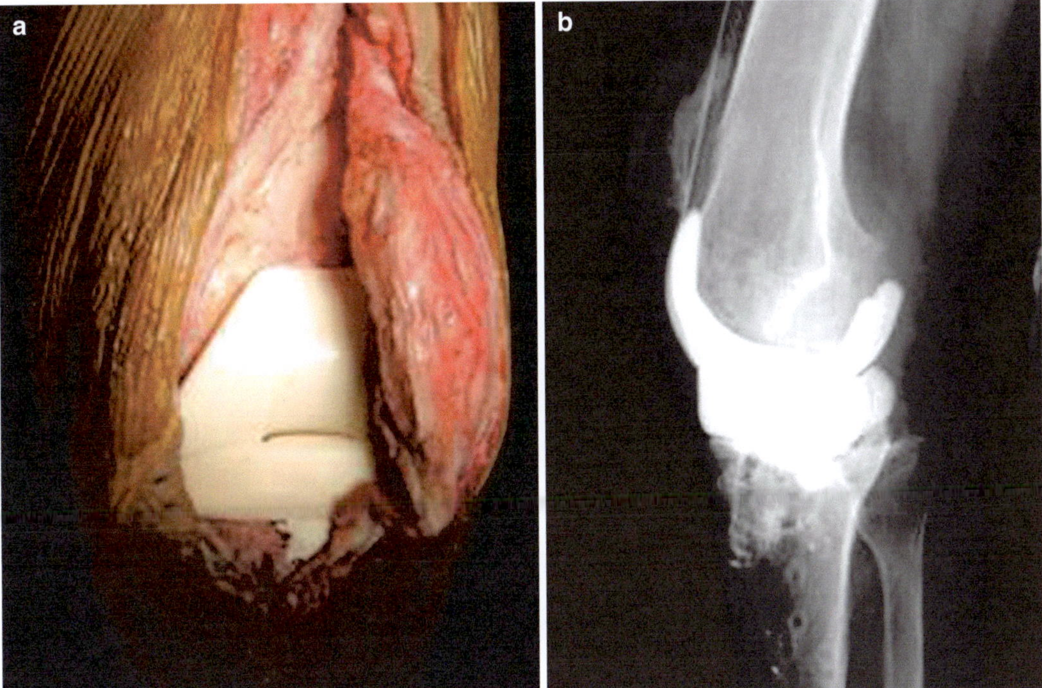

Fig. 22.6 (a) Intraoperative view of an commercially available articulating spacer, (b) radiological lateral view of the same spacer

with articulating spacers (100° versus 92°) [46]. In a review which presented an average of 89.8 % infection free rate in two stage procedures, the rate was higher in the articulating spacer subgroup compared to the static spacer subgroup (91.2 % versus 87 %) [45]. In an another small series of 15 patients, who were treated with the two stage procedure using intraoperatively molded articulating spacers, all cases resulted in infection control for at least 2 years [47]. Although current data shows an advantage of articulating spacers over the static in terms of function and range of motion [37, 40, 48] further research is needed especially related to the newer endoskeleton type spacers.

Limited data is available related to the role of arthrodesis in the infected TKA. It is indicated for infected TKA with deficient extensor mechanisms and in cases with high resistant organisms [23]. Arthrodesis may be an option in patients with recurrent infection or with a history of multiple revision failures (Fig. 22.7).

Amputation is indicated in immunocompromised patients only, or in patients with systematic sepsis or with persistent local infection combined with massive bone loss and continuous pain [23]. It is believed that amputees with the use of an external prosthesis will present better joint function.

The risk of deep infection after revision TKA is greater than that of primary TKA. The rate of infection after revision TKA varies between 1 % and 10 %. Although more studies evaluate the incidence of infection after revision for aseptic loosening, in a review study which included 476 knees, infection relapse occurred in 44 of them (9 %). The infection rate was higher in patients undergoing revision for infection than in patients with aseptic loosening (21–23 % of 91 and 5–21 % of 385) [62]. Thus infection of primary TKA is the most important risk factor for subsequent infection of TKA revisions.

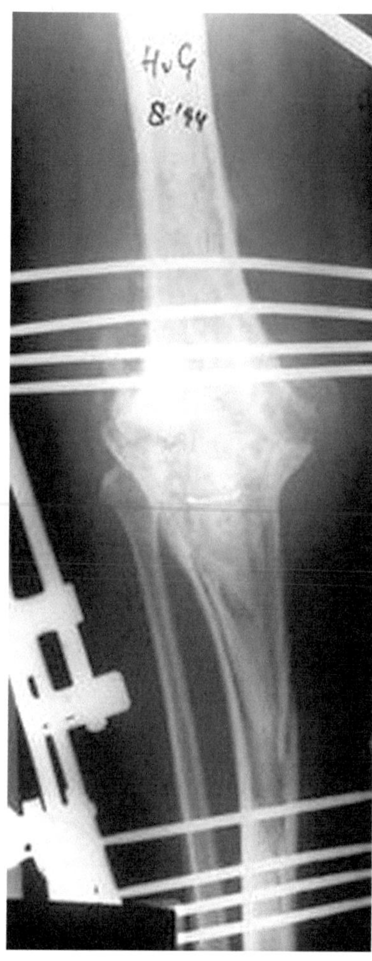

Fig. 22.7 Postoperative radiological AP view of knee arthrodesis using external fixator

References

1. Bozic KJ, Grosso LM, Lin Z, Parzynski CS, Suter LG, Krumholz HM, Lieberman JR, Berry DJ, Bucholz R, Han L, Rapp MT, Bernheim S, Drye EE. Variation in hospital-level risk-standardized complication rates following elective primary total hip and knee arthroplasty. J Bone Joint Surg Am. 2014;96A:640–7.
2. Le DH, Goodman SB, Maloney WJ, Huddleston JI. Current modes of failure in TKA: infection, instability, and stiffness predominate. Clin Orthop. 2014;472:2197–200.
3. Springer BD, Scuderi GR. Evaluation and management of the infected total knee arthroplasty. Instr Course Lect. 2013;62:349–61.
4. Vanhegan IS, Morgan-Jones R, Barrett DS, Haddad FS. Developing a strategy to treat established infection in total knee replacement: a review of the latest evidence and clinical practice. J Bone Joint Surg (Br). 2012;94B:875–81.
5. Poultsides LA, Ma Y, Della Valle AG, Chiu YL, Sculco TP, Memtsoudis SG. In-hospital surgical site infections after primary hip and knee arthroplasty. Incidence and risk factors. J Arthroplasty. 2013;28:385–9.
6. Kurtz SM, Lau E, Watson H, Schmier JK, Parvizi J. Economic burden of periprosthetic joint infection in the United States. J Arthroplasty. 2012;27(8S):61–5.
7. Poultsides LA, Liaropoulos LL, Malizos KN. The socioeconomic impact of musculoskeletal infections. J Bone Joint Surg Am. 2010;92:e13.
8. Bhaveen H, Kapadia BH, McElroy MJ, Issa K, Johnson AJ, Bozic KJ, Mont MA. The economic impact of periprosthetic infections following total knee arthroplasty at a specialized tertiary-care center. J Arthroplasty. 2014;29:929–32.
9. Chen J, Cui Y, Li X, Miao X, Wen Z, Xue Y, Tian J. Risk factors for deep infection after total knee arthroplasty: a meta-analysis. Arch Orthop Trauma Surg. 2013;133:675–87.
10. Simmons TD, Stern SH. Diagnosis and management of the infected total knee arthroplasty. Am J Knee Surg. 1996;9:99–106.
11. Parkinson RW, Kay PR, Rawal A. A case for one-stage revision in infected total knee arthroplasty? Knee. 2011;18:1–4.
12. Bjerke-Kroll BT, Christ AB, McLawhorn AS, Sculco PK, Jules-Elysée KM, Sculco TP. Periprosthetic joint infections treated with two-stage revision over 14 years: an evolving microbiology profile. J Arthroplasty. 2014;29:877–82.
13. Garvin KL, Cordero GX. Infected total knee arthroplasty: diagnosis and treatment. Instr Course Lect. 2008;57:305–15.
14. Burnett RS, Kelly MA, Hanssen AD, Barrack RL. Technique and timing of two-stage exchange for infection in TKA. Clin Orthop. 2007;464:164–78.
15. Moyad TF, Thornhill T, Estok D. Evaluation and management of the infected total hip and knee. Orthopedics. 2008;31:581–8.
16. Mihalko WM, Manaswi A, Cui Q, Parvizi J, Schmalzried TP, Saleh KJ. Diagnosis and treatment of the infected primary total knee arthroplasty. Instr Course Lect. 2008;57:327–39.
17. Leone JM, Hanssen AD. Management of infection at the site of a total knee arthroplasty. J Bone Joint Surg Am. 2005;87A:2335–48.
18. Munjal S, Phillips MJ, Krackow KA. Revision total knee arthroplasty: planning, controversies, and management infection. Instr Course Lect. 2001;50:367–77.
19. McPherson EL, Woodson C, Holtom P, Roidis N, Shufelt C, Patzakis M. Periprosthetic total hip infection. Outcomes using a staging system. Clin Orthop. 2002;403:8–15.
20. Parvizi J. International consensus on periprosthetic joint infection: what was discussed and decided. Am J Orthop. 2013;42:542–3.

21. Francolini I, Donelli G. Prevention and control of biofilm-based medical device related infections. Immunol Med Microbiol. 2010;59:227–38.

22. Costerton JW, Montanaro L, Arciola CR. Biofilm in implant infections: its production and regulation. Int J Artif Organs. 2005;28:1062–8.

23. Kalore NV, Gioe TJ, Singh JA. Diagnosis and management of infected total knee arthroplasty. Open Orthop J. 2011;5:86–91.

24. Windsor RE. Management of total knee arthroplasty infection. Orthop Clin N Am. 1999;22:531–8.

25. Chung JY, Ha CW, Park YB, Song YJ, Yu KS. Arthroscopic debridement for acutely infected prosthetic knee: any role for infection control and prosthesis salvage? Arthroscopy. 2014;30:599–606.

26. Jenny JY, Barbe B, Gaudias J, Boeri C, Argenson JN. High infection control rate and function after routine one-stage exchange for chronically infected TKA. Clin Orthop. 2013;471:238–43.

27. Göksan SB, Freeman MA. One-stage reimplantation for infected total knee arthroplasty. J Bone Joint Surg (Br). 1992;74B:78–82.

28. Buechel FF, Femino FR, D'Alessio J. Primary exchange revision arthroplasty for infected total knee replacement: a long-term study. Am J Orthop. 2004;33:190–8.

29. Von Foerster G, Kluber D, Kabler U. Mid-to long-term results after treatment of 118 cases of periprosthetic infections after knee joint replacement using one-stage exchange surgery. Orthopade. 1991;20:244–52.

30. Bauer T, Piriou P, Lhotellier L, Leclerc P, Mamoudy P, Lortat-Jacob A. Results of reimplantation for infected total knee arthroplasty. 107 cases. Rev Chir Orthop Reparatrice Appar Mot. 2006;92:692–700.

31. Lu H, Kou B, Lin J. One-stage reimplantation for the salvage of total knee arthroplasty complicated by infection. Chin J Surg. 1997;35:456–8.

32. Scott IR, Stockley I, Getty CJ. Exchange arthroplasty for infected knee replacements: a new two-stage method. J Bone Joint Surg (Br). 1993;75B:28–31.

33. Cuckler JM. The infected total knee: management options. J Arthroplasty. 2005;20(4S):33.

34. Sherrell JC, Fehring TK, Odum S, Hansen E, Zmistowski B, Dennos A. Periprosthetic Infection Consortium. The Chitranjan Ranawat Award. Fate of two-stage reimplantation after failed irrigation and débridement for periprosthetic knee infection. Clin Orthop. 2011;469:18–25.

35. Westrich GH, Walcott-Sapp S, Bornstein LJ, Bostrom MP, Windsor RE, Brause BD. Modern treatment of infected total knee arthroplasty with a 2-stage reimplantation protocol. J Arthroplasty. 2010;25:1015–21.

36. Tigani D, Trisolino G, Fosco M, Ben Ayad R, Costigliola P. Two-stage reimplantation for periprosthetic knee infection: influence of host health status and infecting microorganism. Knee. 2013;20:9–18.

37. Ocguder A, Firat A, Tecimel O, Solak S, Bozkurt M. Two-stage total infected knee arthroplasty treatment with articulating cement spacer. Arch Orthop Trauma Surg. 2010;130:719–25.

38. Mahmud T, Lyons MC, Naudie DD, Macdonald SJ, McCalden RW. Assessing the gold standard: a review of 253 two-stage revisions for infected TKA. Clin Orthop. 2012;470:2730–6.

39. Insall JN, Thompson FM, Brause BD. Two-stage reimplantation for the salvage of infected total knee arthroplasty. J Bone Joint Surg Am. 1983;65A:1087–98.

40. Kuzyk PR, Dhotar HS, Sternheim A, Gross AE, Safir O, Backstein D. Two-stage revision arthroplasty for management of chronic periprosthetic hip and knee infection: techniques, controversies, and outcomes. J Am Acad Orthop Surg. 2014;22:153–64.

41. Thabe H, Schill S. Two-stage reimplantation with an application spacer and combined with delivery of antibiotics in the management of prosthetic joint infection. Oper Orthop Traumatol. 2007;19:78–100.

42. Goldman RT, Scuderi GR, Insall JN. Two-stage reimplantation for infected total knee replacement. Clin Orthop. 1996;331:118–24.

43. Haleem AA, Berry DJ, Hanssen AD. Mid-term to long-term follow-up of two-stage reimplantation for infected total knee arthroplasty. Clin Orthop. 2004;428:35–9.

44. Kösters K, van Crevel R, Sturm PD, Willem Schreurs B, de Waal Malefijt MC, van Kampen A, Kullberg BJ. Treatment of knee prosthesis infections: evaluation of 15 patients over a 5-year period. Int Orthop. 2009;33:1249–54.

45. Romano CL, Gala L, Logoluso N, Romanò D, Drago L. Two-stage revision of septic knee prosthesis with articulating knee spacers yields better infection eradication rate than one-stage or two-stage revision with static spacers. Knee Surg Sports Traumatol Arthrosc. 2012;20:2445–53.

46. Pivec R, Naziri Q, Issa K, Banerjee S, Mont MA. Systematic review comparing static and articulating spacers used for revision of infected total knee arthroplasty. J Arthroplasty. 2014;29:553–7.

47. Shaikh AA, Ha CW, Park YG, Park YB. Two-stage approach to primary TKA in infected arthritic knees using intraoperatively molded articulating cement spacers. Clin Orthop. 2014;472:2201–7.

48. Guild GN, Wu B, Scuderi GR. Articulating vs. static antibiotic impregnated spacers in revision total knee arthroplasty for sepsis. A systematic review. J Arthroplasty. 2014;29:558–63.

49. Insall JN, Dorr LD, Scott RD, Scott WN. Rationale of the knee society clinical rating system. Clin Orthop. 1989;248:13–4.

50. Wilde AH, Ruth JT. Two-stage reimplantation in infected total knee arthroplasty. Clin Orthop. 1988;236:23–35.

51. Booth RE, Lotke PA. The results of spacer block technique in revision of infected total knee arthroplasty. Clin Orthop. 1989;248:57–60.

52. Teeny SM, Dorr L, Murata G, Conaty P. Treatment of infected total knee arthroplasty. J Arthroplasty. 1990;5:35–9.

53. Wilson MG, Kelley K, Thornhill TS. Infection as a complication of total knee-replacement arthroplasty. J Bone Joint Surg Am. 1990;72A:878–83.

54. Masri BA, Kendall RW, Duncan CP, Beauchamp CP, McGraw RW, Bora B. Two-stage exchange arthroplasty using a functional antibiotic-loaded spacer in the treatment of the infected knee replacement: the Vancouver experience. Semin Arthroplasty. 1994;5:122–36.
55. Hirakawa K, Stulberg BN, Wilde AH, Bauer TW, Secic M. Results of 2-stage reimplantation for infected total knee arthroplasty. J Arthroplasty. 1998;13:22–8.
56. Fehring TK, Odum S, Calton TF, Mason JB. Articulating versus static spacers in revision total knee arthroplasty for sepsis. The Ranawat award. Clin Orthop. 2000;380:9–16.
57. Durbhakula SM, Czajka J, Fuchs MD, Uhl RL. Antibiotic-loaded articulating cement spacer in the 2-stage exchange of infected total knee arthroplasty. J Arthroplasty. 2004;19:768–74.
58. Hofmann AA, Kane KR, Tkach TK, Plaster RL, Camargo MP. Treatment of infected total knee arthroplasty using an articulating spacer. Clin Orthop. 1995;321:45–54.
59. Hart WJ, Jones RS. Two-stage revision of infected total knee replacements using articulating cement spacers and short- term antibiotic therapy. J Bone Joint Surg (Br). 2006;88B:1011–5.
60. Kurd M, Ghanem E, Steinbrecher J, Parvizi J. Two-stage exchange knee arthroplasty. Does resistance of the infecting organism influence the outcome? Clin Orthop. 2010;468:2060–6.
61. Maheshwari AV, Gioe TJ, Kalore NV, Cheng EY. Reinfection after prior staged reimplantation for septic total knee arthroplasty: is salvage still possible? J Arthroplasty. 2010;25(6S):92–7.
62. Mortazavi SM, Schwartzenberger J, Austin MS, Purtill JJ, Parvizi J. Revision total knee arthroplasty infection: incidence and predictors. Clin Orthop. 2010;468:2052–9.

Kyriakos Avramidis and Theofilos Karachalios

Introduction

Total knee arthroplasty (TKA) is the most common procedure performed for end stage osteoarthritis (OA) in older individuals. Current data from 21 European countries reveal that the annual incidence of TKA is 109 procedures per 100,000 persons, which is more than twice that reported in 1998 [1]. TKA reliably reduces pain and improves function in patients with knee OA and 90 % of patients report reduced pain, improved functional ability and greater health related quality of life after surgery [2]. Moreover, 85 % of patients who undergo TKA report being satisfied with the outcome [2]. Despite the well documented success of this procedure, patients continue to demonstrate physical impairment and functional limitations following TKA compared with individuals without knee disease [3]. One month after TKA quadriceps strength drops to 60 % of preoperative

K. Avramidis, MD, DSc
Orthopaedic Department,
General Hospital of Larissa,
Larissa, Hellenic Republic

T. Karachalios, MD, DSc (✉)
Orthopaedic Department, Faculty of Medicine,
School of Health Sciences,
Center of Biomedical Sciences (CERETETH),
University of Thessalia,
University General Hospital of Larissa,
Mezourlo region, Larissa 41110, Hellenic Republic
e-mail: kar@med.uth.gr

levels, even when traditional postoperative rehabilitation is initiated within 48 h after surgery [4, 5]. This quadriceps weakness persists years after surgery, based on comparisons with age-matched controls [6]. Similarly, functional performance is reported to worsen by 20–25 % 1 month after TKA [7] and reduced function persists with reports of 18 % slower walking speed and 51 % slower stair-climbing speed compared to age-matched controls at 12 months after TKA [3]. Despite these documented impairments and activity limitations, there is little evidence to support the introduction of structured rehabilitation to this population. In 2003, the National Institute of Health (NIH) concluded that "the use of rehabilitation services is perhaps the most understudied aspect of the perioperative management of TKA patients" and "there is no evidence supporting the generalized use of any specific preoperative or postoperative rehabilitation intervention" [2]. Currently, there is no universally accepted rehabilitation protocol for patients after TKA and rehabilitation paradigms are often institution or surgeon specific [8, 9].

In 2007, the most recent meta-analysis on the effectiveness of physical therapy following TKA concluded that physical therapy has no long-term benefits [10]. However, these conclusions were based on only five studies that met the inclusion criteria for the meta-analysis. Potential reasons for the lack of demonstrated efficacy of these trials are the following: (a) none of the included

© Springer-Verlag London 2015
T. Karachalios (ed.), *Total Knee Arthroplasty: Long Term Outcomes*,
DOI 10.1007/978-1-4471-6660-3_23

trials examined the use of a high intensity, long duration rehabilitation program initiated after discharge from hospital, (b) trials in which the intervention consisted of an electrical adjunct to physiotherapy such as the use of continuous passive motion (CPM) or neuromuscular electrical stimulation (NMES) were excluded.

The purpose of this review is to thoroughly evaluate randomized controlled trials (RCTs) and other quality studies in order to determine the effectiveness of structured and systematic postoperative rehabilitation on the short and long term functional recovery of patients after TKA.

Strengthening Interventions

Loss of quadriceps strength after TKA has been documented extensively [4–7]. However, recent studies suggest that hamstring muscle dysfunction [11] and hip abductor muscle weakness [12] are also present after the operation and should be addressed during rehabilitation. Rehabilitation programs which incorporate higher intensity, progressive resistive exercises that target all major muscle groups of the lower extremity have demonstrated superior mid-term [13] and long-term [14–16] strength and functional gains compared with lower intensity programs. Moffet et al. [13] has evaluated the effectiveness of an intensive functional rehabilitation (IFR) program on the functional ability and quality of life (QOL) of patients who underwent primary TKA. Two months after the operation, subjects were randomly assigned to either a group with IFR (n=38) who received 12 supervised rehabilitation sessions combined with home exercises between months 2 and 4 after TKA, or to a control group (n=39) who received standard care. The specific strengthening exercises, performed in a supine or seated position, consisted of maximal isometric pain free contractions (knee extensors and flexors) at different angles of knee flexion and dynamic (concentric-eccentric) contractions against gravity (hip abductors). All participants were evaluated at baseline (2 months after TKA), immediately after IFR (4 months after TKA) and 2 and 8 months later (6 and 12 months after

TKA). The primary outcome measure was the 6 min walk test (6-MWT) at different time intervals, the WOMAC pain score, WOMAC difficulty score and SF-36 Health Survey. Patients in the IFR group walked significantly longer distances in 6 min and had less pain, stiffness and difficulty in performing daily activities compared to controls. Positive changes in QOL (PCS, MCS) in favor of the IFR group were also observed. The authors conclude that IFR was effective in improving short and mid-term functional ability after uncomplicated primary TKA, and suggest that in order to maintain these functional improvements in the long term (1 year post-surgery), more intensive rehabilitation should be introduced during the sub-acute recovery period (2–4 months after TKA). In a recent RCT, Petterson et al. [14] applied a progressive muscle strengthening protocol with or without the addition of NMES commencing 3–4 weeks after TKA and compared these two groups of patients (Exercise group and Exercise-NMES group, 100 patients each) to an embedded cohort of patients (control group) who received "standard rehabilitation" focused on functional training. The active treatment groups received two to three sessions of outpatient physical therapy per week for a total of 6 weeks. Treatment effects were evaluated by a burst superimposition test to assess quadriceps strength, knee range of motion (ROM), timed up and go test (TUG), stair climbing test (SCT) and 6 min walk (6-MW) measurements, SF-36 as well as completion of the knee outcome survey activities of daily living scale (KOS-ADLS) at 3 and 12 months postoperatively. There were no significant differences between the exercise and exercise-NMES groups on any outcome measure at 3 and 12 months (P>0.08); however, both groups significantly improved on all scales from baseline to 3 and 12 months (P<0.001 for all) compared to controls, with the exception of the mental component score (MCS) of the SF-36 which only improved from 0 to 3 months. In other words, strength, activation and function were similar between the exercise and exercise-NMES groups at 3 and 12 months. The standard care group was weaker and exhibited worse function at 12 months compared to both treatment groups. The authors therefore conclude that progressive lower limb muscle strengthening can enhance clinical improvement after TKA, achieving similar short and long term functional recovery approaching the functional level of healthy older adults. The above studies [13, 14] applied high intensity programs 2 and 1 month after surgery, when strength and functional deficits were already profound [3–5], based mainly on concerns related to the assumption that a higher intensity intervention initiated immediately following hospital discharge, could lead to increased pain and swelling and ultimately to poorer ROM and functional outcomes. Bade et al. [16] in another recent RCT, attempts to assess clinical outcomes of a long duration IFR program initiated immediately after discharge from hospital in eight TKA patients. Effects were compared to those of a control group of another eight patients who participated in a lower intensity rehabilitation program. At the 3.5 and 12 week (end of rehabilitation) time points, patients in the IFR group had better functional performance and greater quadriceps strength compared to the control group and this improvement was maintained at 52 weeks. The high intensity program did not impair knee ROM and did not result in any musculoskeletal injuries in this small group of patients. Evgeniadis et al. [17] reports that TKA patients discharged from an 8 week home supervised strengthening exercise program had significantly greater knee flexion and extension active ROM compared to a control group who received only inpatient rehabilitation (mean flexion 98.42 and 80.42° and mean extension −0.8° and −6.42° respectively) 14 weeks after surgery. This improvement of active ROM was accompanied by similar benefits in functional autonomy.

Whole body vibration (WBV) is an exercise mode which has been suggested in order to rehabilitate patients with lower extremity weaknesses and provide an alternative strengthening method in older patients who may not be able to perform standard exercise programs [18]. Johnson et al. [19] investigated the use of WBV as an alternative strengthening regimen in the rehabilitation of individuals after TKA, in comparison with traditional progressive resistance exercise (TPRE). Individuals, 3–6 weeks after TKA, received physical therapy with WBV or TPRE for 4 weeks. Knee extensor strength improved at a level of 84.3 % in the WBV and at a level of 77.3 % in the TPRE group. TUG scores improved at a level of 31 % in the WBV and at a level of 32 % in the TPRE group. There were no significant differences between groups for strength, muscle activation and mobility and no adverse effects were reported in either group. In this study both WBV and TPRE proved equally effective in improving strength and function during rehabilitation after TKA.

Continuous Passive Motion After TKA

The concept of continuous passive motion (CPM) was introduced into orthopaedics by Salter et al. in 1980 [20]. They studied the biologic effect of CPM on the healing of full thickness defects in rabbit knee articular cartilage and found it strikingly beneficial. Salter suggested that immobilization was detrimental to joints, motion was beneficial and CPM minimized forces across damaged joint surfaces. For motion to be continuous, it had to be applied passively, as muscles would fatigue with continuous active movement of a joint [20–22]. Encouraged by these studies, Coutts et al. [23] were the first to introduce continuous passive motion into the postoperative rehabilitation of patients undergoing TKA. They demonstrated improvement in the range of knee motion, reduction in the length of hospital stay and a dramatic decrease in the use of pain medication in a small group of patients receiving CPM for 20 h a day compared to controls who kept their knees immobilized for the first four postoperative days. After this study, the use of CPM devices after TKA increased dramatically and CPM has been widely used as an adjunct to physiotherapy after TKA for the past three decades. Despite this widespread use, however, studies on the effectiveness of CPM have not supported risk and benefit issues and its widespread use remains controversial. Earlier studies (before 2000) recommend its use [24–31], whereas more recent studies have found it to be less valuable in the rehabilitation of TKA [32–37]. Studies presented by Maloney [24], Johnson [25], McInnes [26] and Ververeli [27] have demonstrated a significant increase in the range of motion of the knee, at discharge, due to an increase in active flexion and a decrease in swelling. However, a longer term effect was not evident at 6 weeks, 3 months, 1 and 2 years after operation. At discharge, active knee extension was reported to be less and flexion contracture more in CPM treated knees [25, 27, 38]. This "extensor lag" was found to be transient and was attributed to flexor muscle stiffness and quadriceps muscle weakness of the knees subjected to CPM [38]. In all these studies which report faster knee recovery during the hospital stay, duration of CPM applications varied from 16 to 24 h per day and it was performed during the first 7 days after TKA. Moreover, knees in control groups were immobilized for 3–7 days in a splint, whereas the experimental groups received early postoperative CPM applications [23–29]. These results cannot be applied to contemporary practice because a long period of immobilization is no longer recommended and early movement is always promoted after TKA [35]. CPM is generally applied to patients after TKA during the postoperative hospitalization period (5–10 days) and current recommendations regarding the length of its application in order to attain treatment benefits are between 3 and 5 h in total per day [32]. However, in practice each session cannot last longer than 2 h because patients have to be allowed time for conventional physical therapy interventions, occupational therapy visits, nursing care and radiographic and medical assessments. Furthermore, they need time to achieve all of their rehabilitation goals, in addition to knee flexion, such as transferring and walking with aids, before being discharged [35]. Lenssen et al. [36] has investigated the effectiveness of prolonged CPM use at home for 17 consecutive days after surgery as an adjunct to standardized physiotherapy and found neither long term effects of this intervention nor transfer to better functional performance. Conflicting evidence exists with respect to the use of analgesics

for postoperative pain control in TKA patients using CPM. Colwell and Morris [28] reported a statistically significant decrease in the use of narcotic analgesics in patients using a CPM device in a small RCT study, whereas Pope et al. [29] in a larger, more recent, RCT study comparing three groups of patients (no CPM, CPM of 0–40° and CPM of 0–70°) detected a significant increase of analgesic requirement in the two groups who had CPM. Pope's study also demonstrates significantly increased mean blood drainage postoperatively in the high flexion group who had CPM of 0–70° (1,558 ml) compared with the "no CPM" group (956 ml) and the 0–40° CPM group (1,017 ml).

There is controversy concerning the effect of CPM on the incidence of deep vein thrombosis (DVT) after TKA. Many authors have not found any difference in DVT with CPM applications [27, 32, 39], whereas others have found less DVT in CPM application groups, although this finding may be attributed to the fact that control knees were immobilized [30, 40]. Coutts et al. [30] has presented a multi-center study, in 1983, comparing manipulation rates after TKA in a CPM group (137) and a control group (129) of patients. They reported no manipulations in the active treatment group, while 21 % of the knees in the control group required manipulation. Subsequent studies [27, 31, 41] also support the use of continuous passive motion in order to decrease the rate of manipulation (and its costs) for poor range of motion after TKA. The effects of CPM on the healing process after TKA remain controversial. Wound swelling has been reported to be decreased with the use of CPM after TKA [30, 38]. A wound complication is defined as an infection or other condition that necessitates a change in the postoperative regimen. According to this definition Maloney et al. [24] have reported an increased incidence of wound complications in a series of CPM application after TKA, mainly haematomas, superficial and deep wound infections. Davis [42] report increased aseptic wound drainage with the use of CPM. Conflicting reports by Bennett [43] and Colwell and Morris [28] show no significant difference in wound drainage. Johnson et al., in his landmark paper [25], measured the transcutaneous oxygen tension of knee wounds and found decreased viability of the edges of the wound (particularly the lateral edge) with knee flexion beyond 40° during the first three post-operative days. On the basis of these results, a protocol was designed for CPM to minimize the detrimental effects on wound viability. This protocol included restricting flexion of the knee from 0 to 40° for the first three postoperative days and then slowly increasing the range of motion by daily increments to reach 90° on the sixth day. The CPM machine was removed on the seventh day. In Johnson et al.'s study 102 patients undergoing TKA were randomly assigned to an immediate CPM group which followed the above protocol and a control group which had their knees immobilized in a splint for 7 days. There was no difference in the incidence of infection or wound healing between the two groups, demonstrating that if CPM is not aggressive, the incidence of problems with wound healing will not increase. Speed of CPM made little difference in terms of wound viability, although a setting of one cycle per minute maximized oxygenation without the discomfort associated with faster settings.

Aquatic Therapy

In Europe aquatic therapy, such as pool exercise, is commonly used in the aftercare of patients following TKA. Proponents of water based rehabilitation protocols argue that exercising in warm water may reduce stress on the joint and allow an individual to strengthen their lower extremity using water as resistance, while taking advantage of the weight reducing effects of buoyancy [44]. This weight reduction, in line with to Archimedes law, protects the joints and permits better movement, muscular reinforcement through proprioceptive mechanisms and accelerated mobilization of the operated limb [45]. Resistance to movement can be varied by changing the speed of motion and by increasing water turbulence. Because pool exercises require a continuous balance response, muscular coordination is improved. Patients overall report a sense of

pleasure and pain relief while exercising in water [44, 45]. Liebs et al. [44] has found that water based therapy can be safely started as early as 6 days after TKA, provided the wound is covered with a waterproof adhesive dressing (Op-Site). These authors have also shown that patients randomized to start water based therapy on the sixth postoperative day had better WOMAC, SF-36, and Lequense Knee scores 12 and 24 months after TKA, compared to patients who were randomized to start the same program on the 14th postoperative day. While these results were not statistically different between groups, the effect of the size of the intervention on WOMAC score was similar to the effect of nonsteroidal anti-inflammatory drugs on functional limitations associated with knee OA. The change in WOMAC score also exceeded the minimal clinically important difference cut-off of 24 months following surgery. The authors conclude that early aquatic therapy after TKA led to a clinically important improvement in patient outcomes when compared with late aquatic therapy. However, these authors used only self-reported measures of function and did not compare the outcomes of aquatic based therapy to other land-based rehabilitation programs. Valtonen et al. [46] analyzed the effect of a 12 week progressive aquatic resistance training program on mobility limitations (walking speed and stair ascending time), self-reported function (WOMAC), knee extensor and flexor power assessed isokinetically and quadriceps muscle cross sectional area (CSA) assessed by computed tomography. Fifty patients in the late stages of recovery after TKA (average 10 months postoperatively), were randomized to either an aquatic program group (26) in which progressive strengthening exercises were performed in the pool, or to a control group of patients (24) advised to maintain their usual physical activity level. At the end of the 12 week training program, subjects in the active treatment group had better knee flexion and extension power (48 % and 32 % respectively), greater thigh muscle CSA (3 %), faster habitual walking speed (9 %) and faster stair ascending time (15 %) compared to controls. No differences were found for WOMAC scores between groups.

The authors also evaluated the maintenance of observed aquatic training induced benefits at a follow up of 12 months after the end of the intervention [47]. At this 1 year observation period, knee extensor and flexor powers were still significantly higher (32 % and 50 % respectively) in the active treatment group compared to the control group, while all the significant 12 week improvements in muscle CSA, walking speed and stair ascending time had been lost. The authors suggest that aquatic resistance training should be continued to maintain the training induced benefits on mobility. Harmer et al. [48] randomized 102 patients scheduled for TKA to receive either land based (49) or water based (53) physical therapy, commencing 2 weeks after surgery. Both groups attended 1 h sessions twice a week for 6 weeks. The same therapist supervised both water and land based treatment and the exercise prescription was highly standardized to ensure that the only difference between treatment groups was the medium (water versus land). Patients were evaluated 8 and 26 weeks after TKA and there were no differences between groups for WOMAC score, knee ROM, 6 min walk test and stair climbing power (SCP), although both groups demonstrated significant improvement compared to baseline. The authors conclude that water-based therapy was not particularly advantageous with respect to functional outcome or clinical metrics, although it may be a valid alternative treatment for rehabilitation after TKA.

Balance Training

Impairment of balance is a serious problem in fully recovered TKA patients [49] along with persistent muscle weakness [3, 6]. After TKA patients are at a higher risk of falling and sustaining further orthopaedic injury [50, 51]. During a 6 month observational period of a cohort of patients 6–12 months following their TKA, Matsumoto et al. [50] identified a 32.9 % incidence of fall. Swinkels et al. [51] reported a recent preoperative history of falling to be common (24.2 %) in people undergoing TKA and

approximately 45 % of these patients fell again in the year following surgery. Therefore, resolving balance impairments after TKA, should be an important goal of physical therapy. Two studies with similar methodology have assessed the effectiveness of adding specific balance exercises (agility and perturbation techniques) to a functional training (FT) protocol. Piva et al. [52] has compared the effects of balance training (B) and function training (FT) on mobility outcome in small sample groups. The interventions were 6 weeks of supervised FT or FT + B program, followed by a 4 month home exercise program. Outcome data were collected at baseline, after completion of the supervised program (2 months) and at completion of the 4 month home exercise period (6 months after randomization). Both groups demonstrated clinically important improvements in lower extremity functional status. Differences between groups did not have adequate power to demonstrate statistical significance; however, the degree of improvement seemed higher for gait speed, single leg stance time and stiffness in the FT + B group compared with the FT group. Liao et al. [53] has found that the addition of 8 weeks of balance exercises to a postoperative rehabilitation program significantly improved (at the end of the intervention) functional forward reach, single leg stance, sit to stand test, stair climbing time, 10 min walk time, timed up and go scores and the WOMAC Index scores to a greater extent than a control group which did not receive balance retraining exercises (all P<0.001). It should be noted that Liao et al. had a larger sample size (130 versus 43 patients) and longer intervention (8 versus 6 weeks) than the study by Piva et al. Additionally, patients randomized to receive balance retraining in Liao's study also had longer session duration than subjects of the control group in the same study (up to 90 min versus 60 min). The authors conclude that 8 weeks of additional balance training can improve functional performance in mobility after TKA. Fung et al. [54] tested the use of an integrated Wii Fit™ commercially available motion controlled video game system [55] in the rehabilitation of outpatients following TKA. In addition to standard therapy, subjects randomized to the active treatment group (27) received 15 min of Wii Fit™ gaming activity, while the control group (23) received 15 min of additional lower extremity exercise. There were no differences between groups for active knee flexion and extension, distance covered in the 2 min walk test, numeric pain rating scale, activity specific balance confidence scale, lower extremity functional scale or length of outpatient rehabilitation. These findings suggest that the addition of Wii Fit™ as an alternative to lower extremity strengthening may be an appropriate rehabilitation tool.

Neuromuscular Electrical Stimulation (NMES)

One month after TKA impairment in quadriceps muscle strength is predominantly due to central activation deficits (also referred to as "reflex inhibition"), but is also influenced to a lesser degree by muscle atrophy [4, 5, 56]. Although the neurophysiologic mechanisms for quadriceps muscle voluntary activation deficits are not fully understood, spinal reflex activity from pain or effusion in the knee joint may alter afferent input from the injured joint and result in diminished efferent motor drive to the quadriceps muscle that reduces muscle strength [57]. Early studies by Gibson [58] and Martin [59] demonstrated that neuromuscular electrical stimulation (NMES) can prevent muscle atrophy in patients with knee OA who are awaiting or recovering from TKA. Recent studies by Thomas [60] and Stevens [61] have demonstrated the potential of NMES to mitigate voluntary activation deficits and prevent muscle atrophy early after surgery, thus restoring normal quadriceps muscle function more effectively than voluntary exercise alone. How NMES improves muscle strength is unclear, though some theories have emerged. Firstly, the intensity of the muscle contraction produced during stimulation may be greater than that without NMES (at least 30–50 % of maximal voluntary effort), thus overloading the muscle sufficiently to induce strength gains [60]. Secondly, NMES may alter motor recruitment inducing activation of a greater proportion

of type II muscle fibers which are larger than type I, so greater activation of type II fibers maximizes force production [62]. Results of studies applying NMES to the quadriceps muscle of patients after TKA are promising. Gotlin et al. [63] randomized 40 patients who underwent TKA to either a control group (19) or an NMES group (21). Both groups received conventional physical therapy including CPM to the affected limb, ambulation training, ROM exercises and activities of daily living (ADL) training. Within the first postoperative week, the active treatment group additionally received, twice daily for 1 h during CPM treatment, electrical stimulation (frequency of 35 Hz, stimulation time 15 s followed by a 10 s rest interval) with electrodes placed over the proximal femoral nerve and the distal vastus medialis obliquus (VMO) muscle. Active treatment group patients reduced their extensor lag from 7.5 to 5.7°, whereas control group extensor lag increased from 5.3 to 8.3° in the same time frame. These trends were significantly different (p < 0.01). In addition, NMES patients had a significantly different (p < 0.05) length of hospital stay (7.4–6.7 days). As the greatest loss of quadriceps strength occurs in the first month following TKA [4, 5], Avramidis et al. [64] examined the use of NMES on the quadriceps muscle of the operated limb for the first six postoperative weeks in addition to standard physical therapy and demonstrated a statistically significant improvement in patients' walking speed at 6 weeks (p = 0.0002) as well as a "carry over" effect 6 weeks after discontinuation of treatment (12 weeks after the operation, p < 0.0001). Based on this original study, the same author also attempted to investigate the long term effect of this intervention 1 year after TKA, at which time most of the patients' functional improvement was expected to have occurred [65]. Seventy patients who underwent TKA were randomly assigned to either an NMES group (35) receiving electrical stimulation of the vastus medialis muscle in addition to a traditional physical therapy program or a control group (35) who followed only the same physical therapy protocol, for 6 weeks. NMES was initiated on postoperative day 2 and was applied twice a day for 2 h on each occasion

(4 h total daily treatment) while the patient was lying in bed or sitting. The neuromuscular stimulator was set to 40 Hz, a pulse duration of 300 µs and an 8 s on time followed by an 8 s rest time with the current intensity set at the patient's maximum tolerance. Compared with the control group the NMES group demonstrated faster walking speeds and better scores on the Oxford Knee Score and American Knee Society function score at 6 and 12 weeks following TKA; however, differences between groups were no longer significant at 52 weeks. The NMES group also had significantly better SF-36 physical component (PCS) scores at 6, 12 and 52 weeks postoperatively compared to the control group. These gains were secondary to an initial faster recovery of quadriceps muscle strength and subsequent ability to participate more fully in the voluntary exercise program. No complications were associated with the use of NMES beginning on postoperative day 2, although 3 of the 38 originally recruited patients in the NMES group abandoned use of the stimulator due to discomfort, thus leaving the group with 35 patients who attended subsequent follow up evaluations. In a similar study, Stevens-Lapsley et al. [66, 67] examined the use of NMES to the quadriceps muscle early after TKA utilizing a randomized, unblinded study design. Sixty-six patients undergoing TKA were randomly assigned to receive either standard rehabilitation (control group) or standard rehabilitation plus NMES applied to the quadriceps muscle. Electrical stimulation treatment began on postoperative day 2, continued for 6 weeks and was applied twice per day for 15 isometric contractions on each occasion (a total of only 30 min per day). The stimulator was set to deliver a biphasic current, using a symmetrical waveform, at 50 Hz and a pulse duration of 250 µs, for a 15 s on phase followed by a 45 s rest time with the current intensity set at the patient's maximum tolerance. Data for muscle strength, functional performance and self-report measures (WOMAC Index) were obtained before surgery and at 3.5, 6.5, 13, 26, and 52 postoperative weeks. Compared with the control group, the NMES group demonstrated superior quadriceps strength, hamstring strength, 6 min walking distances,

TUG times, SCT times, and active knee extension at 3.5 weeks after TKA. No differences between groups were noted for changes in the SF-36 (MCS and PCS) and WOMAC scores. At 52 weeks, differences between groups were attenuated but remained significant (favoring NMES) for quadriceps and hamstring muscle strength, TUG, SCT, 6MWT, SF-36 MCS and WOMAC scores. Improvement in active extension ROM tended to be better in the NMES group (p = 0.08). Similarly to the previous study, no adverse events were observed with the utilization of NMES beginning on postoperative day 2. A key observation from the Stevens-Lapsley et al. [66, 67] trial was that patients who were capable of achieving higher stimulation training intensities had greater quadriceps muscle strength and activation gains compared with those utilizing lower intensities. Therefore, increasing the comfort of NMES to accomplish this goal seems to play a role. Electrode size is important because it has a direct effect on current density, with smaller electrodes resulting in higher current density and potentially uncomfortable stimulation before reaching maximum muscle contraction torque. In both Avramidis's and Stevens-Lapsley's studies electrodes were applied to the skin over the vastus medialis muscle and lateral side of the thigh and connected to the "active" and "indifferent" leads respectively. Avramidis et al. [65] utilized 70 × 70 mm electrodes (Pals Plus, Nidd Valley Med., Knaresborough, UK), a shorter rest time (8 s), and longer NMES treatment duration of 2 h per session, whereas Stevens-Lapsley et al. [66, 67] utilized larger 76 × 127 mm electrodes (Supertrodes, SME Inc., Wilmington, USA), as well as longer rest-times (45 s) and shorter NMES treatment times of 15 min per session. These differences may have enabled patients to achieve higher stimulation intensities and, thus, greater strength gains, which may explain why the trial by Stevens-Lapsley et al. [66, 67] observed long term benefits in addition to short term benefits. Though the results of several investigations indicate NMES may be beneficial following TKA, Petterson's recent randomized clinical trial [14] comparing (a) Exercise and (b) Exercise + NMES suggests that NMES (ten contractions, twice per week for 6 weeks) initiated 1 month postoperatively, may not be any more beneficial than exercise alone. Specifically, the authors noted no differences between the exercise and exercise + NMES groups in quadriceps strength, activation or function at 3 and 12 months after TKA. Both groups, however, had better strength, activation and function 12 months postoperatively compared to a cohort receiving less intensive rehabilitation in the community. These results suggest that the timing and frequency of NMES treatment may be critical to patient outcomes. In this study, had the use of NMES commenced immediately after surgery it may have proved more effective, because preventing the early (within the first month) decline of muscle function is likely to be more effective than working to reverse losses after they occur. It is also possible that the frequency of NMES application (two times per week) may not have been sufficient to induce changes in quadriceps muscle strength and activation. In conclusion, early use of NMES (within the first month after TKA) and NMES delivered more than twice per week may be necessary.

Out-Patient Clinic and Home Based Therapy

Physical therapy conducted in an outpatient clinic allows the therapist to directly monitor patient progress and adjust the intervention to the patients' functional status. However, it is more expensive than home based rehabilitation programs and requires that the patient travel to the clinic, which may be difficult for an elderly population. Rajan et al. [68] randomized 120 patients and found no statistically significant benefit of outpatient physiotherapy in knee ROM at 3, 6 months and 1 year after TKA. Mockford et al. [69] randomized 150 patients into a group which received outpatient physiotherapy for 6 weeks and another group receiving no outpatient physiotherapy. No differences between groups were found for flexion and extension ROM, Oxford Knee Score (OKS), Bartlett patellar score (BPS) or SF-12 general health questionnaire 1 year after surgery. The conclusions drawn by Rajan et al. that there is "no need for outpatient physiotherapy after TKA" and by Mockford et al. that "a standard routine course of outpatient physiotherapy does not offer any benefit in the long term to patients undergoing TKA" are not supported by the methodologies and results from these studies. Unfortunately, however, in neither study was there standardization or a description of the protocol or duration of the outpatient physical therapy intervention, and only ROM and self-reported outcomes were assessed to make determinations about the effectiveness of outpatient rehabilitation. Additionally, 1 year after surgery patients in both studies had knee flexion range of motion ($97°$ and $108°$) which was lower than the cut off for functional range of motion ($110°$) and less than the $120°$ reported by Petterson et al. [14], suggesting that these patients were under-rehabilitated. In order to determine the effectiveness of home based therapy monitored via periodic telephone calls from a physical therapist, Kramer et al. [70] randomized 160 patients to receive either clinic based or home based therapy. Both groups were given two booklets of ROM and strengthening exercises with the prescription to perform them at home three times daily until their 12 week follow up, at which time they were advised to continue the home exercises at least once daily, indefinitely. A physical therapist familiar with the protocol evaluated the home based group weekly in order to monitor adherence and compliance with the protocol. The clinic based group attended outpatient therapy between weeks 2 and 12 after surgery, for two sessions per week of 1 h duration each and patients completed the common home exercises only twice on days that they attended clinic sessions. At the 12th and 52nd week follow-up, values for WOMAC, SF-36, 6 m walking, 30 s stair test, knee flexion ROM, and Knee Society clinical rating scale were significantly better compared to baseline in both groups and there was no relative advantage of one group over the other. Madsen et al. [71] compared late clinic based and home based rehabilitation, commencing 4–8 weeks after TKA. They allocated 80 patients undergoing the operation to either group based rehabilitation

(40) or individual, supervised home training (40). The group based rehabilitation consisted of 12 outpatient visits over 6 weeks, including strength-endurance exercises, education and self-management combined with home exercises. The control group performed home exercises, received an initial visit of a physical therapist in which the training program was adjusted to each individual's needs and one or two additional visits during the treatment period to further adjust the program. Three and 6 months after TKA, there were no differences between groups, after adjusting for baseline values, for self-reported measures (Oxford Knee Score, the physical function part of the SF-36, EuroQol-5 Dimensions), impairment metrics (leg extensor power, pain level during the power test) and performance metrics (tandem test for balance, 10 m walking test, 30-s and five times sit to stand tests). The authors conclude that individual, supervised home training and group based rehabilitation programs improved patients' quality of life and physical function equally 6 months after TKA.

Russell et al. [72] has evaluated the equivalence of an internet based tele rehabilitation program compared with conventional outpatient physical therapy for patients following TKA in Australia. Access to rehabilitation may be difficult for patients who live in rural or remote areas and one possible solution is the use of tele rehabilitation technology to enable delivery of such service from a distance. In this study 65 patients were randomized to receive a 6 week program of outpatient physical therapy either in the conventional manner or by means of an Internet based tele rehabilitation program. The primary outcome measure was the WOMAC score and secondary outcomes included the Patient Specific Functional Scale, TUG test, pain intensity, knee flexion and extension, quadriceps muscle strength, limb girth measurements and an assessment of gait. After the 6 week intervention, participants of both groups had significant improvement on all outcome measures (p < 0.01 for all); however, differences between groups were not significant for most of the above outcomes with the exception of the Patient Specific Functional Scale and the stiff-

ness subscale of the WOMAC for which results were better in the tele rehabilitation group (p = 0.04). Despite the lack of between group differences, both groups were under rehabilitated; patients had residual knee flexion contractures and quadriceps lag on active knee extension, indicating significant residual weakness. Moreover, TUG times in both groups were still greater than 12 s at the end of the study, nearly 45 % longer than the TUG times reported by Petterson et al. [14] 3 months after TKA and 30 % longer than the TUG times in the active treatment group reported by Stevens-Lapsley et al. [66, 67] 6.5 weeks after TKA. These results suggest that ROM, strength and functional impairment are not completely resolved with this type of postoperative treatment strategy. The authors also acknowledge a number of limitations in their study, such as an inability to estimate patient compliance with the tele rehabilitation intervention at home and the lack of long term outcomes (only 6 weeks follow-up). Future research is needed to better assess long term effects, as well as the fiscal impact of this alternative mode of remotely delivered physical therapy.

Kauppila et al. [73] has tested whether a 10 day multidisciplinary rehabilitation program was effective in achieving faster and greater functional recovery after TKA. Patients in the active treatment group (44) attended the multidisciplinary program 2–4 months after the surgery. This program involved completing group exercise sessions with a physical therapist and attending lectures from a variety of health care personnel (orthopaedic surgeon, psychologist, social worker and nutritionist). The control group (42) followed usual care. The main measures assessed preoperatively and at 2, 6 and 12 month follow up were the WOMAC index, 15 m walk test, stair test and isometric strength measurement of the knee. The use of rehabilitation services were recorded with a use of a questionnaire. The active treatment group did not achieve functional recovery any faster and neither did their quality of life improve more than conventional care controls. Furthermore, the intervention did not reduce the use of postoperative rehabilitation services. However, patients who undergo TKA often have co morbidities including depression, obesity and cardiovascular impairments and such patients may benefit from a multidisciplinary rehabilitation treatment after surgery. Future studies are needed to test this hypothesis.

Conclusions

Physical therapy and rehabilitation protocols are critical to recovery after TKA. There is a large decrease in quadriceps muscle strength immediately after TKA, which is attributed to activation deficits and atrophy [4, 7]. Progressive strengthening exercise interventions of high intensity and early application of NMES should be used in order to attenuate early quadriceps weakness and the associated impairment. Further work is needed to fully elucidate the relationship between postoperative exercise protocols and outcomes, given that most studies do not accurately describe the "usual care" groups that were included as treatment arms in these randomized trials. Overall, the long term effect of structured physical therapy on the TKA outcomes is unclear.

References

1. Health at a glance 2011: OECD indicators. Paris: OECD Publishing; 2011.
2. NIH Consensus Statement on total knee replacement December 8–10, 2003. J Bone Joint Surg Am. 2004; 86A:1328–35.
3. Walsh M, Woodhouse LJ, Thomas SG, Finch E. Physical impairments and functional limitations: a comparison of individuals 1 year after total knee arthroplasty with control subjects. Phys Ther. 1998;78:248–58.
4. Stevens JE, Mizner RL, Snyder-Mackler L. Quadriceps strength and volitional activation before and after total knee arthroplasty for osteoarthritis. J Orthop Res. 2003;21:775–9.
5. Mizner RL, Petterson SC, Stevens JE, Vandenborne K, Snyder-Mackler L. Early quadriceps strength loss after total knee arthroplasty: the contributions of muscle atrophy and failure of voluntary muscle activation. J Bone Joint Surg Am. 2005;87A:1047–53.
6. Huang CH, Cheng CK, Lee YT, Lee KS. Muscle strength after successful total knee replacement. A 6 to 13 year follow up. Clin Orthop. 1996;328:147–54.
7. Mizner RL, Petterson SC, Snyder-Mackler L. Quadriceps strength and the time course of functional recovery after total knee arthroplasty. J Orthop Sports Phys Ther. 2005;35:424–36.
8. Cameron H, Brotzman S. The arthritic lower extremity: total knee arthroplasty. In: Brotzman SB, Wilk KE, editors. Clinical orthopaedic rehabilitation. 2nd ed. Philadelphia: Mosby; 2003. p. 465–74.
9. Ranawat CS, Ranawat AS, Mehta A. Total knee arthroplasty rehabilitation protocol. What makes the difference? J Arthroplasty. 2003;18:27–30.
10. Minns Lowe CJ, Barker KL, Dewey M, Sackley CM. Effectiveness of physiotherapy exercise after knee arthroplasty for osteoarthritis: systematic review and meta-analysis of randomised controlled trials. Br Med J. 2007;335:812. http//dx.doi.org/10.1136/bmj.39311.460093.BE.
11. Stevens-Lapsley JE, Balter JE, Kohrt WM, Eckhoff DG. Quadriceps and hamstrings muscle dysfunction after total knee arthroplasty. Clin Orthop. 2010;468:2460–8.
12. Piva SR, Teixeira PEP, Almeida GJM, Gil AB, DiGioia AM, Levison TJ, Fitzgerald GK. Contribution of hip abductor strength to physical function in patients with total knee arthroplasty. Phys Ther. 2011;91:225–33.
13. Moffet H, Collet JP, Shapiro SH, Paradis G, Marquis F, Roy L. Effectiveness of intensive rehabilitation on functional ability and quality of life after first total knee arthroplasty. A single-blind randomized controlled trial. Arch Phys Med Rehabil. 2004;85:546–56.
14. Petterson SC, Mizner RL, Stevens JE, Raisis L, Bodenstab A, Newcomb W, Snyder-Mackler L. Improved function from progressive strengthening interventions after total knee arthroplasty. A randomized clinical trial with an imbedded prospective cohort. Arthritis Rheum. 2009;61:174–83.
15. Bade MJ, Stevens-Lapsley JE. Restoration of physical function in patients following total knee arthroplasty. An update on rehabilitation practices. Curr Opin Rheumatol. 2012;24:208–14.
16. Bade MJ, Stevens-Lapsley JE. Early high-intensity rehabilitation following total knee arthroplasty improves outcomes. J Orthop Sports Phys Ther. 2011;41:932–41.
17. Evgeniadis G, Beneka A, Malliou P, Mavromoustakos S, Godolias G. Effects of pre- or postoperative therapeutic exercise on the quality of life, before and after total knee arthroplasty for osteoarthritis. J Back Musculoskelet Rehabil. 2008;21:161–9.
18. Roelants M, Delecluse C, Verschueren SM. Whole-body vibration training increases knee-extension strength and speed of movement in older women. J Am Geriatr Soc. 2004;52:901–8.
19. Johnson AW, Myrer JW, Hunter I, Feland JB, Hopkins JT, Draper DO, Eggett D. Whole-body vibration strengthening compared to traditional strengthening during physical therapy in individuals with total knee arthroplasty. Physiother Theory Pract. 2010;26:215–25.
20. Salter RB, Simmonds DF, Malcolm BW, Rumble EJ, MacMichael D, Clements ND. The biological effect of continuous passive motion on the healing of full-thickness defects in articular cartilage. An experimental investigation in the rabbit. J Bone Joint Surg Am. 1980;62A:1232–51.
21. Salter RB. Motion versus rest: why immobilize joints? J Bone Joint Surg (Br). 1982;64B:251.

22. Salter RB. The physiologic basis of continuous passive motion for articular cartilage healing and regeneration. Hand Clin. 1994;10:211–9.
23. Coutts RD, Kaita J, Barr R, Mason R, Dube R, Amiel D, Woo SLY, Nickel V. The role of continuous passive motion in the postoperative rehabilitation of the total knee patient. Orthop Trans. 1982;6:277–8.
24. Maloney WJ, Schurman DJ, Hangen D. The influence of continuous passive motion on outcome in total knee arthroplasty. Clin Orthop. 1990;256:162–8.
25. Johnson DP. The effect of continuous passive motion on wound healing and joint mobility after knee arthroplasty. J Bone Joint Surg Am. 1990;72A:421–6.
26. McInnes J, Larson MG, Daltroy LH. A controlled evaluation of continuous passive motion in patients undergoing total knee arthroplasty. JAMA. 1992;268:1423–8.
27. Ververeli PA, Sutton DC, Hearn SL. Continuous passive motion after total knee arthroplasty-analysis of costs and benefits. Clin Orthop. 1995;321:208–15.
28. Colwell CW, Morris BA. The influence of continuous passive motion on the results of total knee arthroplasty. Clin Orthop. 1992;276:225–8.
29. Pope RO, Corcoran S, McCaul K, Howie DW. Continuous passive motion after primary total knee arthroplasty. Does it offer any benefits? J Bone Joint Surg (Br). 1997;79B:914–7.
30. Coutts RD, Borden LS, Bryan RS, et al. The effect of continuous passive motion on total knee rehabilitation. Orthop Trans. 1983;7:535–6.
31. Kumar PJ, McPherson EJ, Dorr LD, Wan Z, Baldwin K. Rehabilitation after total knee arthroplasty: a comparison of 2 rehabilitation techniques. Clin Orthop. 1996;331:93–101.
32. Beaupre LA, Davies DM, Jones CA. Exercise combined with continuous passive motion or slider board therapy compared with exercise only. A randomized controlled trial of patients following total knee arthroplasty. Phys Ther. 2001;81:1029–37.
33. Davies DM, Johnston DWC, Beaupre LA, Lier DA. Effect of adjunctive range-of-motion therapy after primary total knee arthroplasty on the use of health services after hospital discharge. Can J Surg. 2003;46:30–6.
34. Leach W, Reid J, Murphy F. Continuous passive motion following total knee replacement: a prospective randomized trial with follow-up to 1 year. Knee Surg Sports Traumatol Arthrosc. 2006;14:922–6.
35. Denis M, Moffet H, Caron F, Quellet D, Paquet J, Nolet L. Effectiveness of continuous passive motion and conventional physical therapy after total knee arthroplasty: a randomized clinical trial. Phys Ther. 2006;86:174–85.
36. Lenssen TAF, Van Steyn MJA, Crijns YHF, Waltjé EMH, Roox GM, Geesink RJT, Van den Brandt PA, De Bie RA. Effectiveness of prolonged use of continuous passive motion (CPM) as an adjunct to physiotherapy, after total knee arthroplasty. BMC Musculoskelet Disord. 2008; 9: doi:10.1186/1471-2474-9-60.
37. Maniar RN, Baviskar JV, Singhi T, Rathi SS. To use or not to use continuous passive motion post-total knee arthroplasty. Presenting functional assessment results in early recovery. J Arthroplasty. 2012;27:193–201.
38. Ritter MA, Gandolf VS, Holston KS. Continuous passive motion versus physical therapy in total knee arthroplasty. Clin Orthop. 1989;244:239–43.
39. Lynch AF, Bourne RB, Rorabeck CH, et al. Deep-vein thrombosis and continuous passive motion after total knee arthroplasty. J Bone Joint Surg Am. 1988;70A:11–4.
40. Vince KG, Kelly MA, Beck J, Insall JN. Continuous passive motion after total knee arthroplasty. J Arthroplasty. 1987;2:281–4.
41. Lachiewicz PF. The role of continuous passive motion after total knee arthroplasty. Clin Orthop. 2000;380:144–50.
42. Davis D. Continuous passive motion for total knee arthroplasty. Phys Ther. 1984;64:709.
43. Bennett LA, Brearley SC, Hart JAL, Bailey MJ. A comparison of 2 continuous passive motion protocols after total knee arthroplasty. A controlled and randomised study. J Arthroplasty. 2005;20:225–33.
44. Liebs TR, Herzberg W, Rüther W, Haasters J, Russlies M, Hassenpflug J. Multicenter randomized controlled trial comparing early versus late aquatic therapy after total hip or knee arthroplasty. Arch Phys Med Rehabil. 2012;93:192–9.
45. Giaquinto S, Ciotola E, Dall'Armi V, Margutti F. Hydrotherapy after total knee arthroplasty. A follow-up study. Arch Gerontol Geriatr. 2010;51:59–63.
46. Valtonen A, Pöyhönen T, Sipilä S, Heinonen A. Effects of aquatic resistance training on mobility limitation and lower-limb impairments after knee replacement. Arch Phys Med Rehabil. 2010;91:833–9.
47. Valtonen A, Pöyhönen T, Sipilä S, Heinonen A. Maintenance of aquatic training-induced benefits on mobility and lower-extremity muscles among persons with unilateral knee replacement. Arch Phys Med Rehabil. 2011;92:1944–50.
48. Harmer AR, Naylor JM, Crosbie J, Russell T. Land-based versus water-based rehabilitation following total knee replacement: a randomized, single-blind trial. Arthritis Rheum. 2009;61:184–91.
49. Gage WH, Frank JS, Prentice SD, Stevenson P. Postural responses following a rotational support surface perturbation, following knee joint replacement: frontal plane rotations. Gait Posture. 2008;27:286–93.
50. Matsumoto H, Okuno M, Nakamura T, Yamamoto K, Hagino H. Fall incidence and risk factors in patients after total knee arthroplasty. Arch Orthop Trauma Surg. 2012;132:555–63.
51. Swinkels A, Newman JH, Allain TJ. A prospective observational study of falling before and after knee replacement surgery. Age Ageing. 2009;38:175–81.
52. Piva SR, Gil AB, Almeida GJM, DiGioia AM, Levison TJ, Fitzgerald GK. A balance exercise program appears to improve function for patients with total knee arthroplasty: a randomized clinical trial. Phys Ther. 2010;90:880–94.

53. Liao CD, Liou TH, Huang YY, Huang YC. Effects of balance training on functional outcome after total knee replacement in patients with knee osteoarthritis: a randomized controlled trial. Clin Rehabil. 2013;27:697–709.

54. Fung V, Ho A, Shaffer J, Chung E, Gomez M. Use of Nintendo Wii Fit™ in the rehabilitation of outpatients following total knee replacement: a preliminary randomised controlled trial. Physiotherapy. 2012;98:183–8.

55. Company history – Wii. Available at: http://www.nintendo.com/corp/history.jsp

56. Mizner RL, Stevens JE, Snyder-Mackler L. Voluntary activation and decreased force production of the quadriceps femoris muscle after total knee arthroplasty. Phys Ther. 2003;83:359–65.

57. Hurley MV. Quadriceps weakness in osteoarthritis. Curr Opin Rheumatol. 1998;10:246–50.

58. Gibson JNA, Morrison WL, Scrimgeour CM, Smith K, Stoward PJ, Rennie MJ. Effects of therapeutic percutaneous electrical stimulation of atrophic human quadriceps on muscle composition, protein synthesis and contractile properties. Eur J Clin Invest. 1989;19:206–12.

59. Martin TP, Gundersen LA, Blevins FT, Coutts RD. The influence of functional electrical stimulation on the properties of vastus lateralis fibres following total knee arthroplasty. Scand J Rehabil Med. 1991;23:207–10.

60. Thomas AC, Stevens-Lapsley JE. Importance of attenuating quadriceps activation deficits after total knee arthroplasty. Exerc Sport Sci Rev. 2012;40:95–101.

61. Stevens JE, Mizner RL, Snyder-Mackler L. Neuromuscular electrical stimulation for quadriceps muscle strengthening after bilateral total knee arthroplasty: a case series. J Orthop Sports Phys Ther. 2004;34:21–9.

62. Young A. The relative isometric strength of type I and type II muscle fibres in the human quadriceps. Clin Physiol. 1984;4:23–32.

63. Gotlin RS, Hershkowitz S, Juris PM, Gonzalez EG, Scott N, Insall JN. Electrical stimulation effect on extensor lag and length of hospital stay after total knee arthroplasty. Arch Phys Med Rehabil. 1994;75:957–9.

64. Avramidis K, Strike PW, Taylor PN, Swain ID. Effectiveness of electric stimulation of the vastus medialis muscle in the rehabilitation of patients after total knee arthroplasty. Arch Phys Med Rehabil. 2003;84:1850–3.

65. Avramidis K, Karachalios T, Popotonasios K, Sacorafas D, Papathanasiades AA, Malizos KN. Does electric stimulation of the vastus medialis muscle influence rehabilitation after total knee replacement? Orthopedics. 2011;34:175.

66. Stevens-Lapsley JE, Balter JE, Wolfe P, Eckhoff DG, Kohrt WM. Early neuromuscular electrical stimulation to improve quadriceps muscle strength after total knee arthroplasty: a randomized controlled trial. Phys Ther. 2012;92:210–26.

67. Stevens-Lapsley, Balter JE, Wolfe P, Eckhoff DG, Schwartz RS, Schenkman M, Kohrt WM. Relationship between intensity of quadriceps muscle neuromuscular electrical stimulation and strength recovery after total knee arthroplasty. Phys Ther. 2012;92:1187–96.

68. Rajan RA, Pack Y, Jackson H, Gillies C, Asirvatham R. No need for outpatient physiotherapy following total knee arthroplasty. A randomized trial of 120 patients. Acta Orthop Scand. 2004;75:71–3.

69. Mockford BJ, Thompson NW, Humphreys P, Beverland DE. Does a standard outpatient physiotherapy regime improve the range of knee motion after primary total knee arthroplasty? J Arthroplasty. 2008;23:1110–4.

70. Kramer JF, Speechley M, Bourne R, Rorabeck C, Vaz M. Comparison of clinic- and home-based rehabilitation programs after total knee arthroplasty. Clin Orthop. 2003;410:225–34.

71. Madsen M, Larsen K, Madsen IK, Søe H, Hansen TB. Late group-based rehabilitation has no advantages compared with supervised home-exercises after total knee arthroplasty. Dan Med J. 2013;60:A4607.

72. Russell TG, Buttrum P, Cert G, Wootton R, Jull GA. Internet-based outpatient telerehabilitation for patients following total knee arthroplasty. A randomized controlled trial. J Bone Joint Surg Am. 2011;93A:113–20.

73. Kauppila AM, Kyllönen E, Ohtonen P, Hämäläinen M, Mikkonen P, Laine V, Siira P, Mäki- Heikkilä P, Sintonen H, Leppilahti J, Arokoski JPA. Multidisciplinary rehabilitation after primary total knee arthroplasty: a randomized controlled study of its effects on functional capacity and quality of life. Clin Rehabil. 2010;24:398–411.

Mid and Long Term Functional Outcome of Total Knee Arthroplasty

24

Nikolaos Rigopoulos and Theofilos Karachalios

Total knee arthroplasty (TKA) is a surgical procedure performed throughout the world in high numbers and at a high cost for health systems. Many countries have published national guidelines for the selection of a cost effective implant. The major criterion for this selection is the long term survival of the artificial joint. On the other hand, the evaluation of functional outcome and quality of life is also an important issue if the operation has to be proved cost effective. However, there is no general agreement related to the use of functional outcome tools in evaluating TKA [1].

Although the majority of patients report substantial gains in functional outcomes following primary TKA, the degree of improvement varies widely. In order to evaluate the potential role of

N. Rigopoulos, MD
Orthopaedic Department, Center of Biomedical Sciences (CERETETH), University of Thessalia, Larissa, Hellenic Republic

T. Karachalios, MD, DSc (✉)
Orthopaedic Department,
Center of Biomedical Sciences (CERETETH),
University of Thessalia, Larissa, Hellenic Republic

Orthopaedic Department, Faculty of Medicine,
School of Health Sciences,
Center of Biomedical Sciences (CERETETH),
University of Thessalia,
University General Hospital of Larissa,
Mezourlo region, Larissa 41110, Hellenic Republic
e-mail: kar@med.uth.gr

preoperative pain due to other musculoskeletal conditions on postoperative functional outcomes, authors have attempted to quantify bilateral knee and low back pain before primary TKA and evaluate its effect on postoperative physical functional outcome. They concluded that the degree of functional improvement depends on the burden of musculoskeletal pain in other weight bearing joints [2–4].

There are several assessment tools which can be used in order to evaluate TKA functional outcomes. The majority of these functional scales are not patient oriented. Usually, there is a person (medical personnel), other than the patient, who performs the test by clinical examination alone or by a combination of clinical examination and the administration of a questionnaire of physical activities. However, patient satisfaction scores do not always correlate with clinical functional parameters recorded by the medical personnel [5, 6].

Mahomed et al. [7] developed a validated, self-administered satisfaction scale (very satisfied, somewhat satisfied, somewhat dissatisfied, very dissatisfied) which assesses overall satisfaction in terms of pain relief and the ability to perform daily and leisure activities. Wylde et al. [8] utilized this satisfaction scale in a comparison study of fixed versus mobile bearing TKAs (250 knees). While the authors found no differences in satisfaction between the two types of implants, they did note surprisingly low satisfaction rates for specific activities (66 % "very satisfied" for

© Springer-Verlag London 2015

T. Karachalios (ed.), *Total Knee Arthroplasty: Long Term Outcomes*,
DOI 10.1007/978-1-4471-6660-3_24

pain relief, 52 % for return to normal activities of daily living and 44 % for the ability to perform leisure activities) [8].

Thomsen et al. [9] investigated whether the achievement of a higher degree of knee flexion after TKA would result in a better patient perceived outcome. High flex compared to non high flex TKA showed increased knee flexion, but no significant differences were found in patient perceived outcomes. It was suggested that improved knee flexion (more than 110°) has little relevance for the patients due to the fact that pain free range of motion and high patient satisfaction were achieved with both types of TKA's [9]. Boese et al. [10] have also investigated contemporary high flexion TKA knee designs which claim to provide more than 120° of flexion. Although a high degree of flexion is necessary for some activities of daily living there were no significant mid-term improvements in terms of function, patients' overall satisfaction, flexion gained or lost, and the need for further surgery [10]. Chang et al. [11] assessed alterations in physical activity profiles of Korean patients after TKA and tried to determine whether postoperative physical activity level is influenced by patient sociodemographic factors and postoperative functional outcomes. They conclude that regular participation in physical activity should be encouraged to improve patient satisfaction [11].

Outcome measures used to evaluate an intervention, such as TKA, should be valid (measure the proper outcome), reproducible (the same value should be obtained on repeated assessments of a stable patient), and responsive to changes in a patient's condition [12]. For assessing TKA, validated outcomes tools include those that are related to general health (SF-36, SF-12, Nottingham Health Profile, Sickness Impact Profile, & EuroQol), disease specific (WOMAC, Oxford Knee Score) and patient specific (MACTAR). A number of tests are available to assess functional outcomes after TKA. For functional capacity, in order to assess patients undergoing TKA, the 6 min walk and 30-s stair climb are commonly used. Other functional capacity tools include the KOOS, which is based on the WOMAC score but it has been expanded to

include the outcomes of pain, activities of daily living, sport and recreation function, and knee related quality of life. Other functional outcomes of interest include the International Knee Documentation, the Lower Extremity Functional Scale, and the UCLA activity level rating [1]. The short form – 36 Health Survey (SF-36) is a 36 item questionnaire which has been used extensively and validated as a measurement of general health status. It generates scores in eight dimensions, namely physical functioning, role limitation due to physical problems, role limitation due to emotional problems, social functioning, mental health, energy/vitality, bodily pain, and general health perception. Other similar assessment tools have the disadvantage that they have been used up to 2 years post operatively and the sustainability of these outcomes in the longer term remains unknown. However, there are published efforts to evaluate changes in the SF-36 over a period of 5 years and at the same time to validate the effects of age and gender on the scores [13]. The SF-36 has been criticized when applied on an individual basis, but its extensive use in outcome analysis and its proven validity and reliability make it useful for comparison between different conditions. Sample size and duration of follow-up are always important. A designated person (nurse, student etc) should be responsible for the administration and collection of the questionnaires, ensuring the consistency and completeness of the database. Details about health status and outcomes may be lost with a simpler questionnaire (e.g. SF-12). The Oxford knee score (OKS) is a validated and widely accepted disease specific patient reported outcome measure, but there is limited evidence regarding long term trends in the score. Williams et al. [14] reviewed 5,600 individual OKS questionnaires (1,547 patients) from a prospectively collected TKA database in order to determine the trends in OKS over a 10 year period following TKA. The maximum post operative OKS was observed at 2 years, following which a gradual but significant decline was observed over the 10 year assessment. A similar trend was observed for most of the individual OKS components. Kneeling ability initially improved in the first year but was then followed by rapid deterioration. Pain severity exhibited the greatest improvement, although residual pain was reported in over two thirds of patients post-operatively. Peak improvement in night pain component did not occur until year 4. Post operative OKS was lower in women younger than 60 years and in those with a BMI >35 [14].

The Knee Society clinical score (KSS), the Knee Society Functional Score, the Western Ontario, the McMaster Universities Index of Osteoarthritis score and the Hospital for Special Surgery score (HSS) are disease specific tools also widely used for the clinical assessment of TKA surgery. A long term survival analysis of a consecutive series of patients with hydroxyapatite-coated cementless TKAs was performed by a single surgeon between 1992 and 1995. All patients were invited for a clinical outcome review which was based on the Knee Society clinical score (KSS) and an independent radiological analysis. Of 471 TKAs performed on 356 patients, 432 TKAs on 325 patients were followed for a mean of 16.4 years (15–18) [15]. Long et al. [16] also evaluated functional outcome after TKA in young and active patients. There is also a meta-analysis of revision rates and functional outcome in TKA using only long term results from a wide base of articles. All the above papers concluded, using the Knee Society Knee Score, the Knee Society Function Score, the Hospital for Special Surgery Score and the New Jersey Orthopedic Hospital Knee Evaluation System, that TKA is a successful treatment for osteoarthritis of the knee with an expected revision rate of less than 5 % within 10 years and a long lasting functional improvement of more than 30 % on any assessment score [15–17].

To date, no single functional outcome tool has emerged as a gold standard for TKA research although there is considerable agreement that validated outcome tools that are responsive, reliable, and reproducible should be used. The widely used Knee Society clinical rating scale has not been validated. As a consequence, the WOMAC and Oxford 12 disease specific scores are the most frequently used outcomes tools. When comparisons with other medical interventions are needed, the general health outcomes such as the SF-12, SF-36, or EuroQol can be useful [1]. Recently there has been an evolving effort from various authors to evaluate functional outcome after TKA using assessment tools that are mainly patient oriented with each patient being asked to complete a self administered, validated Total Knee Function Questionnaire. However, this is a very difficult task when trying to evaluate mid or long term functional results because of the problem of recall bias. Therefore, in most articles mid and long term functional results are presented as combined data derived from both patient oriented questions and clinical assessment tools. Bourne et al. [18] re-examined patient's satisfaction using historic TKA implants. Despite substantial advances in primary TKA, numerous studies suggest only 82–89 % of primary TKA patients are satisfied. A cross sectional study of patient satisfaction was performed after 1,703 primary TKAs in the province of Ontario. The satisfaction questionnaire included three questions: (1) Overall, how satisfied are you with the results of your TKA? (2) How satisfied are you with your most recent TKA surgery for reducing pain (walking on a flat surface, going up or down stairs, sitting or lying down)? and (3) How satisfied are you with your most recent TKA surgery for improving your ability to perform five functions (going up stairs, getting in/out of a car or on/off a bus, rising from bed, lying in bed, performing light domestic duties)? A question concerning overall satisfaction was used to determine a two category satisfaction outcome by combining patients who answered very dissatisfied, dissatisfied, or neutral into one group, and patients who answered satisfied or very satisfied into the second group. This two category outcome (satisfied, not satisfied/neutral) was used as the measure of overall satisfaction for all statistical analyses. Data confirmed that approximately one in five (19 %) primary TKA patients were not satisfied with the outcome. Satisfaction in terms of pain relief varied from 72 % to 86 % and of function from 70 % to 84 % for specific activities of daily living. The strongest predictors of patient dissatisfaction after primary TKA were expectations not met (10.79 greater risk), a low WOMAC (2.59 greater risk) at 1 year, preoperative pain at rest (2.49 greater risk) and a postoperative complication requiring hospital readmission (1.99 greater risk) [18].

Patient oriented tests seem to be more efficient than unvalidated scoring systems in which the patient is asked about their level of pain and return to specific activities, followed by the surgeon objectively measuring range of motion and joint stability. Increasing evidence is emerging that patients and doctors do not always agree on ratings of quality of life improvements after therapeutic interventions.

The use of new designs and high flexion TKAs can provide a very satisfactory range of motion during the first postoperative period. However, long term functional results do not defer when the design factor is considered. It seems that overall health status, co-existing musculoskeletal diseases, patient's expectations not being met, efficient surgical technique and participation in physical activities of daily living are the most important factors affecting mid and long term functional results after TKA.

References

1. Bourne RB. Measuring tools for functional outcomes in total knee arthroplasty. Clin Orthop. 2008;466:2634–8.
2. Ng CY, Ballantyne JA, Brenkel IJ. Quality of life and functional outcome after primary total hip replacement. A five-year follow-up. J Bone Joint Surg Br. 2007;89B:868–73.
3. Ayers DC, Li W, Oatis C, Rosal MC, Franklin PD. Patient-reported outcomes after total knee replacement vary on the basis of preoperative coexisting disease in the lumbar spine and other nonoperatively treated joints: the need for a musculoskeletal comorbidity index. J Bone Joint Surg Am. 2013;95A:1833–7.
4. Clement ND, MacDonald D, Simpson AH, Burnett R. Total knee replacement in patients with concomitant back pain results in a worse functional outcome and a lower rate of satisfaction. Bone Joint J. 2013;95B:1632–9.
5. Janse AJ, Gemke RJ, Uiterwaal CS, van der Tweel I, Kimpen JL, Sinnema G. Quality of life: patients and doctors don't always agree: a meta-analysis. J Clin Epidemiol. 2004;57:653–61.
6. Mantyselka P, Kumpusalo E, Ahonen R, Takala J. Patients' versus general practitioners' assessments of pain intensity in primary care patients with non-cancer pain. Br J Gen Pract. 2001;51:995–7.
7. Mahomed NN, Liang MH, Cook EF, Daltroy LH, Fortin PR, Fossel AH, Katz JN. The importance of patient expectations in predicting functional outcomes after total joint arthroplasty. J Rheumatol. 2002;29:1273–9.
8. Wylde V, Learmonth I, Potter A, Bettinson K, Lingard E. Patient reported outcomes after fixed- versus mobile-bearing total knee replacement: a multi-centre randomised controlled trial using the Kinemax total knee replacement. J Bone Joint Surg Br. 2008;90B:1172–9.
9. Thomsen MG, Husted H, Otte KS, Holm G, Troelsen A. Do patients care about higher flexion in total knee arthroplasty? A randomized, controlled, double-blinded trial. BMC Musculoskelet Disord. 2013;14:127.
10. Boese CK, Gallo TJ, Plantikow CJ. Range of motion and patient satisfaction with traditional and high-flexion rotating-platform knees. Iowa Orthop J. 2011;31:73–7.
11. Chang MJ, Kim SH, Kang YG, Chang CB, Kim TK. Activity levels and participation in physical activities by Korean patients following total knee arthroplasty. BMC Musculoskelet Disord. 2014;15:24.
12. Irrang JJ, Anderson AF, Boland AL, Harner CD, Kurosaka M, Neyret P, Richmond JC, Shelborne KD. Development and validation of the International Knee Documentation Committee subjective knee form. Am J Sports Med. 2001;29:600–13.
13. McGuigan FX, Hozack WJ, Moriarty L, Eng K, Rothman RH. Predicting quality-of-life outcomes following total joint arthroplasty. J Arthroplasty. 1995;10:742–7.
14. Williams DP, Blakey CM, Hadfield SG, Murray DW, Price AJ, Field RE. Long-term trends in the Oxford knee score following total knee replacement. J Bone Joint Surg Br. 2013;95B:45–51.
15. Melton JT, Mayahi R, Baxter SE, Facek M, Glezos C. Long-term outcome in an uncemented, hydroxyapatite-coated total knee replacement: a 15- to 18-year survivorship analysis. J Bone Joint Surg Br. 2012;94B:1067–70.
16. Long WJ, Bryce CD, Hollenbeak CS, Benner RW, Scott WN. Total knee replacement in young, active patients: long-term follow-up and functional outcome: a concise follow-up of a previous report. J Bone Joint Surg Am. 2014;96B:e159.
17. Lützner J, Hübel U, Kirschner S, Günther KP, Krummenauer F. Long-term results in total knee arthroplasty. A meta-analysis of revision rates and functional outcome. Chirurg. 2011;82:618–24.
18. Bourne RB, Davis AM, Charron KDJ. Who is satisfied and who is not? Clin Orthop. 2010;468:57–63.

Long Term Outcome of Total Knee Arthroplasty. The Effect of Navigation

Aristides Zimbis and Theofilos Karachalios

Introduction

Total knee arthroplasty (TKA) is an effective procedure which relieves pain, restores knee function, and improves the quality of life of patients with end stage knee arthritis [1–6]. Further improvement of its results seems difficult. Ten year survival rates are reported to be higher than 90 % in large patient series and registers [7]. Total knee arthroplasty outcomes are highly dependent on surgical technique, specifically limb alignment, and implant positioning. Proper alignment of the femoral and tibial components is an important predictor of postoperative pain, polyethylene liner wear, stability, and

implant longevity [8–11]. Implant malposition is also associated with postoperative pain, decreased function and/or higher revision rates. More than 50 % of TKA revisions are performed within 2 years after surgery and a common reason is component malposition [12]. In addition, when TKA is performed in lower volume hospitals (hospital volume of 25–50 TKAs/year), a higher TKA revision rate at 5–8 years has been reported. Numerous studies have demonstrated that poor clinical outcomes and decreased implant longevity in TKA are often associated with inaccurate placement of either the tibial or the femoral implant [9, 13–18]. Choong et al. [19] found that more accurate component placement correlates with better knee function and improved quality of life. Some investigators have reported that even in major arthroplasty centers, optimal postoperative alignment of the components can only be obtained in 70–80 % of patients using conventional techniques with either intra or extramedullary alignment rods. Computer assisted navigation techniques, including image based and image free systems, have been recently developed and used in order to improve the positioning of the components and the axis of the limb in TKAs performed for both deformed and normally aligned knees [20–25]. Effective soft tissue balancing is also a determinant of TKA long term outcome [15, 26]. Common reason for TKA failure is patella component or extensor mechanism failure in combination with femoral and tibial

A. Zimbis, MD, DSc
Orthopaedic Department, Center of Biomedical Sciences (CERETETH), University of Thessalia, Larissa, Hellenic Republic

School of Health Sciences, Faculty of Medicine, University of Thessalia, Larissa, Hellenic Republic

T. Karachalios, MD, DSc (✉)
Orthopaedic Department, Center of Biomedical Sciences (CERETETH), University of Thessalia, Larissa, Hellenic Republic

Orthopaedic Department, Faculty of Medicine, School of Health Sciences, Center of Biomedical Sciences (CERETETH), University of Thessalia, University General Hospital of Larissa, Mezourlo region, Larissa 41110, Hellenic Republic
e-mail: kar@med.uth.gr

T. Karachalios (ed.), *Total Knee Arthroplasty: Long Term Outcomes*,
DOI 10.1007/978-1-4471-6660-3_25

components, alignment failure [18, 27, 28]. In cases with extraarticular femoral deformities, it is difficult to perform distal femoral cuts using intramedullary alignment rods and instrumentation for extramedullary alignment is not reliable in the coronal and sagittal planes. Instead, computer assisted navigation can help surgeons to perform TKA in such difficult cases [29].

Computer assisted navigated TKA was first performed in 1997 [30] and its use and technology have evolved rapidly. Navigation in TKA has been recognized as a useful technique in patients undergoing TKA with extraarticular deformity [31] and its clinical applications in primary TKA are now expanding in order to include knees with less deformity [20]. Navigated TKA is gaining popularity [32, 33] and combines the technology of computer assisted orthopaedic surgery with conventional TKA in an attempt to improve clinical, radiographic, and functional scores in patients undergoing TKA by reducing radiographic outliers. Significant interest has been shown in the development of computer-assisted surgery (CAS) using imageless navigation systems [25, 34–36]. Augmented reality systems are based on a display technique that combines information taken from the real environment with data generated by the computer, augmenting the real scene with additional information and enhancing the user' s perception of the world.

The purpose of this review is to present navigation principles, systems which are currently in clinical use and evaluate recent literature concerning the effect of these modern techniques on the long term outcome of THA.

Basic Principles and Techniques

Surgical navigation systems are augmented reality systems which provide the surgeon with accurate visual and numerical information on spatial relationship of patient's anatomic structures and surgical tools during surgery, updated in real-time. The augmentation can be carried out in several ways. Some systems show in the virtual scene the three dimensional model of the anatomy reconstructed either from preoperative CT or MRI studies of the patient, or adapting generic existing models to the patient under evaluation. Other systems do not visualize the 3D model of the anatomy but show the model information required for the task with lines and points determined from direct measurement of limb dynamics and of bone surface. In general surgical navigation systems include three main components [37]. An **intra-operative** position tracking system (that is the device used to monitor relevant object in the operating field, collecting in real time data relating to their location and orientation; depending on the technology they use, these tracking systems can be mechanical, optical, electromagnetic or ultrasonic) (Fig. 25.1). A **display device** showing the virtual scenario, updated in real time (Fig. 25.2). A **control software** which processes data collected by the tracking system to update the position of the objects in the virtual scenario and produces the images to be shown by the display device. These images have to be provided at a sufficient frame rate in order to avoid flickering images. Moreover the system must be able to update them as much frequently as is possible, because the longer is the delay in processing the tracker's data to display new images, the worse is the accuracy of the virtual environment in reproducing the real world (Fig. 25.3).

All these systems allow a preoperative or intraoperative planning of the surgery based on patient's specific information, permitting the simulation of different surgical strategies and to choose the optimal one. In case of preoperative planning, during the intervention, the planned strategy can be displayed in the virtual scenario and integrated with intraoperative information. During the intervention, providing visual and numerical information of the position of surgical tools and patient's anatomy is updated in real-time, these systems give to the surgeon an accurate visual feedback, guiding him towards the completion of the planned strategy. These systems have the ability to provide more visual information in the surgical field than is available to the naked eye and help in solving the problems of visualization especially in case of minimally invasive surgery. It is well known that less invasive

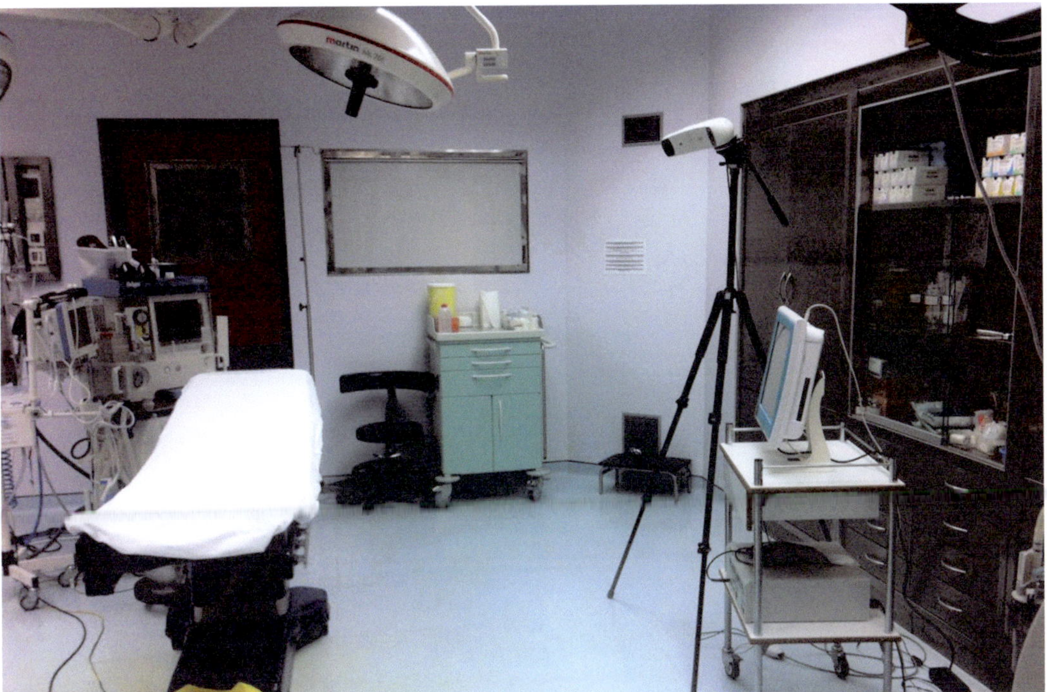

Fig. 25.1 The detector device used to monitor relevant object in the operating field, collecting real time data relating to their location and orientation is shown. It detects the joint and the instruments position and need to have visual contact with them. Depending on the technology they use, these tracking systems can be mechanical, optical, electromagnetic or ultrasonic

surgery contribute to rather better patient outcomes, but minimization of invasiveness generally results in a lack of surgeon's perception and dexterity. Showing the structural anatomy of the patient together with surgical tools, these augmented reality navigation systems allow the surgeon to accurately localize anatomical areas and to reach predefined positions watching at the display device.

Several orthopaedic procedures lends themselves well to the use of augmented reality navigation systems. Most common tasks developed by existing navigation systems are: joint replacement, arthroscopic surgery, fracture treatment and spinal surgery.

As proposed in Picard et al. [38], surgical navigation systems can be divided in: (a) **systems using preoperative models**. They can be either from preoperative three dimensional anatomy models reconstructed from CT/MRI images of the femur and of the tibia of the patient (patient specific) or generic anatomical model of the part in exam (non patient specific). By examining the imaging modalities on which the existing systems are based, one can identify two antithetic trends. The first one is patient oriented and tends to exploit the most advanced devices and techniques to reach excellent quality standards. CT and MRI based systems generally go in this direction and are very powerful, accurate and expensive. The other trend is focused on simplicity and accessibility. Conventional X-ray and fluoroscopy based systems are often less accurate, but affordable for most potential users. The choice of a specific imaging modality is frequently linked with that of a particular registration approach [39]. The image based navigation system has the advantage of precise preoperative planning, but the additional radiation, cost of preoperative CT scans, and additional time for preoperative planning do not improve accuracy [40]. (b) **Systems using intraoperative models**. They help the surgeon to achieve the planned implant. The knee joint, the data collection probe, and the

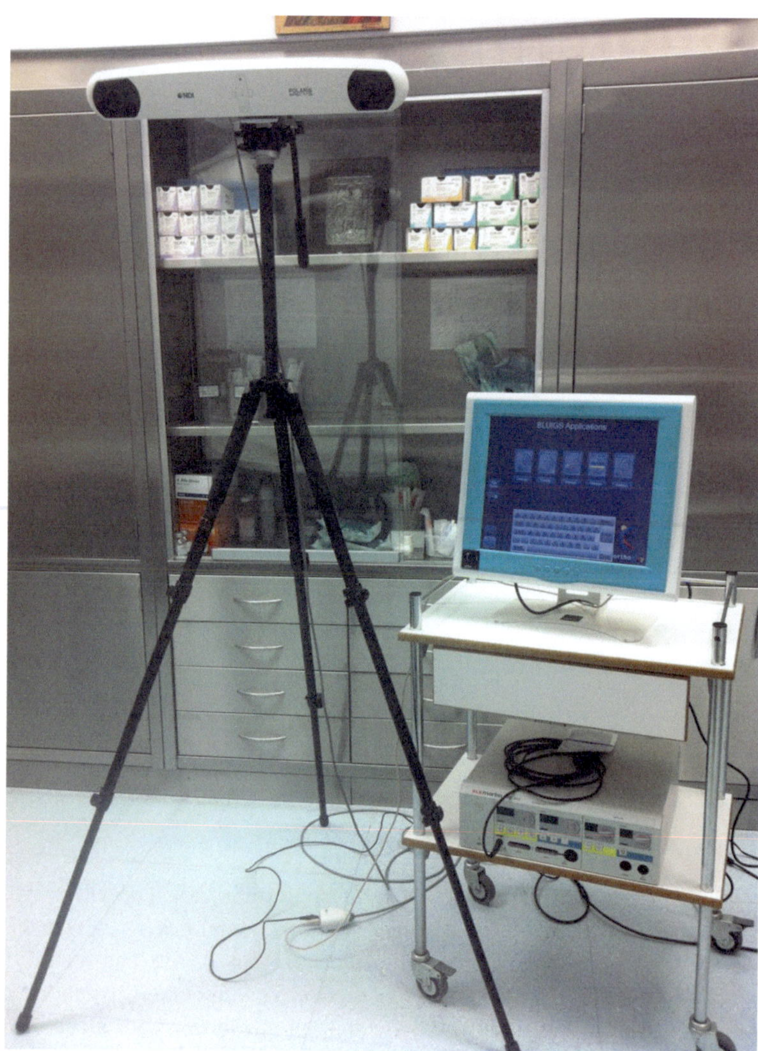

Fig. 25.2 The display device showing the virtual scenario, updated in real time is shown

implant insertion tool are sensorized with securely affixed optical targets and, after the registration and calibration process performed using a particular procedure, they can be localized and tracked in real time (Fig. 25.4). They use intraoperatively acquired medical images to determine the model (image based), and systems using models derived from information determined with direct measurement of the bone surface or limb dynamics (non image based). During surgery, using the localizer, the surgeon collects points on tibial and femoral surfaces, and statistical information about the shape variation of the femur are used to interpolate the data points. The positions of all sensorized objects, including the patient's anatomy, are tracked in real time by an optoelectronic localizer and reproduced in the virtual scene. Then, through the registration process, the system matches the ideal fitting between acquired points and the generic model. Using a statistical method to build the model has the advantage of requiring less data points to obtain a sufficient interpolation accuracy, reducing intraoperative time required for data acquisition [41]. Finally, to be accepted by surgeons, equipment have to be small unobtrusive, user friendly, safe and compatible to the surgical environment. Adding any equipment in the operating

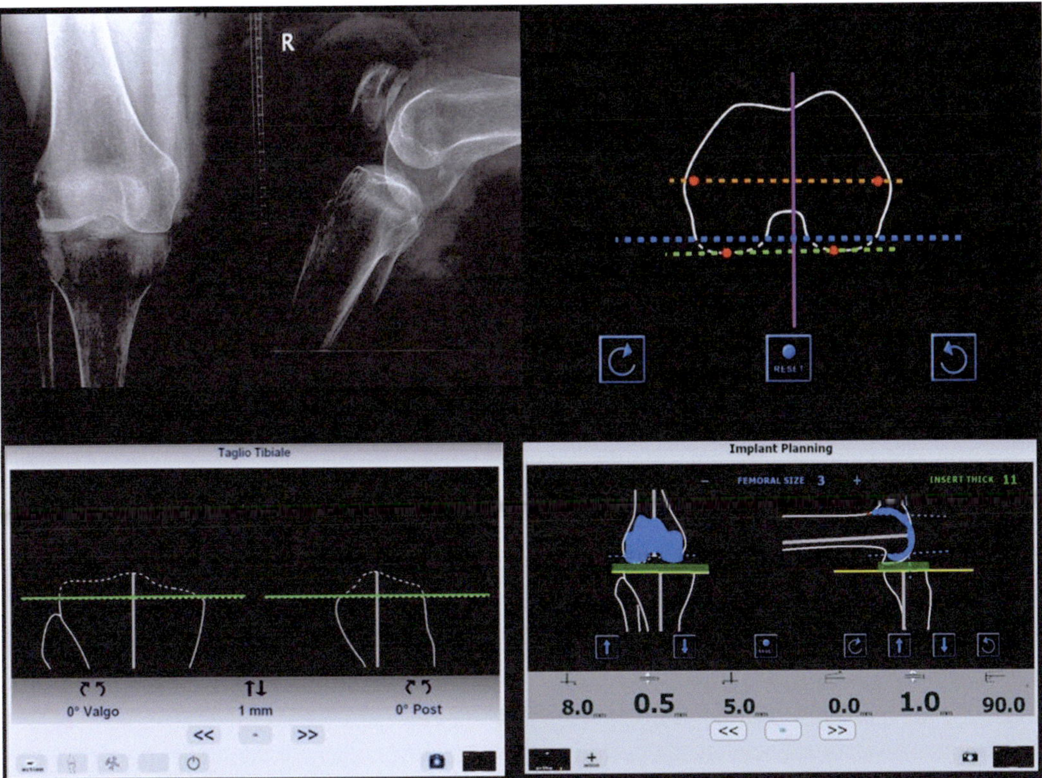

Fig. 25.3 When data collected and processed by the tracking system is completed a virtual scenario is produced. The images appear at the display device and the surgeon can perform the preoperative planning for the orientation of osteotomy and for prosthesis template

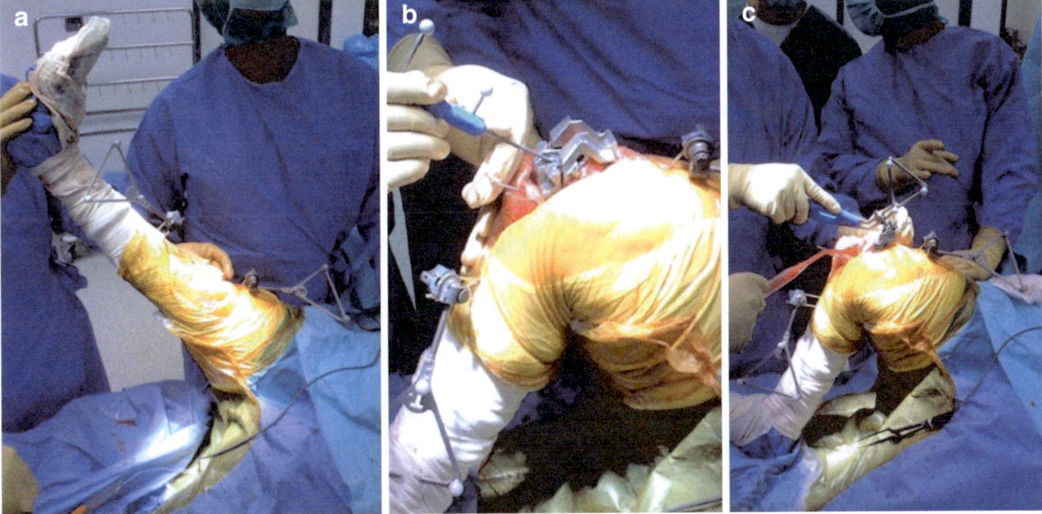

Fig. 25.4 At the patient side the surgeon has to place bone markers on femur and tibia. (**a**) After that, using the data collection probe, he has to define a list of specific landmarks. (**b**) Finally according to his preoperative planning he can use the sensorized cutting blocks and perform the osteotomies, while they can be localized and tracked in real time (**c**)

room increases the risk of infection, so any part of the system that comes into contact with the sterile field must be easily sterilized or draped. The digitalization of the bony landmarks is one of the crucial steps in navigation. Problems of reproducibility with intraoperative termination of these landmarks have been described to especially appear with the femoral epicondyles [42, 43].

Clinical Data

In order to evaluate the advantages of navigated TKA over conventional TKA we need to look very critically at the percentage of radiographic outliers in coronal and sagittal plane alignment, the accuracy in component axial rotation, the improvement of flexion extension gap and ligament balancing, the operative times once experience is gained, the costs, the complication rates, the duration of learning curves, the postoperative functional scores and the survival of TKA implants as a result of application of a new surgical technique.

According to recent literature, several studies have demonstrated that computer assisted navigated TKA achieves straight mechanical leg axis in coronal plane (on full length standing radiographs of the lower extremity) within the range of 3° of deviation [44–67]. Moreover the number of limb alignment outliers is reduced compared to traditional mechanical instrumented TKA [35, 40, 46, 49, 63, 68–70]. However, all studies between image based navigation and conventional techniques [40] groups were similar in early clinical outcomes as range of motion, knee scores, and postoperative complication rates at the final follow up. There were no statistical significant differences between the study groups. Moreover many of the reports supporting navigated TKA include small cohorts with a relative short follow up and present low levels of evidence [40, 71].

Improved alignment in navigated TKA in the coronal plane and a reduction in radiographic outliers have been demonstrated in most of the reports which compare the two groups. Despite this fact, an improvement in clinical function scores, revision rates, or improved survival for TKA performed with navigation compared to conventional techniques has not been demonstrated [69]. There are many studies which do not provide functional follow up data, but only report less than 2 years clinical outcome and radiographic data. Clearly these studies, although providing useful feedback to surgeons about radiographic and alignment results, do not add to the body of evidence in favor of navigated TKA in terms of the question of long term functional improvements and lower revision rates. Generally there is no evidence from mid to longer term studies which supports functional improvements or reduced revision rates for navigated TKA. On the other hand, even published meta-analyses studies cannot agree on the concept of whether there is evidence to support any functional improvements in navigated TKA [69]. Different methods of statistical analyses, incomplete power calculations, and cohort studies combined together lead to confusing and contradictory results.

Moreover, many of the studies have been performed in high volume surgical centers by surgeons with an interest or even conflict of interest with industry and the development of navigation technology and who perform many TKA procedures already. Although, there is evidence to support improvements in coronal plane alignment, however, sagittal plane and axial/rotational alignment have been less well studied. The accuracy to adjust the rotational alignment of the femoral component is a further prerequisite to avoid malfunctioning in TKAs. It is well known that even small deviations of rotational alignment of the components have a considerable influence on patellar tracking, stability and on the overall biomechanics of the joint [42]. Diagnosis of malrotation is challenging enough since it usually requires computed tomography (CT), bony landmarks (usually the femoral epicondyles) and special software to reduce the imaging artifacts which can provoke imprecision with and without navigation [42, 43].

Computer assisted navigation systems have been designed in order to increase precision of the implantation of TKAs [46, 49, 68]. This could not explain the fact that the improvements in coronal alignment (with fewer outliers) have not produced improved clinical knee scores, implant survival, better TKA function, or durability. It may be attributed to three potential causes: (1) better alignment in two planes is mitigated by the remaining errors in the axial (rotational) plane either because of an incorrect definition of the navigation system landmarks or by the shear malalignment of the components in the axial plane; (2) alignment goals of a neutral mechanical axis are not the correct target, and individual adjustments need to be made based on each patient's anatomic variability; and (3) the groups studied are too small (insufficient power) and/or the clinical scoring systems measuring functional status are not refined enough and suffer early ceiling effects, not allowing to prove superiority.

Navigated TKA requires additional steps to be taken in the operative room for computer processing, pin and tracker placement, array registering of data points, and analysis of intraoperative data. This increase in operating room time is variable and ranges between an increase of 8–63 min and to a nearly double or more than double the procedure time, with a higher incidence of complications because of small but consistent errors in navigation landmarking, compared to conventional TKA [46, 69, 72, 73]. Surgeons may rely on the navigation, perform minimal or not enough bone resections, and prolong operating room times even further. Soft tissue balancing can not be directed from computer assisted navigation systems. Another potential source of error is when the use of the navigation system is limited to the bone cuts and is stopped before final cementing of the implants. Finally, the volume of the operations performed by the surgeon and the experience in using computer navigation technology might be contributing factors [69].

Several authors have studied major complications related to computer navigation and TKA. They present different results: Bauwens et al. [46] found no difference in infection and thromboembolic events. Church et al. [74] performed a double blind randomized study to compare the incidence of fat embolic phenomena between navigated and non navigated knee prosthesis and demonstrated a significant reduce in embolic events in the CAS group. Fat and bone marrow is a potential activator of the clotting system and is thought to be an important factor for deep venous thrombosis.

In all studies comparing navigated TKA to conventional TKA, the cost of using a navigated TKA system is a factor that is well recognized yet difficult to quantify. Cost is often addressed indirectly with an increase in operative and procedure time for navigated TKA [75]. The use of computer assisted navigation causes costs, including the cost of the navigation system and a prolonged operative time [76]. These costs are justified if there is a benefit for the patient. It has been suggested that the use of a navigation system might be cost effective if there are decreased revision rates [77]. However, improved long term function, lower revision rates and/or survival, are not supported by any currently available evidence data [69].

TKA is one of the most successful procedures in terms of functional improvement, quality of life and cost effectiveness [78, 79]. It is therefore difficult for any new technique to further improve these results. Although many of these studies do show improvement in radiographic outliers, they correctly suggest that these improvements have not yet translated to improved knee function, quality of life, and survival of the implant [71]. One can argue that it may take a longer time to show a possible difference [71]. These findings are not sufficient enough in order to conclude that surgical navigation has to be abandoned. Surgeons, who perform relatively few TKAs, should also be cautious about adopting navigated TKA. Navigation is not a substitute for meticulous intraoperative surgical technique and training in TKA.

The established roles for navigated TKA include use in patients with extra articular deformity or retained implants and hardware that does not allow for traditional extra or intramedullary alignment guides. In addition, its use in resident teaching to provide immediate feedback regarding the accuracy of cutting guide placement may be helpful. In order to effectively evaluate clinical outcomes of navigated TKA, future clinical trials should be designed in order to follow patients in short and mid terms documenting improved clinical function and in long terms establishing whether lower revision rates are achieved. For the above reasons the main questions for knee arthroplasty surgeons still remaining to be answered is how to create, modify, and identify knee functional assessment tools, imaging techniques, and reliable component alignment parameters to determine the benefits of navigated TKA. Therefore, more sensitive evaluation tools may be necessary.

References

1. Lombardi AV, Berend KR, Walter CA, Aziz-Jacobo J, Cheney NA. Is recovery faster for mobile-bearing unicompartmental than total knee arthroplasty? Clin Orthop. 2009;467:1450–7.
2. Horwitz MD, Awan S, Chatoo MB, Stott DJ, Powles DP. An 8- to 10-year review of the Rotaglide total knee replacement. Int Orthop. 2009;33:111–5.
3. Parsch D, Kröger M, Moser MT, Geiger F. Follow-up of 11–16 years after modular fixed-bearing TKA. Int Orthop. 2009;33:431–5.
4. Ang DC, Tahir N, Hanif H, Tong Y, Ibrahim SA. African Americans and Whites are equally appropriate to be considered for total joint arthroplasty. J Rheumatol. 2009;36:1971–6.
5. Kashyap SN, Van Ommeren JW, Shankar S. Minimally invasive surgical technique in total knee arthroplasty: a learning curve. Surg Innov. 2009;16:55–62.
6. Erak S, Rajgopal V, Macdonald SJ, McCalden RW, Bourne RB. Ten-year results of an inset biconvex patella prosthesis in primary knee arthroplasty. Clin Orthop. 2009;467:1781–92.
7. Pradhan NR, Gambhir A, Porter ML. Survivorship analysis of 3234 primary knee arthroplasties implanted over a 26-year period: a study of eight different implant designs. Knee. 2006;13:7–11.
8. Berger RA, Crossett LS, Jacobs JJ, Rubash HE. Malrotation causing patellofemoral complications after total knee arthroplasty. Clin Orthop Relat Res. 1998;356:144–53.
9. Jeffery RS, Morris RW, Denham RA. Coronal alignment after total knee replacement. J Bone Joint Surg Br. 1991;73B:709–14.
10. Wasielewski RC, Galante JO, Leighty RM, Natarajan RN, Rosenberg AG. Wear patterns on retrieved polyethylene tibial inserts and their relationship to technical considerations during total knee arthroplasty. Clin Orthop. 1994;299:31–43.
11. Czurda T, Fennema P, Baumgartner M, Ritschl P. The association between component malalignment and postoperative pain following navigation-assisted total knee arthroplasty: results of a cohort/nested case-control study. Knee Surg Sports Traumatol Arthrosc. 2010;18:863–9.
12. Sharkey PF, Hozack WJ, Rothman RH, Shastri S, Jacoby SM. Insall Award paper. Why are total knee arthroplasties failing today? Clin Orthop. 2002;307:13–6.
13. Fang DM, Ritter MA, Davis KE. Coronal alignment in total knee arthroplasty: just how important is it? J Arthroplasty. 2009;24:39.
14. Lotke PA, Ecker ML. Influence of positioning of prosthesis in total knee replacement. J Bone Joint Surg Am. 1977;59A:77.
15. Longstaff LM, Sloan K, Stamp N, et al. Good alignment after total knee arthroplasty leads to faster rehabilitation and better function. J Arthroplasty. 2009;24:570.
16. Bargren JH, Blaha JD, Freeman MA. Alignment in total knee arthroplasty. Correlated biomechanical and clinical observations. Clin Orthop. 1983;287:173–8.
17. Tew M, Waugh W. Tibiofemoral alignment and the results of knee replacement. J Bone Joint Surg Br. 1985;67B:551.
18. Moreland JR. Mechanisms of failure in total knee arthroplasty. Clin Orthop. 1988;226:49–64.
19. Choong PF, Dowsey MM, Stoney JD. Does accurate anatomical alignment result in better function and quality of life? Comparing conventional and computer-assisted total knee arthroplasty. J Arthroplasty. 2009;24:560.
20. Hernandez-Vaquero D, Suarez-Vazquez A, Sandoval-Garcia MA, Noriega-Fernandez A. Computer assistance increases precision of component placement in total knee arthroplasty with articular deformity. Clin Orthop. 2010;468:1237–41.
21. Stiehl JB. Comparison of tibial rotation in fixed and mobile bearing total knee arthroplasty using computer navigation. Int Orthop. 2009;33:679–85.
22. van Strien T, van der Linden-van der Zwaag E, Kaptein B, van Erkel A, Valstar E, Nelissen R. Computer assisted versus conventional cemented total knee prostheses alignment accuracy and micromotion of the tibial component. Int Orthop. 2009;33:1255–61.
23. Dattani R, Patnaik S, Kantak A, Tselentakis G. Navigation knee replacement. Int Orthop. 2009;33:7–10.
24. Kamat YD, Aurakzai KM, Adhikari AR, Matthews D, Kalairajah Y, Field RE. Does computer navigation in total knee arthroplasty improve patient outcome at midterm follow- up? Int Orthop. 2009;33:1567–70.
25. Minoda Y, Kobayashi A, Iwaki H, Ohashi H, Takaoka K. TKA sagittal alignment with navigation systems and conventional techniques vary only a few degrees. Clin Orthop. 2009;467:1000–6.
26. Kim KK, Heo YM, Won YY, Lee WS. Navigation-assisted total knee arthroplasty for the knee retaining femoral intramedullary nail, and distal femoral plate and screws. Clin Orthop Surg. 2011;3:77–80.
27. Engh GA, Dwyer KA, Hanes CK. Polyethylene wear of metal-backed tibial components in total and unicompartmental knee prostheses. J Bone Joint Surg Br. 1992;74B:9–17.

28. Kilgus DJ, Moreland JR, Finerman GA, Funahashi TT, Tipton JS. Catastrophic wear of tibial polyethylene inserts. Clin Orthop. 1991;273:223–31.

29. Shao J, Zhang W, Jiang Y. Computer-navigated TKA for the treatment of osteoarthritis associated with extra-articular femoral deformity. Orthopedics. 2012;35:794–9.

30. Delp SL, Stulberg SD, Davies B, Picard F, Leitner F. Computer assisted knee replacement. Clin Orthop. 1998;354:49–56.

31. Bottros J, Klika AK, Lee HH, Polousky J, Barsoum WK. The use of navigation in total knee arthroplasty for patients with extra-articular deformity. J Arthroplasty. 2008;23:74–8.

32. Australian Orthopaedic Association National Joint Replacement Registry. Computer assisted surgery in primary total knee replacement between 2006 and 2008. Adelaide: Australia AOA NJRR; 2010.

33. Graham DJ, Harvie P, Sloan K, Beaver RJ. Morbidity of navigated vs conventional total knee arthroplasty: a retrospective review of 327 cases. J Arthroplasty. 2011;26:1224–7.

34. Molli RG, Anderson KC, Buehler KC, et al. Computer-assisted navigation software advancements improve the accuracy of total knee arthroplasty. J Arthroplasty. 2011;26:432–8.

35. Mason JB, Fehring TK, Estok R, et al. Meta-analysis of alignment outcomes in computer-assisted total knee arthroplasty surgery. J Arthroplasty. 2007;22:1097.

36. Brin YS, Nikolaou VS, Joseph L, et al. Imageless computer assisted versus conventional total knee replacement. A Bayesian meta-analysis of 23 comparative studies. Int Orthop. 2011;35:331–9.

37. Nikou C, Di Gioia A, Blackwell M, Jaramaz B, Kanade T. Augmented reality imaging technology for orthopaedic surgery. Oper Tech Orthop. 2000;10:82–6.

38. Picard F, Moody J, Jaramaz B, Di Gioia A, Nikou C, La Barca RS. A classification proposal for computer-assisted knee systems. In: Proceedings of Medical Image Computing and Computer-Assisted Intervention- MICCAI. 2000. p. 1145–51.

39. Woodard EJ, Leon SP, Moriarty TM, Quinones A, Zamani AA, Jolesz FA. Initial experience with intraoperative magnetic resonance imaging in spine surgery. Spine. 2001;26:410–7.

40. Tao C, Gouyou Z, Xianlong Z. Clinical and radiographic outcomes of image-based computer-assisted total knee arthroplasty: an evidence-based evaluation. Surg Innov. 2011;18:15–20.

41. Klos TVS, Banks AZ, Banks SA, Cook FF. Computer assisted anterior cruciate ligament reconstruction. In: Nolte LP, Ganz R, editors. Computer assisted orthopaedic surgery CAOS. Gottingen: Hogrefe & Huber; 1998. p. 184–9.

42. Jerosch J, Peuker E, Philipps B, Filler T. Interindividual reproducibility in perioperative rotational alignment of femoral components in knee prosthetic surgery using the transepicondylar axis. Knee Surg Sports Traumatol Arthrosc. 2002;10:194–7.

43. van der Linden-van der Zwaag HM, van der Zwaag HM, Valstar ER, van der Molen AJ, Nelissen RG. Transepicondylar axis accuracy in computer assisted knee surgery: a comparison of the CT-based measured axis versus the CAS determined axis. Comput Aided Surg. 2008;13:200–6.

44. Anderson KC, Buehler KC, Markel DC. Computer assisted navigation in total knee arthroplasty: comparison with conventional methods. J Arthroplasty. 2005;20:132–8.

45. Bathis H, Shafizadeh S, Paffrath T, Simanski C, et al. Are computer assisted total knee replacements more accurately placed? A meta-analysis of comparative studies. Orthopade. 2006;35:1056–65.

46. Bauwens K, Matthes G, Wich M, Gebhard F, et al. Navigated total knee replacement. A meta-analysis. J Bone Joint Surg Am. 2007;89A:261–9.

47. Bertsch C, Holz U, Konrad G, Vakili A, et al. Early clinical outcome after navigated total knee arthroplasty. Comparison with conventional implantation in TKA: a controlled and prospective analysis. Orthopade. 2007;36:739–45.

48. Bolognesi M, Hofmann A. Computer navigation versus standard instrumentation for tka: a single-surgeon experience. Clin Orthop Relat Res. 2005;440:162–9.

49. Chauhan SK, Scott RG, Breidahl W, Beaver RJ. Computer- assisted knee arthroplasty versus a conventional jig-based technique. A randomised, prospective trial. J Bone Joint Surg Br. 2004;86B:372–7.

50. Chin PL, Yang KY, Yeo SJ, Lo NN. Randomized control trial comparing radiographic total knee arthroplasty implant placement using computer navigation versus conventional technique. J Arthroplasty. 2005;20:618–26.

51. Decking R, Markmann Y, Fuchs J, Puhl W, et al. Leg axis after computer-navigated total knee arthroplasty: a prospective randomized trial comparing computer-navigated and manual implantation. J Arthroplasty. 2005;20:282–8.

52. Decking R, Markmann Y, Mattes T, Puhl W, et al. On the outcome of computer-assisted total knee replacement. Acta Chir Orthop Traumatol Cech. 2007;74:171–4.

53. Dutton AQ, Yeo SJ, Yang KY, Lo NN, et al. Computer-assisted minimally invasive total knee arthroplasty compared with standard total knee arthroplasty. A prospective, randomized study. J Bone Joint Surg Am. 2009;90A:2–9.

54. Ensini A, Catani F, Leardini A, Romagnoli M, et al. Alignments and clinical results in conventional and navigated total knee arthroplasty. Clin Orthop. 2007;457:156–62.

55. Haaker RG, Stockheim M, Kamp M, Proff G, et al. Computer-assisted navigation increases precision of component placement in total knee arthroplasty. Clin Orthop. 2005;433:152–9.

56. Holm S. A simple sequentially rejective multiple test procedure. Scand J Stat. 1979;6:65–70.

57. Gøthesen O, Espehaug B, Havelin LI, Petursson G, Hallan G, Strøm E, Dyrhovden G, Furnes O. Functional

outcome and alignment in computer-assisted and conventionally operated total knee replacements: a multicentre parallel-group randomised controlled trial. Bone Joint J. 2014;96B:609–18.

58. Kim SJ, MacDonald M, Hernandez J, Wixson RL. Computer assisted navigation in total knee arthroplasty: improved coronal alignment. J Arthroplasty. 2005;20(S3):123–31.

59. Molfetta L, Caldo D. Computer navigation versus conventional implantation for varus knee total arthroplasty: a case-control study at 5 years follow-up. Knee. 2008;15:75–9.

60. Picard F, Deakin AH, Clarke JV, Dillon JM, et al. Using navigation intraoperative measurements narrows range of outcomes in TKA. Clin Orthop. 2007;463:50–7.

61. Seon JK, Park SJ, Lee KB, Li G, et al. Functional comparison of total knee arthroplasty performed with and without a navigation system. Int Orthop. 2009;33(4):987–90.

62. Song EK, Seon JK, Yoon TR, Park SJ, et al. Functional results of navigated minimally invasive and conventional total knee arthroplasty: a comparison in bilateral cases. Orthopedics. 2006;29(S10):S145–7.

63. Sparmann M, Wolke B, Czupalla H, Banzer D, et al. Positioning of total knee arthroplasty with and without navigation support. A prospective, randomised study. J Bone Joint Surg Br. 2003;85B:830–5.

64. Spencer JM, Chauhan SK, Sloan K, Taylor A, et al. Computer navigation versus conventional total knee replacement: no difference in functional results at 2 years. J Bone Joint Surg Br. 2007;89B:477–80.

65. Stockl B, Nogler M, Rosiek R, Fischer M, et al. Navigation improves accuracy of rotational alignment in total knee arthroplasty. Clin Orthop. 2004;426:180–6.

66. Stulberg B, Zadzilka J. Navigation matters: initial experience with navigation for bilateral total knee arthroplasty. Tech Knee Surg. 2008;7:166–71.

67. Victor J, Hoste D. Image-based computer-assisted total knee arthroplasty leads to lower variability in coronal alignment. Clin Orthop. 2004;428:131–9.

68. Stulberg S, Loan P, Sarin V. Computer-assisted navigation in total knee replacement: results of an initial experience in thirty-five patients. J Bone Joint Surg Am. 2002;84A:90–8.

69. Stephen R, Burnett J, Barrack RL. Computer-assisted total knee arthroplasty is currently of no proven clinical benefit: a systematic review. Clin Orthop. 2013;471:264–76.

70. Matziolis G, Krocher D, Weiss U, Tohtz S, Perka C. A prospective, randomized study of computer-assisted and conventional total knee arthroplasty. J Bone Joint Surg Am. 2007;89A:236–43.

71. Ishida K, Matsumoto T, Tsumura N, Kubo S, Kitagawa A, Chin T, et al. Mid-term outcomes of computer-assisted total knee arthroplasty. Knee Surg Sports Traumatol Arthrosc. 2011;19:1107–12.

72. Bathis H, Perlick L, Tingart M, Luring C, Zurakowski D, Grifka J. Alignment in total knee arthroplasty. A comparison of computer- assisted surgery with the conventional technique. J Bone Joint Surg Br. 2004;86B:682–7.

73. Kim YH, Kim JS, Hong KS, Kim YJ, Kim JH. Prevalence of fat embolism after total knee arthroplasty performed with or without computer navigation. J Bone Joint Surg Am. 2008;90A:1238.

74. Church JS, Scadden JE, Gupta RR, Cokis C, et al. Embolic phenomena during computer-assisted and conventional total knee replacement. J Bone Joint Surg Br. 2007;89B:481–5.

75. Hiscox CM, Bohm ER, Turgeon TR, Hedden DR, Burnell CD. Randomized trial of computer-assisted knee arthroplasty: impact on clinical and radiographic outcomes. J Arthroplasty. 2011;26:125964.

76. Cerha O, Kirschner S, Gunther KP, Lützner J. Cost analysis for navigation in knee endoprosthetics. Orthopade. 2009;38:1235–40.

77. Slover JD, Tosteson AN, Bozic KJ, Rubash HE, Malchau H. Impact of hospital volume on the economic value of computer navigation for total knee replacement. J Bone Joint Surg Am. 2008;90A:1492–500.

78. NIH Consensus Statement on total knee replacement. J Bone Joint Surg Am. 2004;86A:1328–35.

79. Rasanen P, Paavolainen P, Sintonen H, Koivisto AM, Blom M, Ryynanen OP, Roine RP. Effectiveness of hip or knee replacement surgery in terms of quality-adjusted life years and costs. Acta Orthop Scand. 2007;78:108–15.

Quality of Life and Patient Satisfaction After Total Knee Arthroplasty Using Contemporary Designs

Zoe H. Dailiana, Ippolyti Papakostidou, and Theofilos Karachalios

Introduction

As medical and public health advances have led to enhanced treatments of existing diseases, and to delayed mortality, researchers have changed the way of examining health, looking beyond causes of mortality and morbidity and assessing the relationship of health to the quality of an individual life. The Constitution of the World Health Organization (WHO) defines health as "A state of complete physical, mental, and social well-being not merely the absence of disease ...", and thus the measurement of health and health care effects must include the changes in the frequency and severity of diseases as well as an estimation of well-being after appraising improvement in the quality of life (QoL) related to health care. Although there are generally satisfactory ways of measuring the frequency and severity of diseases this is not the case in the measurement of well-being and QoL [1]. QoL is a global concept that has different philosophical, political and health-related definitions. WHO defines QoL as individuals' perception of their position in life in the context of the culture and value systems in which they live and in relation to their goals, expectations, standards and concerns. This broad concept is affected by a person's physical health, psychological state, level of independence, social relationships, personal beliefs, and relationship to salient features of his environment [2]. When QoL is considered in the context of health and disease, it is commonly referred to as health-related quality of life (HRQoL), to differentiate it from other aspects of quality of life. Since health is a multidimensional concept, HRQoL is also multidimensional and incorporates domains related to the physical, mental and emotional, and social functioning of an individual (Table 26.1) [3].

For decades, surgical prosthetic interventions were objectively assessed through operative complications, the survival and lifetime of implanted materials, morbidity and mortality rates. More recently other subjective scales have been added to follow up evaluation protocols. Moreover, it has been shown that for complete assessment of the benefits of a surgical intervention, it is essential to

Z.H. Dailiana, MD, DSc (✉) • I. Papakostidou, RN, DSc
Department of Orthopaedic Surgery,
Faculty of Medicine, School of Health Sciences,
University of Thessalia, 3 Panepistimiou St, Biopolis,
Larissa 41500, Hellenic Republic
e-mail: dailiana@med.uth.gr

T. Karachalios, MD, DSc
Department of Orthopaedic Surgery,
Faculty of Medicine, School of Health Sciences,
University of Thessalia, 3 Panepistimiou St, Biopolis,
Larissa 41500, Hellenic Republic

Orthopaedic Department, Faculty of Medicine,
School of Health Sciences, Center of Biomedical
Sciences (CERETETH), University of Thessalia,
University General Hospital of Larissa,
Mezourlo region, Larissa 41110, Hellenic Republic
e-mail: kar@med.uth.gr

© Springer-Verlag London 2015
T. Karachalios (ed.), *Total Knee Arthroplasty: Long Term Outcomes*,
DOI 10.1007/978-1-4471-6660-3_26

Table 26.1 Core components of multidimensional HRQoL assessment

Physical
Functional
Psychological/emotional
Social/occupational

provide evidence of its impact in terms of health status and HRQoL [4]. These terms refer to experiences of illness such as pain and fatigue, and broader aspects of the individual's physical, emotional, and social well-being. Unlike conventional medical indicators, these broader impacts of illness and treatment need to be assessed and reported by the patient [5]. The measurement of QoL provides objective evaluations of how and how much the disease influences a patient's life and how he or she copes with it. These evaluations may be used as a baseline of outcome measures and should provide a framework to determine the impact of any change on patients' QoL [6]. In this review we present the impact of total knee arthroplasty (TKA) on patient satisfaction and quality of life.

HRQoL Assessment

According to recent publications, there is an increasing interest in the use of HRQoL measures. There have been two fundamental types: generic instruments and disease specific instruments.

Generic health instruments include single indicators, health profiles and utility measures. These measures attempt to capture important aspects or dimensions of HRQoL and are applicable across a broad range of conditions and populations. Because of its broad scope, the sensitivity of this type of measure is inferior to one reported with specific instruments [7]. Unlike generic health measures, *disease-specific measures* focus on symptoms and disabilities specific to the condition such as osteoarthritis of the knee. At the expense of a comprehensive health evaluation, specific instruments tend to be more responsive to change within that defined domain.

One challenge of measuring HRQoL, particularly in joint arthroplasties, is to select measures that are responsive to change. Research in this area has shown that both generic and disease-specific measures are needed to thoroughly evaluate the effect of joint replacements [7]. It should be noted that in the international literature the terms QoL and HRQoL are used interchangeably, although it is probably more appropriate to use the latter term in health. In this section the term QoL is used to describe the HRQoL.

Because TKA is a high-volume, high-cost medical intervention, numerous HRQoL outcomes have been developed to allow investigators to quantify preoperative to postoperative improvements in the health status of patients undergoing TKA. The most commonly used outcomes tools are: the Oxford Knee Score (OKS) [8], the Knee Society Clinical Rating Scale (KSS) [9], the Knee Injury and Osteoarthritis Outcome Score (KOOS) [10], the Western Ontario and McMaster Universities Osteoarthritis Index (WOMAC) [11], and the Medical Outcomes Study 36-Item Short-Form Health Survey (SF-36) [12]. The SF-36 is the only generic scale identified to measure outcomes of TKA; the other scales are specific to knee replacement or osteoarthritis. With the exception of the KSS that is completed by the clinician, the WOMAC, OKS, KOOS and SF-36 scales are self-reported. The Oxford Knee Score (OKS) is the questionnaire in most widespread use in knee outcome research in the UK. Since April 2009 the Department of Health has required the routine collection of the OKS for every knee replacement undertaken within the NHS. This is known as Patient-Reported Outcome Program (PROMs) [13].

QoL Following TKA

Based on existing research evidence, TKA is a safe and cost-effective treatment for alleviation of pain and restoration of physical function in patients not responding to nonsurgical treatment. Overall, TKA has been shown to be a very successful, relatively low-risk therapy despite variations in patient health status and characteristics, type of prosthesis implanted, orthopaedic surgeon, and surgical facilities [14]. Although following TKA, patients show marked improvement in pain and physical function, time to recovery can vary. Clinically important improvements were reported with TKA at 6 months after surgery in terms of pain, stiffness, and/or function subscales of OKS, WOMAC and SF-36 [12, 15–19]. This evidence is supported by the English PROMs (Patient-Reported Outcome Measures) Programme, which uses 6-month outcome data to compare the results of hospitals that perform TKAs [13]. Further support was documented in a systematic review of three randomised controlled trials (RCTs) and six prospective cohort studies containing 4,369 patients in total, which report that most of the improvement shown on the OKS occurs in the first 6 months after TKA although there is erratic evidence of a minimally important difference occurring between 6 and at 12 months [20]. In a multicenter RCT involving 116 surgeons and 2,352 patients and using as primary outcome measures the OKS, SF-12 and EQ-5D (a standardised instrument for use as a measure of health outcome), the improvements in functional status and QoL scores were observed at 3 months after TKA [21]. A slow pattern of improvement can be observed up to 1 year using disease/joint specific and generic questionnaires [12, 22–25]. Generic health measures showed a smaller magnitude of change, which is to be expected given the construct of these measures that evaluate overall health and include the effect of other health conditions. The largest changes were seen in the domains that were primary related to total joint arthroplasty: pain and physical function [26].

While TKA provides pain relief and an improved QoL, physical function may decline over time without any identifiable medical or device complication [27–29]. In a review of 5,600 individual OKS questionnaires from a prospectively-collected knee replacement database, a gradual but significant decline was observed over a 10-year assessment [29]. Progression of arthritis at other sites, especially in the lumbar spine [30], the effect of aging [28, 31], and an increasing number of patients with a medical infirmity were the most common causes of decline of functional capacity.

Pain and Function Limitations After TKA

While a majority of patients report improvement in pain and function scores, a substantial number of individuals do not meet the level of improvement expected [32].

Chronic pain is the primary reason for people electing to undergo TKA and therefore pain relief is a key outcome after surgery [33]. However, some patients feel that TKA was not successful in relieving their pain; the percentage of these patients was found to be 13 % at 6 months postoperatively [34]. At 12 months postoperatively, the prevalence of medically unexplained chronic pain was found to be 13 % in a sample of 116 patients [35]. In this study, one in eight patients scored greater than 40 on a 100 VAS pain scale, despite having normal radiographic and clinical findings. Mid-term results have also uncovered a high prevalence of chronic pain after TKA [32]. Five years after TKA 6 % of patients reported medically unexplained moderate to severe chronic pain [36]. Seven years after TKA, 30 % of patients reported developing moderate to severe pain at some time interval since their initial recovery from surgery [37]. Much of the chronic pain and associated disability experienced by patients after TKA is medically unexplained. In a series of 27 patients that underwent an exploration of TKA for severe unexplained pain, only 45 % were found to have implant-related problems [38]. There is now evidence that there is a possible biological factor in the maintenance of chronic pain after TKA, through a dysfunction of pain modulation in the central nervous system known as central sensitization [39, 40].

Improvements in functional ability after TKA are also variable [32]. The restoration of unimpaired functional ability after TKA is rare, with only 33 % of people reporting no functional limitations with their replaced knee [41]. Nearly one fifth of TKA patients felt that their surgery was not successful in enabling them to resume their regular physical activities [34]. One year after TKA, patients still experienced substantial functional impairment compared with their age and gender matched peers, especially going upstairs, bending to the floor, walking and climbing stairs [30]. In a French national longitudinal survey, comprised of 202 subjects with TKA, people with TKA reported significantly greater difficulties than the general population with bending forward, walking more than 500 m and carrying 5 kg for 10 m [42]. In another study, patients reporting some difficulty with activities because of their knee function were three times more following TKA, compared to individuals with healthy knee function [43]. Poor functional ability in some TKA patients could be a reflection of limitations imposed by medical co-morbidities rather than the replaced knee. However, comparisons with the general population suggest otherwise. People with knee arthroplasty do not reach the level of mobility reported by the general population [34, 43–46]. One year post TKA, patients still experience substantial functional limitations compared with their age and gender matched peers [30, 43, 47]. In a 7-year matched pair cohort study of TKA patients and healthy controls, patients had significantly lower physical function than controls [48]. Similarly, the French Handicap, Disability and Dependence survey, which included interviews of nearly 17,000 individuals, found that people with joint replacement had greater limitations and reported worse health than people without a joint replacement [49]. The underlying causes of these differences are unclear. Although it is likely that much of these differences are a reflection of the biomechanical deficiencies of contemporary TKA designs, other potential factors include alteration of the remaining soft tissues and the absence of the native cruciate ligaments. Related factors include the general condition of the soft tissues in patients with TKAs, including the presence of scar tissue, changes attributable to osteoarthritis, and a possible reduction in muscular tone and lower limb strength [43].

Factors Predicting PROMs After TKA

A variety of factors predicting TKA outcomes have been evaluated, including gender, age, obesity, medical factors, implant design, and surgical technique.

Gender

The current data regarding gender are contradictory. The 2003 NIH consensus statement concludes gender was not strongly associated with short-term functional outcomes as assessed by the WOMAC, SF-36, or KSS [14]. In a large prospective study of 7,326 primary TKAs there were equal pain relief and walking improvements for both sexes during a 5-year follow-up period [50]. In four prospective studies of less than 300 patients each, gender was not associated with any difference in prevalence of substantial pain up to six [51–53] and 12 months post TKA [35]. On the contrary, a multinational randomized study of 860 TKA patients reported worse pain in women on the WOMAC pain scale at 1 and 2 years post TKA, but no age differences [54]. In a large retrospective observational study, women were 45 % more likely to report moderate to severe pain 2 years after primary TKA [55].

Age

Data related to the effect of age on PROMs are also contradictory. While some studies report better outcomes in older patients [36, 55, 56], others have reported similar outcomes in all age groups [35, 51–53, 57] or poorer in older age [54, 58, 59]. It is unclear whether the potentially better outcome in older patients is due to less demand on the replaced joint (e.g. higher pain tolerance or less scar formation with less stiffness) or to different levels of expectations compared to younger patients. On the other hand, older patients are likely to have more co-morbidities and less room for improvement than younger people. Well selected elderly patients can derive as much benefit from TKA as younger recipients [60].

Obesity

The correlation between knee osteoarthritis and obesity has been recognized for several years [61]. The negative effects of obesity following total joint arthroplasty, such as increased morbidity and mortality, have also been well documented in the literature. However, the association between obesity and outcome after TKA is disputed and little is known about whether specific body mass indices can be used as cut offs to determine which patients are most at risk for having a poor postoperative outcome [62]. Some studies indicate that obese individuals experience lower quality of life and performance after TKA [63–66]. In a large data set, including 1,011 primary TKAs, the effect of obesity was investigated in five groups of patients based on BMI 1 year postoperatively. It was concluded that the performance of the obese individuals quantified by the WOMAC and SF-36 outcomes tools was significantly lower. Additionally, 1-year follow up indicated that higher BMI negatively affected the ascending and descending capabilities of these individuals [63]. In a prospective study including 535 primary TKAs with a mean follow up of 9.2 years, the Hospital for Special Surgery (HSS) scores were significantly lower in obese individuals compared to peer-matched non-obese patients [64]. In another prospective study, 445 consecutive primary TKAs were followed up to 9 years. Clinical outcomes of non-obese (BMI <30) were compared to obese (BMI >30) patients. Significant improvements in outcome were seen and sustained in all groups 9 years after TKA. However, lower function scores were seen at all follow-up periods prior to 9 years in the highly obese subset with BMI >35 [65]. In a systematic review of the literature identifying 24 studies with a mean 5-year follow-up, the postoperative mean objective and function KSS were significantly lower in morbidly obese patients compared to non-obese. However, obese patients did not have significantly lower KSS (objective and function scores) compared to non-obese. Morbidly obese patients also had significantly lower implant survivorship than obese and non-obese patients [62]. There are, however, other investigations reporting contradictory findings with no significant differences observed between obese and non-obese individuals in regard to the outcome of TKA [67–70]. They report that body weight did not adversely influence the outcome of TKA in the short term [68, 69] or in the long term although there was a trend for obesity to influence

the rate of aseptic loosening [67, 70]. The degree of functional improvement following TKA in the obese population remains controversial. It appears that obese patients have similar satisfaction rates as the non-obese population following total joint arthroplasty. As BMI increases (>40), however, the functional improvement becomes less and/or occurs more gradually and is tempered by the associated increased complication profile [71].

Medical Factors

Medical factors that are highly predictive of a poor outcome after TKA include a greater number of co-morbidities and a worse pre-operative status i.e. high pain and disability [72]. Depressive symptoms are also significant predictors of both pain and functional limitations after TKA [35, 73]. Low self-efficacy is related to higher intensity pain in arthritis [74], and expectations for complete pain relief after TKA exert a strong influence on achieving better function and less pain postoperatively [75]. Physical and psychological issues may influence the success of TKA, and understanding patient differences could facilitate the decision making process before, during, and after surgery, thereby achieving the greatest benefit from TKA [14].

Implant Design

Despite the increased success of TKA, questions have arisen regarding the materials and implant designs that are most effective for specific patient populations. Implant design has evolved over time, with improvement in success rates [14]. A number of knee prosthesis designs are on the market today, however their relative merits are generally unclear. The mobile bearing compared to the fixed bearing design has the theoretical advantages of decreased wear and improved kinematics, which should result in an improvement in functional outcome and a decrease in long-term failure rate. The main theoretical disadvantage is instability and dislocation of the bearing [76]. According to many RCTs, meta-analysis and systemic reviews, no statistically significant differences could be identified in any of the PROMs between patients who received the fixed-bearing or the mobile-bearing knee post-operatively [77–80]. The polyethylene components of modern prosthetic designs appear to be quite durable [14]. Another common variation is the design of the tibial component. Use of a metal-backed base plate has theoretical advantages in that it distributes load more evenly across the bone implant interface than an all polyethylene tibia, and thus should decrease the risk of loosening. Limited comparisons between non-metal backed and metal backed components have been performed, and no definitive difference has been reported [81, 82]. There is considerable variability in patellar resurfacing; many surgeons routinely use it while others choose patellar retention. Although there is no clear evidence as to which approach is best, the role of soft tissue balancing and patella-friendly prosthetic designs is recognized.

Surgical Technique

Technical factors in performing TKA surgery may influence both short and long term clinical outcomes. Navigation systems have been developed to improve the accuracy of alignment of the components in TKA. Proper alignment of the prosthesis appears to be critical in minimizing long term wear, risk of osteolysis and loosening of the prosthesis. Computer navigation may eventually reduce the risk of substantial malalignment and improve soft tissue balance and patellar tracking [83, 84]. However, the technology is expensive, increases operating room time, and the benefits on PROMs remain unclear [14]. Minimally invasive surgery (MIS) is widely promoted as a possible improvement over conventional TKA. It allows for faster recovery time, less pain, less need for assistive devices, better knee flexion during the early post-operative period, and improvements in function [85, 86]. However, concerns have risen over potentially increased complications associated with delayed wound healing and infections,

and the learning curve required for successful accomplishment of MIS techniques [87]. Poor visualization during surgery could also affect long-term outcomes (e.g. component malalignment) [85, 86, 88]. A systematic review of RCTs comparing MIS and conventional TKA found that MIS resulted in longer operating times, early improvements in KSS (6 and 12 weeks, but not after 6 months), early improvements in knee range of motion (6 days after TKA), and a greater incidence of delayed wound healing and infection, although no greater incidence in overall complications and component malalignment [85]. Again, the benefits on PROMs remain unclear. A meta-analysis of RCTs comparing clinical and radiological outcomes following MIS and conventional TKA found that knee flexion was significantly greater following MIS and that there were trends for statistically significant improvements in quadriceps muscle strength during early follow-up, but not at later follow-up [86]. In a systematic review of the published literature on MIS TKA, patients tended to have decreased postoperative pain, rapid recovery of quadriceps function, reduced blood loss, improved range of motion (mostly reported as a short-term gain) and shorter hospital stay compared with patients undergoing standard TKA. However, an increased tourniquet time and increased incidence of component malalignment in the MIS TKA groups is also reported [88].

Patient Satisfaction

The concept of satisfaction is most widely employed in consumer marketing and can be defined as "an attitude like judgment following an act, based on a series of product-consumer interactions" [89]. In the health service industries, patient satisfaction is perhaps the most important criterion of success and it has been used as a healthcare performance indicator for clinical care [90–92]. Quantifying satisfaction in a valid way is a challenge because is not straightforward to assess, and non-validated instruments can provide misleading data.

Satisfaction with TKA

Patient satisfaction with the outcome of TKA is becoming increasingly used as a measure of the patient's perception of TKA success and it has been recognized as an important measure of outcome because there is a well- documented discrepancy between clinician and patient ratings of health status [93–98]. On the other hand, the higher rates of success for this procedure have led younger and more active patients to undergo TKA, expecting to be more active and pain free after surgery. Therefore, it is important to evaluate patient satisfaction after TKA in more detail, although we do not have a gold standard method to measure it by. While the majority of patients are satisfied with the outcome following TKA, and show good improvement in function afterwards, some are dissatisfied with the outcome. Despite on-going advances in primary TKA patient selection, in implant design and surgical techniques, the rate of dissatisfaction following TKA ranges from 5.5 % to 19 % with patients citing either a lack of pain relief or lack of functional improvement [93, 99–106]. The Swedish Arthroplasty Registry has reported that 2–17 years after TKA, 81 % of the 25,000 patients were satisfied with the outcome of their surgery, 8 % were not satisfied and 11 % undecided [99]. The National Joint Registry for England and Wales found that 82 % of patients were satisfied at just over 1 year after primary TKA [106]. Other studies have found that 14–19 % of patients were dissatisfied with the outcome 1 year after primary TKA [14, 93, 100, 107]. Satisfaction with the outcome of TKA can vary depending on the domain being assessed. For example, in a cohort of 407 patients (523 knees), 73 % of patients were very satisfied with pain relief, but only 50 % of patients were very satisfied with their ability to perform leisure activities 10 years after TKA [41]. In another cohort of 1,703 primary TKA patients, satisfaction with pain relief varied from 72 % to 86 % and with function from 70 % to 84 % for specific activities of daily living 1 year after surgery [93]. In a small prospective study (n = 112) with 7 years of follow-up, 86 % of patients were satisfied with

TKA, 80 % would undergo the operation again, and 56 % did regular physical activity and had better WOMAC pain and functional scores [108]. Determining which factors affect patient satisfaction after TKA is a very important clinical issue and depends on many factors, including pain relief and functional ability achieved postoperatively, the fulfilment of pre- surgical expectations and mental wellbeing [100, 109]. Achievement of pain relief and functional status are the most important predictors of satisfaction [100–111]. While pain relief is very relevant to patient satisfaction, it is not the sole driver. It is quite possible for patients to report good levels of pain relief and overall dissatisfaction or vice versa. Marrying of expectations and resultant perception of outcome has been suggested as a model for understanding satisfaction response. The failure to meet optimistic expectations is associated with dissatisfaction following joint arthroplasty, with the expectations of kneeling, squatting and ease of climbing stairs amongst the least frequently met expectations [100, 111].

On the other hand, older patients demonstrate poorer functional outcomes, but exhibit high levels of satisfaction, perhaps due to lower preoperative expectations [45, 112, 113]. Psychological issues such as depression and a tendency to catastrophize have also a negative effect on both outcomes and satisfaction [114, 115].

Conclusions

Primary TKA is most commonly performed for advanced knee osteoarthritis. Satisfactory outcomes of primary TKA in most patients are strongly supported by more than 20 years of follow up data. There appears to be rapid and substantial improvement in the patient's pain, functional status, and overall health related quality of life in approximately 90 % of patients.

Current data regarding the effect of age, gender and obesity on patient reported outcome measures remain contradictory, although older patients are likely to have less room for improvement than younger people, and lower BMI is associated with greater satisfaction and better functional outcome. Physical and psychological issues may influence the success of TKA, and understanding patients' differences could help us achieve the greatest benefit from TKA.

Despite on- going advances in primary TKA patient selection, in implant design and surgical techniques, the dissatisfaction rate following TKA ranges from 5.5 % to 19 % with patients citing either a lack of pain relief or functional improvement.

References

1. The WHOQOL Group. The development of the World Health Organization quality of life assessment instrument (the WHOQOL). In: Orley J, Kuyken W, editors. Quality of life assessment: international perspectives. Heidelberg: Springer Verlag; 1994.
2. WHOQOL Group. Development of the WHOQOL: rationale and current status. Int J Ment Health. 1994;23:24–56.
3. Ferrans CE. Definitions and conceptual models of quality of life. In: Lipscomb J, Gotay CC, Snyder C, editors. Outcomes assessment in cancer. Cambridge, UK: Cambridge University Press; 2005. p. 14–30.
4. Garratt A, Schmidt L, Mackintosh A, Fitzpatrick R. Quality of life measurement: bibliographic study of patient assessed health outcome measures. Br Med J. 2002;324(7351):1417.
5. Fitzpatrick R, Davey C, Buxton MJ, Jones DR. Evaluating patient-based outcome measures for use in clinical trials. Health Technol Assess. 1998;2:1–74.
6. Higginson IJ, Carr AJ. Measuring quality of life. Using quality of life measures in the clinical setting. Br Med J. 2001;322:1297–300.
7. Fitzpatrick R, Fletcher A, Gore S, Jones D, Spiegelhalter D, Cox D. Quality of life measures in health care, I: applications and issues in assessment. Br Med J. 1992;305(6861):1074–7.
8. Murray DW, Fitzpatrick R, Rogers K, Pandit H, Beard DJ, Carr AJ, Dawson J. The use of the Oxford hip and knee scores. J Bone Joint Surg Br. 2007;89B:1010–4.
9. Insall JN, Dorr LD, Scott RD, Scott WN. Rationale of the Knee Society clinical rating system. Clin Orthop. 1989;248:13–4.
10. Roos EM, Roos HP, Lohmander LS, Ekdahl C, Beynnon BD. Knee injury and Osteoarthritis Outcome Score (KOOS) – development of a self-administered outcome measure. J Orthop Sports Phys Ther. 1998;28:88–96.
11. Bellamy N, Buchanan WW, Goldsmith GH, Campbell J, Stitt LW. Validation study of WOMAC: a health status instrument for measuring clinically important patient relevant outcomes to antirheumatic drug therapy in patients with osteoarthritis of hip or knee. J Rheumatol. 1988;15:1833–40.
12. Escobar A, Quintana JM, Bilbao A, Arostegui I, Lafuente I, Vidaurreta I. Responsiveness and clinically important differences for the WOMAC and SF-36 after total knee replacement. Osteoarthritis Cartilage. 2007;15:273–80.
13. Guidance on the routine collection of Patient Reported Outcome Measures (PROMs). For the NHS in England 2009/10; 2008. Available at: http://www.mstrust.org.uk/competencies/downloads/NHS-PROMS.pdf
14. NIH Consensus Development conference on total knee replacement. National Institutes of Health Consensus Development Conference Statement December 8–10, 2003. Available at: http://consensus.nih.gov/2003/2003totalkneereplacement117html.htm
15. Jones CA, Voaklander DC, Suarez-Alma ME. Determinants of function after total knee arthroplasty. Phys Ther. 2003;83:696–706.
16. Escobar A, Quintana JM, Bilbao A, Azkarate J, Guenaga JI, Arenaza JC, Gutierrez LF. Effect of patient characteristics on reported outcomes after total knee replacement. Rheumatology. 2007;46:112–9.
17. Xie F, Lo NN, Pullenayegum EM, O'Reilly DJ, Goeree R, Lee HP. Evaluation of health outcomes in osteoarthritis patients after total knee replacement: a two-year follow-up. Health Qual Life Outcomes. 2010;8:87.
18. Clement ND, Macdonald D, Howie CR, Biant LC. The outcome of primary total hip and knee arthroplasty in patients aged 80 years or more. J Bone Joint Surg Br. 2011;93B:1265–70.
19. Ko Y, Narayanasamy S, Wee H-L, Lo NN, Yeo SJ, Yang KY, Yeo W, Chong HC, Thumboo J. Health-related quality of life after total knee replacement or unicompartmental knee arthroplasty in an urban Asian population. Value Health. 2011;14:322–8.
20. Browne JP, Bastaki H, Dawson J. What is the optimal time point to assess patient-reported recovery after hip and knee replacement? A systematic review and analysis of routinely reported outcome data from the English patient-reported outcome measures programme. Health Qual Life Outcomes. 2013;11:128.
21. KAT Trial Group, Johnston L, MacLennan G, McCormack K, Ramsay C, Walker A. The Knee Arthroplasty Trial (KAT) design features, baseline characteristics, and two-year functional outcomes after alternative approaches to knee replacement. J Bone Joint Surg Am. 2009;91A:134–41.
22. Hamilton D, Henderson GR, Gaston P, MacDonald D, Howie C, Simpson AH. Comparative outcomes of total hip and knee arthroplasty: a prospective cohort study. Postgrad Med J. 2012;88(1045):627–31.
23. Bachmeier CJM, March LM, Lapsley HM, Tribe KL, Courtenay BG, Brooks PM. A comparison of outcomes in osteoarthritis patients undergoing total hip and knee replacement surgery. Osteoarthritis Cartilage. 2001;9:137–46.

24. Terwee CB, Van Der Slikke RM, Van Lummel RC, Benink RJ, Meijers WG, de Vet HC. Self-reported physical functioning was more influenced by pain than performance-based physical functioning in knee-osteoarthritis patients. J Clin Epidemiol. 2006;59: 724–31.

25. Nunez M, Nunez E, Segur JM, Maculé F, Sanchez A, Hernández MV, Vilalta C. Health-related quality of life and costs in patients with osteoarthritis on waiting list for total knee replacement. Osteoarthritis Cartilage. 2007;15:258–65.

26. Jones CA, Pohar S. Health-related quality of life after total joint arthroplasty: a scoping review. Clin Geriatr Med. 2012;28:395–429.

27. Nilsdotter AK, Toksvig-Larsen S, Roos EM. A 5 year prospective study of patient-relevant outcomes after total knee replacement. Osteoarthritis Cartilage. 2009;17:601–6.

28. Ritter MA, Thong AE, Davis KE, Berend ME, Meding JB, Faris PM. Long-term deterioration of joint evaluation scores. J Bone Joint Surg Br. 2004;86B:438–42.

29. Williams DP, Blakey CM, Hadfield SG, Murray DW, Price AJ, Field RE. Long-term trends in the Oxford knee score following total knee replacement. Bone Joint J. 2013;95B:45–51.

30. Benjamin J, Johnson R, Porter S. Knee scores change with length of follow-up after total knee arthroplasty. J Arthroplasty. 2003;18:867–71.

31. Meding JB, Meding LK, Ritter MA, Keating EM. Pain relief and functional improvement remain 20 years after knee arthroplasty. Clin Orthop. 2012;470:144–9.

32. Wylde V, Dieppe P, Hewlett S, Learmonth ID. Total knee replacement: is it really an effective procedure for all? Knee. 2007;14:417–23.

33. Hawker G, Wright J, Coyte P, Paul J, Dittus R, Croxford R, Katz B, Bombardier C, Heck D, Freund D. Health-related quality of life after knee replacement. J Bone Joint Surg Am. 1998;80A:163–73.

34. Jones CA, Voaklander DC, Johnston DW, Suarez-Almazor ME. Health related quality of life outcomes after total hip and knee arthroplasties in a community based population. J Rheumatol. 2000;27: 1745–52.

35. Brander VA, Stulberg SD, Adams AD, Harden RN, Bruehl S, Stanos SP, Houle T. Predicting total knee replacement pain: a prospective, observational study. Clin Orthop. 2003;461:27–36.

36. Elson DW, Brenkel IJ. Predicting pain after total knee arthroplasty. J Arthroplasty. 2006;21:1047–53.

37. Murray DW, Frost SJD. Pain in the assessment of total knee replacement. J Bone Joint Surg Br. 1998;80B:426–31.

38. Mont MA, Serna FK, Krackow KA, Hungerford DS. Exploration of radiographically normal total knee replacements for unexplained pain. Clin Orthop. 1996;454:216–20.

39. Neugebauer V, Schaible HG. Evidence for a central component in the sensitization of spinal neurons with joint input during development of acute arthritis in cat's knee. J Neurophysiol. 1990;64:299–311.

40. Kosek E, Ordeberg G. Abnormalities of somatosensory perception in patients with painful osteoarthritis normalize following successful treatment. Eur J Pain. 2000;4:229–38.

41. Wright RJ, Sledge CB, Poss R, Ewald FC, Walsh ME, Lingard EA. Patient-reported outcome and survivorship after Kinemax total knee arthroplasty. J Bone Joint Surg Am. 2004;86A:2464–70.

42. Dechartres A, Boutron I, Nizard R, Poiraudeau S, Roy C, Baron G, Ravaud P, Ravaud JF. Knee arthroplasty: disabilities in comparison to the general population and to hip arthroplasty using a French national longitudinal survey. PLoS One. 2008;3(7):e2561.

43. Noble PC, Gordon MJ, Weiss JM, Reddix RN, Conditt MA, Mathis KB. Does total knee replacement restore normal knee function? Clin Orthop. 2005;463:157–65.

44. Linsell L, Dawson J, Zondervan K, Rose P, Carr A, Randall T, Fitzpatrick R. Pain and overall health status in older people with hip and knee replacement: a population perspective. J Public Health. 2006;28:267–73.

45. Rat AC, Guillemin F, Osnowycz G, Delagoutte JP, Cuny C, Mainard D, Baumann C. Total hip or knee replacement for osteoarthritis: mid- and long-term quality of life. Arthritis Care Res. 2010;62:54–62.

46. Dowsey MM, Nikpour M, Dieppe P, Choong PF. Associations between pre-operative radiographic changes and outcomes after total knee joint replacement for osteoarthritis. Osteoarthritis Cartilage. 2012;20:1095–102.

47. Weiss JM, Noble PC, Conditt MA, Kohl HW, Roberts S, Cook KF, Gordon MJ, Mathis KB. What functional activities are important to patients with knee replacements? Clin Orthop. 2002;460:172–88.

48. Cushnaghan J, Coggon D, Reading I, Croft P, Byng P, Cox K, Dieppe P, Cooper C. Long-term outcome following total hip arthroplasty: a controlled longitudinal study. Arthritis Rheum. 2007;57:1375–80.

49. Boutron I, Poiraudeau S, Ravaud JF, Baron G, Revel M, Nizard R, Dougados M, Ravaud P. Disability in adults with hip and knee arthroplasty: a French national community based survey. Ann Rheum Dis. 2003;62:748–54.

50. Ritter MA, Wing JT, Berend ME, Davis KE, Meding JB. The clinical effect of gender on outcome of total knee arthroplasty. J Arthroplasty. 2008;23:331–6.

51. Jones CA, Voaklander DC, Johnston DW, Suarez-Almazor ME. The effect of age on pain, function, and quality of life after total hip and knee arthroplasty. Arch Intern Med. 2001;161:454–60.

52. Fortin PR, Clarke AE, Joseph L, Liang MH, Tanzer M, Ferland D, Phillips C, Partridge AJ, Bélisle P, Fossel AH, Mahomed N, Sledge CB, Katz JN. Outcomes of total hip and knee replacement: preoperative functional status predicts outcomes at six months after surgery. Arthritis Rheum. 1999;42:1722–8.

53. Papakostidou I, Dailiana ZH, Papapolychroniou T, Liaropoulos L, Zintzaras E, Karachalios TS, Malizos KN. Factors affecting the quality of life after total knee arthroplasties: a prospective study. BMC Musculoskelet Disord. 2012;13:116.

54. Lingard EA, Katz JN, Wright EA, Sledge CB. Predicting the outcome of total knee arthroplasty. J Bone Joint Surg Am. 2004;86A:2179–86.

55. Singh JA, Gabriel S, Lewallen D. The impact of gender, age, and preoperative pain severity on pain after TKA. Clin Orthop. 2008;466:2717–23.

56. Fitzgerald JD, Orav EJ, Lee TH, Marcantonio ER, Poss R, Goldman L, Mangione CM. Patient quality of life during the 12 months following joint replacement surgery. Arthritis Rheum. 2004;51:100–9.

57. Roth ML, Tripp DA, Harrison MH, Sullivan M, Carson P. Demographic and psychosocial predictors of acute perioperative pain for total knee arthroplasty. Pain Res Manag. 2007;12:185–94.

58. Kennedy LG, Newman JH, Ackroyd CE, Dieppe PA. When should we do knee replacements? Knee. 2003;10:161–6.

59. Santaguida PL, Hawker GA, Hudak PL, Glazier R, Mahomed NN, Kreder HJ, Coyte PC, Wright JG. Patient characteristics affecting the prognosis of total hip and knee joint arthroplasty: a systematic review. Can J Surg. 2008;51:428–36.

60. Brander VA, Malhotra S, Jet J, Heinemann AW, Stulberg SD. Outcome of hip and knee arthroplasty in persons aged 80 years and older. Clin Orthop. 1997;345:67–78.

61. Niu J, Zhang YQ, Torner J, Nevitt M, Lewis CE, Aliabadi P, Sack B, Clancy M, Sharma L, Felson DT. Is obesity a risk factor for progressive radiographic knee osteoarthritis? Arthritis Rheum. 2009;61:329–35.

62. McElroy MJ, Pivec R, Issa K, Harwin SF, Mont MA. The effects of obesity and morbid obesity on outcomes in TKA. J Knee Surg. 2013;26:83–8.

63. Stickles B, Phillips L, Brox WT, Owens B, Lanzer WL. Defining the relationship between obesity and total joint arthroplasty. Obes Res. 2001;9:219–23.

64. Jackson MP, Sexton SA, Walter WL, Walter WK, Zicat BA. The impact of obesity on the mid-term outcome of cementless total knee replacement. J Bone Joint Surg Br. 2009;91B:1044–8.

65. Collins RA, Walmsley PJ, Amin AK, Brenkel IJ, Clayton RA. Does obesity influence clinical outcome at nine years following total knee arthroplasty? J Bone Joint Surg Br. 2012;94B:1351–5.

66. Dowsey MM, Liew D, Stoney JD, Choong PF. The impact of pre-operative obesity on weight change and outcome in total knee replacement: a prospective study of 529 consecutive patients. J Bone Joint Surg Br. 2010;92B:513–20.

67. Foran JRH, Mont MA, Rajadhyaksha AD, Jones LC, Etienne G, Hungerford DS. Total knee arthroplasty in obese patients: a comparison with a matched control group. J Arthroplasty. 2004;19:817–24.

68. Deshmukh RG, Hayes JH, Pinder IM. Does body weight influence outcome after total knee arthroplasty? A 1-year analysis. J Arthroplasty. 2002;17:315–9.

69. Nunez M, Lozano L, Nunez E, Sastre S, Luis Del Val J, Suso S. Good quality of life in severely obese total knee replacement patients: a case-control study. Obes Surg. 2011;21:1203–8.

70. Krushell RJ, Fingeroth RJ. Primary total knee arthroplasty in morbidly obese patients: a 5- to 14-year follow-up study. J Arthroplasty. 2007;22:77–80.

71. Workgroup of the American Association of Hip and Knee Surgeons (AAHKS. Evidence based committee obesity and total joint arthroplasty. A literature based review. J Arthroplasty. 2013;28:714–21.

72. Mahomed NN, Liang MH, Cook EF, Daltroy LH, Fortin PR, Fossel AH, Katz JN. The importance of patient expectations in predicting functional outcomes after total joint arthroplasty. J Rheumatol. 2002;29:1273–9.

73. Faller H, Kirschner S, Konig A. Psychological distress predicts functional outcomes at three and twelve months after total knee arthroplasty. Gen Hosp Psychiatry. 2003;25:372–3.

74. Keefe FJ, Kashikar-Zuck S, Robinson E, Salley A, Beaupre P, Caldwell D, Baucom D, Haythornthwaite J. Pain coping strategies that predict patients' and spouses' ratings of patients' self-efficacy. Pain. 1997;73:191–9.

75. Lingard EA, Sledge CB, Learmonth ID, The Kinemax Outcomes G. Patient expectations regarding total knee arthroplasty: differences among the United States, United Kingdom, and Australia. J Bone J Surg Am. 2006;88A:1201–7.

76. O'Connor JJ, Goodfellow JW. Theory and practice of meniscal knee replacement: designing against wear. Proc Inst Mech Eng H. 1996;210:217–22.

77. Wylde V, Learmonth I, Potter A, Bettinson K, Lingard E. Patient-reported outcomes after fixed-versus mobile-bearing total knee replacement: a multi-centre randomised controlled trial using the kinemax total knee replacement. J Bone Joint Surg Br. 2008;90B:1172–9.

78. Harrington MA, Hopkinson WJ, Hsu P, Manion L. Fixed- vs mobile-bearing total knee arthroplasty. Does it make a difference? – a prospective randomized study. J Arthroplasty. 2009;24:24–7.

79. Oh KJ, Pandher DS, Lee SH, Sung Joon Jr SD, Lee ST. Meta-analysis comparing outcomes of fixed-bearing and mobile-bearing prostheses in total knee arthroplasty. J Arthroplasty. 2009;24:873–84.

80. Smith H, Jan M, Mahomed N, Davey J, Gandhi R. Meta-analysis and systematic review of clinical outcomes comparing mobile bearing and fixed bearing total knee arthroplasty. J Arthroplasty. 2011;26:1205–13.

81. Najibi S, Iorio R, Surdam JW, Whang W, Appleby D, Healy WL. All-polyethylene and metal-backed tibial components in total knee arthroplasty: a matched

pair analysis of functional outcome. J Arthroplasty. 2003;18:9–15.

82. Cheng T, Zhang G, Zhang X. Metal-backed versus all-polyethylene tibial components in primary total knee arthroplasty. Acta Orthop Scand. 2011;82:589–95.

83. Cheng T, Zhao S, Peng X, Zhang X. Does computer-assisted surgery improve postoperative leg alignment and implant positioning following total knee arthroplasty? A meta-analysis of randomized controlled trials? Knee Surg Sports Traumatol Arthrosc. 2012;20:1307–22.

84. Zhang GQ, Chen JY, Chai W, Liu M, Wang Y. Comparison between computer-assisted-navigation and conventional total knee arthroplasties in patients undergoing simultaneous bilateral procedures: a randomized clinical trial. J Bone Joint Surg Am. 2011;93A:1190–6.

85. Cheng T, Liu T, Zhang G, Peng X, Zhang X. Does minimally invasive surgery improve short-term recovery in total knee arthroplasty? Clin Orthop. 2010;468:1635–48.

86. Smith TO, King JJ, Hing CB. A meta-analysis of randomised controlled trials comparing the clinical and radiological outcomes following minimally invasive to conventional exposure for total knee arthroplasty. Knee. 2012;19:1–7.

87. King J, Stamper DL, Schaad DC, Leopold SS. Minimally invasive total knee arthroplasty compared with traditional total knee arthroplasty. Assessment of the learning curve and the postoperative recuperative period. J Bone Joint Surg Am. 2007;89A:1497–503.

88. Kolisek FR, Bonutti PM, Hozack WJ, Purtill J, Sharkey PF, Zelicof SB, Ragland PS, Kester M, Mont MA, Rothman RH. Clinical experience using a minimally invasive surgical approach for total knee arthroplasty: early results of a prospective randomized study compared to a standard approach. J Arthroplasty. 2007;22:8–13.

89. Fournier SB, Mick DG. Rediscovering satisfaction. J Mark. 1999;63:5–19.

90. Doyle C, Lennox L, Bell D. A systematic review of evidence on the links between patient experience and clinical safety and effectiveness. Br Med J Open. 2013;3(1):e001570.

91. Mira JJ, Tomás O, Virtudes-Pérez M, Nebot C, Rodríguez-Marín J. Predictors of patient satisfaction in surgery. Surgery. 2009;145:536–41.

92. Tisnado DM, Rose-Ash DE, Malin JL, Adams JL, Ganz PA, Kahn KL. Financial incentives for quality in breast cancer care. Am J Manag Care. 2008;14:457–66.

93. Bourne RB, Chesworth BM, Davis AM, Mahomed NN, Charron KD. Patient satisfaction after total knee arthroplasty: who is satisfied and who is not? Clin Orthop. 2010;468:57–63.

94. Kwon SK, Kang YG, Kim SJ, Chang CB, Seong SC, Kim TK. Correlations between commonly used clinical outcome scales and patient satisfaction after total knee arthroplasty. J Arthroplasty. 2010;25:1125–30.

95. Baumann C, Rat AC, Mainard D, Cuny C, Guillemin F. Importance of patient satisfaction with care in predicting osteoarthritis specific health-related quality of life one year after total joint arthroplasty. Qual Life Res. 2011;20:1581–8.

96. Becker R, Doring C, Denecke A, Brosz M. Expectation, satisfaction and clinical outcome of patients after total knee arthroplasty. Knee Surg Sports Traumatol Arthrosc. 2011;19:1433–41.

97. Janse AJ, Gemke RJ, Uiterwaal CS, van der Tweel I, Kimpen JL, Sinnema G. Quality of life: patients and doctors don't always agree: a meta-analysis. J Clin Epidemiol. 2004;57:653–61.

98. Gioe TJ, Pomeroy D, Suthers K, Singh JA. Can patients help with long-term total knee arthroplasty surveillance? Comparison of the American Knee Society Score self-report and surgeon assessment. Rheumatology (Oxford). 2009;48:160–4.

99. Robertsson O, Dunbar M, Pehrsson T, Knutson K, Lidgren L. Patient satisfaction after knee arthroplasty: a report on 27,372 knees operated on between 1981 and 1995 in Sweden. Acta Orthop Scand. 2000;71:262–7.

100. Scott CE, Howie CR, MacDonald D, Biant LC. Predicting dissatisfaction following total knee replacement: a prospective study of 1217 patients. J Bone Joint Surg Br. 2010;92B:1253–8.

101. Jorn LP, Johnsson R, Toksvig-Larsen S. Patient satisfaction, function and return to work after knee arthroplasty. Acta Orthop Scand. 1999;70:343–7.

102. Kane RL, Saleh KJ, Wilt TJ, Bershadsky B, Cross 3rd WW, MacDonald RM, Rutks I. Total knee replacement. Evid Rep Technol Assess (Summ). 2003;86:1–8.

103. Katz JN, Phillips CB, Baron JA, Fossel AH, Mahomed NN, Barrett J, Lingard EA, Harris WH, Poss R, Lew RA, Guadagnoli E, Wright EA, Losina E. Association of hospital and surgeon volume of total hip replacement with functional status and satisfaction three years following surgery. Arthritis Rheum. 2003;48:560–8.

104. Mahomed N, Sledge C, Daltroy L, Fossel A, Katz J. Self-administered satisfaction scale for joint replacement arthroplasty. J Bone Joint Surg Br. 1998;80B(S1):9.

105. National Joint Registry for England and Wales: Summary report the 2nd annual report. September 2005. Available at http://www.njrcentre.org.uk/njrcentre/portals/0/documents/england/reports/njr_ar_2.pdf

106. Dailiana Z, Papakostidou I, Varitimidis S, Liaropoulos L, Zintzaras E, Karachalios TS, Michelinakis E, Malizos KN. Patient-reported quality of life after primary major joint arthroplasty: a prospective comparison of hip and knee arthroplasty (submitted for publication).

107. Noble PC, Conditt MA, Cook KF, Mathis KB. The John Insall Award: patient expectations affect satisfaction with total knee arthroplasty. Clin Orthop. 2006;452:35–43.

108. Núñez M, Lozano L, Núñez E, Segur JM, Sastre S, Maculé F, Ortega R, Suso S. Total knee replacement and health-related quality of life: factors influencing long-term outcomes. Arthritis Rheum. 2009;61:1062–9.

109. Culliton SE, Bryant DM, Overend TJ, Macdonald SJ, Chesworth BM. The relationship between expectations and satisfaction in patients undergoing primary total knee arthroplasty. J Arthroplasty. 2012;27:490–2.

110. Matsuda S, Kawahara S, Okazaki K, Tashiro Y, Iwamoto Y. Postoperative alignment and ROM affect patient satisfaction after TKA. Clin Orthop. 2013;471:127–33.

111. Scott CE, Bugler KE, Clement ND, MacDonald D, Howie CR, Biant LC. Patient expectations of arthroplasty of the hip and knee. J Bone Joint Surg Br. 2012;94B:974–81.

112. Baker PN, van der Meulen JH, Lewsey J, Gregg PJ, National Joint Registry for England and Wales. The role of pain and function in determining patient satisfaction after total knee replacement. Data from the National Joint Registry for England and Wales. J Bone Joint Surg Br. 2007;89B:893–900.

113. Bremner-Smith AT, Ewings P, Weale AE. Knee scores in a 'normal' elderly population. Knee. 2004;11:279–82.

114. Sullivan M, Tanzer M, Reardon G, Amirault D, Dunbar M, Stanish W. The role of presurgical expectancies in predicting pain and function one year following total knee arthroplasty. Pain. 2011;152:2287–93.

115. Lavernia CJ, Alcerro JC, Brooks LG, Rossi MD. Mental health and outcomes in primary total joint arthroplasty. J Arthroplasty. 2012;27:1276–82.

Index

A

Advance medial pivot (AMP) TKA
bone stock preservation, primary and revision, 148
clinical wear rates
polyethylene particles, 146, 147
PS and AMP, 146
synovial fluid, 146
complication rates, reduction, 144
cruciate retaining/substituting designs, 144
implant geometry, 144
normal knee kinematics and stability
antero-posterior, design features, 145, 146
A/P sliding and rotation, 145
articulating convex, 144
ball-in-socket design, 144, 145
circular femoral condyles, 145
femoro-tibial articulation, 145
four-bar-link mechanism, 144
paradoxical motion, 145, 146
rollback, 144
static and dynamic, 145
tibia pivots, 144
patellofemoral joint kinematics
articulation design features, 148
high complication rates, 146
trochlear groove femoral component, 146, 148
radiological results, 144
ROM, optimization
designs comparison, 145–146
multicenter study group, 145–146
tibiofemoral joint kinematics, 144
American Knee Society Score (AKSS), 43
AMP TKA. *See* Advance medial pivot (AMP) TKA
Aquatic therapy
observation period, 232
pool exercise, aftercare of patients, 231
WOMAC score, 231
Arthritic knee, 1, 70, 71, 75
Arthrodesis
external fixator, 223, 224
infected TKA management strategies, 219, 220, 223
infection and periprosthetic fractures, 179
Arthroscopic debridement and retention of implants, 220
Articulating spacers, 222, 223

Augmentation
deficient lateral condyle, 74
polyethylene liner molding, 170
reality systems, 246
Australian Orthopaedic Association National Joint
Replacement Registry, 150

B

Balance training
functional training (FT) protocol, 232
physical therapy, 232
Wii Fit™, 232–233
The Blauth prosthesis, 25, 179, 182
Body mass index (BMI)
bilateral TKA, 60, 62
obesity, classification, 56–57
osteoarthritis, 56
tibial tray, implantation, 86
in women younger, 243
Bone resection
anterior referencing systems, 91
malrotation, 91–92
posterior referencing systems, 91
RH's designs, 181
rotational positioning, 92–93
tibial tray rotation, 93
Whiteside line, 92, 93
Bristol Knee Score rating system, 44

C

CAS. *See* Computer assisted surgery (CAS)
CCK. *See* Condylar contained (CCK) TKAs
Cemented fixation
deformation and degradation over time, 156
Genesis II TKA, 155
osteolysis, 155
Cementless fixation
aseptic loosening, 156
cam/post configuration theory, 158
cost-effectiveness, 159
critical evaluation, 157
decades, 155

© Springer-Verlag London 2015
T. Karachalios (ed.), *Total Knee Arthroplasty: Long Term Outcomes*,
DOI 10.1007/978-1-4471-6660-3

Cementless fixation (*cont.*)
  early HA coated design, 155, 156
  longevity, 158
  meta-analysis, 157
  methodology, 158–159
  obesity, 158
  periprosthetic bone loss, 158
  porous, 158
  Regenerex, 158
  rheumatoid arthritis, 158
  structural and material characteristics, 158, 159
  survival rate, 157
  tantalum trabecular metal technology, 158
  tibial tray malalignment, 157
  titanium foam, 158
  tritanium dimensionised matrix, 158
  valgus/varus deformity, 158
Chondrosarcoma, 193, 195
Cobalt chromium hinged TKA, 40
Cochrane database report, 157
Computer assisted surgery (CAS)
  axis correction, 96
  combined femoral and tibial deformity, 72
  imageless navigation systems, 246
  infrared camera and appropriate software, 96
  intramedullary alignment systems, use of, 96–97
  limb mechanical axis malalignment, 96
  reconstruction, 72–73
  restoration, mechanical axis, 96
Condylar Constrained Implant, 170, 171
Condylar contained (CCK) TKAs
  bilateral implants, 172
  protection against varus/valgus instability, 170
  risk of instability and postoperative pain, 173
  The Sheehan prosthesis, 179, 182
Consolidated Standards of Reporting Trials
     (CONSORT), 213
Constrained knee designs
  bilateral CCK implants, 171, 172
  CCK prosthesis implanted, severely deformed femur,
     173
  cemented stems, 174–175
  complex revision cases, 169
  Condylar Constrained Implant, 170, 171
  excessive femoral rollback, wear and aseptic
     loosening, 170
  'extrinsic' and 'intrinsic' stability, 169
  flexion-extension, 169
  intercondylar stabilizing designs, 170
  kinematic conflict, 169
  knee balance and degree of constraint, 172, 173
  non-/semi-constrained design, 170
  residual instability, 174
  The St. George knee, 169–170
  surgical considerations, 174, 175
  traditional long cemented stems, 171
Continuous passive motion (CPM)
  conventional physical therapy, 233
  DVT after TKA, 230
  hospitalization period, postoperative, 230
  narcotic analgesics, 230

orthopaedics, 229
  physiotherapy after TKA, 229
  postoperative rehabilitation of
     patients, 229
  wound complications, 230–231
Cruciate retaining (CR) designs
  description, 109
  instability/rupture after TKA, 113
  ligaments and tibial constraint, 13
  mobile bearings, 15
  PS *vs.* CR TKAs, 114, 128–131
Cruciate sacrificing (CS) designs, 13

D
2D–3D CT registration techniques, 152
Dislocation safety factor (DSF), 115
Distal femur endoprostheses
  bone resection, 194
  cemented fixation, 195–196
  uncemented fixation, 196–197
  vessel identification and protection, 194, 195
The Duocondylar TKA, 32, 35

E
Early clinical outcomes
  ACL-PCL, 148–149
  designs, 148
  flexion, 149
  hypothesis, 149
  knee scores and range of motion, 149
  level I study, 149
  MP, 148–149
  PFC Sigma mobile bearing, 149
  prostheses, 148
  radiological survey, 149
Effect of age, in TKA
  in elderly patients, 51
  on PROMs, 258
  in younger patients
    arthroscopic debridement, 50
    Oxford knee and EuroQol scores, 50
    proximal tibial osteotomy, 50
    socioeconomic factors, 51
    survival rate, 50
The Eftekhar Mark II, 3, 22, 23
Endo–Modell prostheses, 181, 183, 186, 187
Enhanced recovery protocols (ERP), 106
Enneking classification system, 194
Evaluation scales
  AKSS, 43
  aseptic technique and antibiotic prophylaxis, 40
  disability, 40
  generic measures, 42
  health status tools, reliability, 40–41
  individual risk factors, 40
  inter positional arthroplasty, 39, 40
  measurement tool, validity
    construct, 41–42
    external and internal, 41

OKS (*see* The Oxford knee score (OKS))
responsiveness, 42
The Ewald TKA, 32
Ewing's sarcoma, 193
Extensor mechanism impingement,
95, 96, 111
Extraarticular femoral deformities, 246

F
Femur and tibial cut alignment
extramedullary alignment
systems, 93, 94
intramedullary alignment
systems, 93, 94
intramedullary *vs.* extramedullary instrumentation, 94
transesophageal echocardiography, 94
in varus knees, 93
The Finn rotating knee, 183, 184
Fixation components
cemented, 155
cementless, 155
Cochrane database report, 157
hybrid, 155
Flexion contracture
angle of flexion, 76
computer assisted surgery, 76
knee extension, 230
postoperative range of motion, 76
for PS TKA, 112
residual functional disability, 75–76
stair ascending and descending, 76
surgical techniques, 75
and tibial loosening, 24
The Freeman–Swanson TKA, 33, 35
The French GUEPAR prosthesis, 179, 180
French Handicap, Disability and Dependence survey, 258
Functional outcomes, TKA
assessment tools, 242
36 Health Survey (SF-36), 242
interventions, 242
KSS, 243
OKS, 242–243
postoperative physical, 241
and quality of life (QOL), 241
self-administered satisfaction scale, 241
socio-demographic factors and postoperative, 242

G
Geometric knee arthroplasty, 3, 22
Global Modular Reconstruction System (GMRS), 199
Gluck's surgical interventions, 39–40
The Guepar prosthesis, 3, 23, 25, 180
Gunston polycentric knee, 3

H
HA. *See* Hydroxyapaptite (HA)
Health-related QoL (HRQoL) assessment
disease-specific measures, 256
generic health instruments, 256
outcomes tools, 256
36 Health Survey (SF-36)
generic health status tool, 42
NMES group, 234
TKA outcomes, 256
WOMAC pain score, 228
High Activity Arthroplasty Score (HAAS), 44
Hinge designs. *See* Rotating hinge (RH) prostheses
Hospital for Special Surgery knee rating
system, 43
The Hospital of Special Surgery (HSS),
4, 32, 52, 56, 62, 118, 186,
187, 243, 259
HRQoL. *See* Health-related QoL (HRQoL)
assessment
Human knee kinematics
classical theory, 10
development of theories, 9, 10
dome shaped designs, 14
femoral component designs, 13
joints of, 7
mobile bearing, 13
modern theory, 10–12
motion capture systems, 9
patellofemoral kinematics, 15
PCL, 10
primary total condylar, percentage of,
13, 14
rigid body, 7–9
tibiofemoral kinematics, 14–15
traditional J curve/instantaneous centres, 13
unloaded and loaded knees, 143
Hydroxyapaptite (HA)
bioactive coatings, 157
implant–bone interfaces, 157
radiostereometric analysis, 157
tibial fixation, 158

I
IFR. *See* Intensive functional rehabilitation (IFR)
program
Infected TKA management strategies, 218, 219
Infection, knee megaprosthesis
amputation, 201
bone resection, length of, 201
coagulase-negative Staphylococcus, 200
distal femur uncemented stem, 200
iodine-coated, 201
massive allograft transplantation, 201
silver coated, 200–201
Intensive functional rehabilitation (IFR)
program, 228, 229
Inter positional arthroplasty, 39, 40
Intraoperative models
bony landmarks, digitalization, 250
image based and systems models, 248
planned implant, 247
surgeons, 248, 250
Intra-operative position tracking system, 246, 247

In vivo kinematic analysis, medial-pivot knee
   anteroposterior translation, 151, 152
   2D–3D CT registration techniques, 152
   extensor mechanism, 151
   fluoroscopic analysis, 151
   moderate and deep flexion, 151–152
   openchain model, 151
   patellofemoral, 152
   tibio-femoral joint motion, 152

J

Joint line elevation, 89, 90, 95–96, 114
Juvenile idiopathic arthritis (JIA), 49, 52–53, 63

K

KMFTR. *See* Kotz Modular Femur Tibia Reconstruction
   (KMFTR) System
The Knee Injury and Osteoarthritis Outcome score
   (KOOS), 50, 242, 256
Knee joint deformity
   fixed flexion deformity, 69–70
   malalignment, 69
   in neutral knee, 69
The Knee Society clinical score (KSS)
   accuracy and validity, 44
   clinical assessment, TKA surgery, 243
   and independent radiological analysis, 243
   satisfaction questionnaires, 243
   tested clinical scores, 139
   unvalidated scoring systems, 244
   WOMAC and Oxford 12 disease specific scores, 243
Knee Society Radiological Evaluation System, 43–44
The Kodama–Yamamoto TKA, 30
Kotz Modular Femur Tibia Reconstruction (KMFTR)
   System
   distal femoral resections, 196, 197
   HMRS and GMRS, 199
   uncemented stems and fixed hinge system, 194
KSS. *See* The Knee Society clinical score (KSS)

L

The Leeds TKA, 31
Legion HK, hinge design, 185
Ligaments retaining/substituting designs
   age-matched controls, 112
   CR/PS prosthesis, 112
   Mechanoreceptors, 112
   PCL, 111–112
   ROM and tibial spine, 112
   tibial surface, 112
Long term follow up, RP TKRs
   cemented and uncemented group results, 136–137
   CT scans, 139
   durability, cemented LCS, 138
   fixed and mobile-bearing, 138
   function scores, 138

Kaplan–Meier survivorship analysis, 137
   knees, 138
   KSS scores, 139
   LCS, 136
   osteolysis, 137
   parameters, 138–139
   patella resurfacing, 139
   patients, 138
   pre-op and post-op hospitals, 138
   radiographic evaluation, 138
   revisions, 139
   survival rate, 139
   systematic reviews and meta-analyses, 139
   tested clinical scores, 139
Low Contact Stress (LCS)
   meniscal bearing TKR, 137
   rotating platform TKRs, 136
   Swedish knee registry, 139

M

Malignant bone tumors
   amputation, 193
   chondrosarcoma and osteosarcoma, 193
   compress implants, 194
   Ewing's sarcoma, 193
   KMFTR prosthesis, 194
   tumor endoprosthesis, failure of, 194
Malrotation diagnosis, 250
Medial Pivot TKA designs, 143
Mid/long-term clinical outcomes
   AGC outcomes, 128
   alumina ceramic femoral component, 151
   anteroposterior condylar contact point, 151
   arthroplasty, 126
   cumulative success rate, 149
   double-high tibial insert, 150
   evaluation scores, 149
   factors, 126
   flexion gaps, 151
   Genesis I, 128
   Genesis II, 126, 130
   INBS II and LCS TKA designs, 149
   kneeling, 151
   knee society score and flexion, 149
   literature, 126, 127
   metal backed patellar components, 127
   patella, 126
   posterior cruciate ligament, 151
   postoperative varus deformity, 151
   pre and postoperative clinical scores, 150
   prosthetic infection and periprosthetic fractures
      treatment, 126
   radiographs, 151
   radiological results, 149, 150
   range of motion, 150
   survival rate, 126, 149
   tibial and patellar component, 126
   total condylar TKAs, 128

valgus–varus balancing, 149
varus and valgus deformity, 127
Miller–Galante II total knee replacement, 3, 23, 210–211
Minimally invasive surgery (MIS)
    adequate knee exposure, 102
    advantages, 101, 103
    blood loss, 105
    clinical scores, 104
    complications, 105–106
    and conventional techniques, 103–106
    conventional TKA, 260
    definition, 102–103
    dissatisfied, 101
    level I/II, 103
    medial parapatellar approach, 101
    midterm/long term results, 106
    mini lateral approach, 104
    mini midvastus, 103
    mini-subvastus, 103
    MMP, 103
    operative time, 106
    orthopaedic community, 106
    pain, 104
    patella dislocation without eversion, 102
    postoperative pain and functional recovery, 101
    QS-TKA, 103
    quadriceps muscle strength, 104–105
    radiographic alignment, 105
    RCT, 103
    ROM, 104
    scepticism, 102, 106
    small instruments, 102
    unicompartmental knee replacement, 101
    vastus lateralis, 103
Mobile bearing knee
    definition, 13
    and low conforming fixed-bearing designs, 165
    TKAs, 165
    total condylar knee, 36
Modern theory
    3D imaging techniques, 11
    distal femoral condyle, circularity, 11
    knee motion, phases of, 11
    patella degrees of freedom, 12
    The "Screwhome" arc of motion, 11
    tibial rotation, 12
    tibiofemoral flexion, 12

N

Navigated TKA. *See also* Surgical navigation systems
    augmented reality systems, 246
    extraarticular femoral deformities, 246
    femoral and tibial components, 245
    image based and image free systems, 245
    implant malposition, 245
    soft tissue balancing, 245
Neuromuscular electrical stimulation (NMES)
    Avramidis's and Stevens–Lapsley's studies, 234
    electrical stimulation, vastus medialis muscle, 233–234
    motor recruitment, 233
    muscle contraction intensity, 233
    reflex inhibition, 233
    voluntary activation deficits, 233
New Jersey Orthopaedic Hospital Score (NJOH), 43
The Noiles prosthesis, 181, 184, 186

O

Obesity
    aseptic loosening, 60
    bilateral TKA, 60, 61
    BMI levels, 56–57
    in cementless TKA, 158
    complications, 56
    component malposition
        alignment, 57
        intramedullary tibial cutting guide, 59–60
        subcutaneous tissues with extended midline incision, 58, 59
        tourniquet placement, 58, 59
    definition, 56
    with osteoarthritis, 55–56
    periprosthetic joint infection, 57
    postsurgical complications, 57
    PROMs after TKA, 258–259
    spinal anesthesia, on obese patient, 56, 57
    weight loss after TKA, 60
    WOMAC scores, 60, 62
OKS. *See* The Oxford knee score (OKS)
One stage exchange procedure, 220, 221
Osteoarthritis (OA)
    biomechanical factors, 56
    BMI levels, 56
    prevalence, obesity, 55–56
    valgus deformity, 73–75
    varus deformity, 70, 71, 88
    WOMAC, 43
    in younger patient, 50
Osteolysis, 155
Osteosarcoma, 193
Out-patient clinic and home based therapy
    future research, 236
    internet based tele rehabilitation program, 236
    multidisciplinary rehabilitation program, 236–237
    patients' functional status, 235
    ROM and self-reported outcomes, 235
    sessions, 235
Oxford knee score, 139
The Oxford knee score (OKS), 42–43, 235, 242–243, 256, 257

P

Paradoxical motion, 145
Patellar buttons, 3–4, 31, 34, 163
Patellar clunk syndrome, 113, 116–117, 208

Patella resurfacing
  anatomical issues, 206
  blood supply preserving approach, 208
  cartilage degeneration, 211
  complications, 208
  component alignment, 207
  CONSORT, 213
  extensor mechanism dysfunction, 206
  femoral component designs, 207–208
  Hospital for Special Surgery score, 210
  inflammatory arthropathy population, 210
  intact patella vascularization, preservation, 206–207
  metal backed patella designs, 209
  Miller–Galante II total knee replacement, 210–211
  nonsurfaced, asymptomatic TKA, 208, 209
  normal patellar thickness restoration, 206, 207
  optimal femoral, tibial and patellar component orientation, 207
  painful patellofemoral joint, 205
  proponents, 209
  radiological appearance, 205, 206
  randomised trials, 212–213
  RCT of Kinemax TKAs, 211
  RCTs and quasi-RCTs, 213
  resurfaced, asymptomatic TKA, 208
  revision rates, 209
  soft tissue impingement, 207
  surgical technique errors, 206
  symmetrical patellar facets creation, 206
  tibial tuberosity transfer, 207
  tilt and instability, bilateral TKA, 207, 208
  tracking restoration, 207
Patellofemoral joint
  duocondylar TKA, 35
  Endo-Modell prosthesis, 181, 183
  patellar complications, 205
  restoration, 146–148
  scoring systems, 44–45
  surgical technique, 206
Patellofemoral kinematics, 15
Patient-reported outcome measures (PROMs)
  age, 258
  definition, 256
  gender, 258
  implant design, 259–260
  medical factors, 259
  obesity, 258–259
  vs. other outcome scores, 45
  patient's point of view, 45
  surgical technique, 260
  survival analysis, 45
Patient satisfaction
  clinician and patient ratings, health status, 261
  definition, 260
  pain relief and functional status, 261
  psychological issues, 261
  The Swedish Arthroplasty Registry, 261
Patient specific cutting guides, 97
PCL. *See* Posterior cruciate ligament (PCL)

Periprosthetic joint infection, 57, 217
Polycentric and geometric TKAs
  The Blauth prosthesis, 25
  concepts and techniques, 21
  The Eftekhar Mark II, 23
  Geotibial and Geopatellar knee designs, 23
  The Guepar hinge, 23
  The Guepar prosthesis, 25
  minimally constrained components, 22
  patellar pain, flexion contracture and tibial loosening, 24
  proper axial alignment, 24
  radiolucent lines, development, 26
  rheumatoid and degenerative arthritis, 24
  The Seehan prosthesis, 25
  thinner polyethylene insertion, 22
Polyethylene effect
  after primary surgery, 165, 166
  after surgery and uncemented TKA, 164
  causes, UHMWPE failure, 165
  cultural and socioeconomic factors, 163
  highly cross linked polyethylenes, 165
  in vitro analyses report, 166
  low-wear TKAs, 165
  metal-backed modular components, 163
  mobile-bearing TKAs, 165
  randomized controlled trials, 165, 167
  UHMWPE, 163–164
Posterior cruciate ligament (PCL)
  abnormal knee biomechanics, 130–131
  arthritic process, 126
  AS/ultra-congruent TKA, 125
  CR bearings, 13
  CR TKA, 125
  debatable issue, 125
  deficient knees, 119
  femoral box designs, 119
  four-bar linkage system, 125
  instability failures, 114
  intraoperative findings, 109
  knee arthroplasty design, 125
  mechanoreceptors, 125
  meta-analyses, 119
  multiple confounding factors, 109
  no clear benefits/drawbacks, 109
  orthopedic surgeons, 109
  posterior cruciate condylar knee, 34
  posterolateral and posteromedial structures, 125
  postoperative knee flexion, 119
  PS TKA, 125
  roll-back, 109, 125
  severe knee deformity, 129
  single tibial insert, 32
  sparing and substituting types, 109
  stages, 126
  tibia and femur, 125
  tibial femoral rotation, 14
Posterior stabilized (PS) design
  advantages, 109

criticisms, total condylar prosthesis, 110
description, 13
dislocation risk component, 109
dual-cam mechanism, 109
GMK sphere system, 111
history, 110
Insall-Burstein, 110–111
intramedullary instruments, 110
knee flexion, 111
medial pivot TKA, 111
patella, 110
post and cam mechanism, 109
tibial plateau components, 110
tibial polyethylene component, 110
total condylar implant, 110
translation and dislocation, 110
variations, 109
Posterior tibial slope, 95
PROMs. *See* Patient-Reported Outcome Program
 (PROMs)
Proximal tibia resections
 cemented fixation, 198–199
 characteristics, 197
 description, 197, 198
 functional performance during gait, 197
 Trevira attachment tube, 198
 uncemented fixation, 199–200
PS design. *See* Posterior stabilized (PS)
PS TKA
 advantages
  knee kinematics, 113
  polyethylene wear, 114
  posterior cruciate ligament rupture, 114
  ROM, 113–114
  surgical exposure and ligament balancing, 113
 cam-post articulations, 119
 disadvantages
  dislocations, 115
  intercondylar fractures, 115–116
  patellar clunk syndrome, 116–117
  patellar fractures, 116
  synovial entrapment, 116–117
  tibial spine wear, 114–115
 HA-coated versions, 119
 HSS knee score, 118
 IB I metal-backed TKAs, 118
 indications and contraindications, 112–113
 Insall-Burstein I and II prosthesis, 117, 118
 knee flexion, 118
 metal-backed tibial components, 118
 modularity, 118
 polyethylene wear, 118
 radiographic assessment, 119
PS *vs.* CR TKAs
 abnormal knee biomechanics, 130–131
 arthritic process, 129
 clinical outcomes, 128
 cruciate retainers and substituters, 128
 I² heterogeneity, 129

implant survival and patient satisfaction, 128
Kinematic-KMS TKA, AP radiograph, 128
literature, 127, 128, 130
meta-analysis reports, 128
PCL, 129
PFC, AP and lateral radiograph, 128, 129
proprioception, 130
prosthesis, 129
retaining and balancing, PCL, 131
ROM and knee flexion, 129
surgeon, 129–130
surgical technique, 129

Q
Quality of life (QoL). *See also* Patient satisfaction
 chronic pain, 257
 The Constitution of WHO, definition, 255
 English PROMs Programme, 257
 evaluations, 256
 French Handicap, Disability and Dependence
  survey, 258
 health and disease context, 255
 HRQoL assessment, 256
 multidimensional assessments,
  components, 255, 256
 pain relief and physical function, 257
 safe and cost-effective treatment, 256
 unimpaired functional ability after TKA, 257–258

R
Range of motion (ROM), 104, 145–146
Regenerex, 158
Rehabilitation effect
 end stage osteoarthritis (OA), 227
 IFR program, 228
 limb muscle strengthening, 229
 6 min walk test (6-MWT), 228
 NIH, 227
 physical impairment and functional
  limitations, 227
 treatment effects, 228
 WBV, 229
Restoration, limb mechanical axis
 bilateral severe valgus and varus knee deformity, 86
 bilateral valgus knee deformities, 86, 87
 extension and flexion gaps, 89, 90
 and joint line elevation, 89, 90
 residual instability, 90
 tibial tray, alignment, 86
 varus placement, tibial component, 86, 87
RH. *See* Rotating hinge (RH) prostheses
Rheumatoid arthritis (RA)
 duocondylar implant, 25
 effect of diagnosis, 51–53
 erythrocyte sedimentation rate levels, 52
 multisystem disease characteristics, 51
 primary RH TKA, 186

Rigid body
  anatomical reference landmarks and 3D image
      registration, 9
  bone geometry and soft tissue envelope, 8
  bones of, 7–8
  cadaveric bone samples, 8
  erroneous process, 8
  mathematical models, 9
  medical imaging techniques, 9
  x-ray technology, 8
ROM. *See* Range of motion (ROM)
Rotating hinge (RH) prostheses
  Blauth prosthesis, 179, 182
  condylar designs, 179
  Endo–Modell prostheses, 181, 183, 187
  Engelbrecht, developer, 187
  etiology, 189
  The Finn rotating knee, 183, 184
  fixed hinge designs, 186
  The French GUEPAR prosthesis, 179, 180
  indications, 186
  Legion HK, 185
  modular segmental kinematic rotating
      hinge, 181, 184
  The Noiles prosthesis, 181, 184, 186
  RH prostheses, 179
  salvage knee surgery, 189
  The Sheehan prosthesis, 179, 182
  soft tissue and collateral ligament releases, 189
  The Solution RT rotating hinge, 184, 185, 188
  S-ROM modular knee, 183, 184, 188
  The Stanmore prosthesis, 179, 180
  St. Georg prosthesis, 179, 181
  trochlea design, 187
  VCC, 188–189
Rotating platform TKR
  advantages
    floated tibial tray, 135
    malalignment, 136
    mobile-bearing designs, 135
    optimal tibial surface coverage, 136
    paradoxical anterior/natural posterior femoral
        translation, 135
  bone-implant interface, 135
  decades, 136
  dual articulation, 136
  hinged designs, 135
  hybrid LCS®, 136, 137
  implant loosening and polyethylene wear, 135
  meticulous soft tissue balancing, 139
  mobile-bearing, 136
  optimum surgical technique, 139
  polyethylene instability and dislocation, 136
  short and mid-term results, 136
  tibio-femoral bearing surfaces, 135

S
The "Screwhome" arc of motion, 11
Second generation TKAs
  anatomical, 31
  aseptic loosening, 34

  clinical improvement, 34
  description, 30
  The duocondylar, 32, 35
  The Ewald TKA, 32
  Freeman–Samuelson design, 36
  The Freeman–Swanson, 33
  Kinemax TKA, 35
  The Kodama–Yamamoto, 30
  LCS, 34
  The Leeds, 31
  mobile bearing knee, 34
  total condylar (TC), 33
  The UCI TKA, 30
The Sheehan prosthesis, 23, 179, 182
Short-form 36 (SF-36)
  accuracy and validity, 44
  description, 42
  limitations, 42
  scores, in dimensions, 242
  strengthening interventions, 228
SLR. *See* Straight leg raise test (SLR)
Soft tissue balancing, 113, 172, 245
The Solution RT rotating hinge, 184, 185, 188
Special Surgery knee score, 138–139
Spine-cam mechanism, 114, 116
Sporting activities, 64–65
S-ROM modular knee, 183, 184, 188
SSI. *See* Surgical site infection (SSI)
The Stanmore prosthesis, 179, 180
St. Georg prosthesis, 179, 181
Straight leg raise test (SLR), 104
Surgical morbidity, 80–81
Surgical mortality, 80
Surgical navigation systems
  advantages, 250
  augmented reality systems, 246
  CAS, 250–251
  clinical outcomes, 251–252
  complications, 251
  control software, 246, 249
  coronal plane alignment, 250
  cost effective, 251
  display device, 246, 248
  functional improvement, quality of life, 251
  intraoperative models, 247–250
  intra-operative position tracking, 246, 247
  limb alignment outliers, 250
  malrotation diagnosis, 250
  operative room, 251
  preoperative models, 247
  preoperative planning, 246
  tasks, 247
  visual and numerical information, 246
Surgical site infection (SSI)
  advantages, 220
  aggressive biological behaviors, 218
  amputation, 223
  articulating spacer, 222, 223
  average cost of in hospital care, 217
  with biofilm formation, infected TKA, 217, 218
  classification systems, 218
  clinical outcome studies

one stage exchange procedure, 220, 221
two stage exchange procedure, 221
custom made antibiotic static spacer, 222
diagnosis, 218
disadvantages, 222
implant salvage, TKA with early postoperative, 220
infected tissue debridement extensor mechanism
    defects, 218, 219
infectious disease consultant, 218, 220
knee arthrodesis, external fixator, 223, 224
knee soft tissue envelop, 218, 219
management strategies, 218–219
periprosthetic infection rate, 217
risk factors, 217
Surgical techniques
    CAS, 72–73
    direct lateral approach, 102
    grafting techniques, 72
    mini medial parapatellar, 102
    mini-midvastus, 102
    mini-subvastus, 102
    osteotomies and ligament balancing, 101
    posteromedial capsulotomy, 72
    quadriceps-sparing, 102
    quadriceps tendon, 103
    tibial component, downsizing and lateralizing, 72
Survival analysis, 45
The Swedish Arthroplasty Registry, 261
Swedish knee registry, 139
Synovial entrapment, 116–117

T
Tantalum trabecular metal technology, 158
Tibiofemoral kinematics, 13–15
Titanium foam, 158
Total Condylar knee (TC), 4
Total knee arthroplasty (TKA)
    activity level, 62–65
    bone deformity
        valgus osteoarthtitic knee, femoral diaphyseal, 69,
        71
        varus osteoarthritic knee, tibial metaphyseal, 69,
        70
    clinical benefits, 49
    complication and mortality rates, 81–82
    costs, 81
    effect of body weight (*see* Obesity)
    eligibility criteria, 80
    factors, 143
    history
        anatomical total condylar knee, 3
        anatomic and functional approaches, 3
        bone cement, use of, 3
        functional approach, to knee design, 4
        geometric designs, 3
        Guepar prosthesis, 3
        implants, 4, 5

interposition arthroplasty, 2
intramedullary stems, 2
mobile bearing arthroplasties, 4
patellar buttons, 3–4
resection arthroplasty, 2
indication and aim, surgery, 1
inter-related elements, 85
osteoarthritis, 143
outcome measures (*see* Evaluation scales)
patient outcomes, 79–80
predictors, TKA outcome, 49–50
revision, evaluation of, 85
revision surgery, 81
steps and stages, 1–2
surgical factors, 55
Tritanium dimensionised matrix, 158
Two stage exchange procedure, 221

U
The UCI TKA, 30, 35
Ultrahighmolecular-weight polyethylene (UHMWPE)
    failure causes, 164–165
    total joint arthroplasty, 163–164

V
Valgus knee deformity
    bone deformities and soft tissues contractures, 88–89
    cruciate retaining implants, 74
    distal femoral anatomy, 73
    inside-out release technique, 74
    knee joint, 88
    lateral parapatellar approach, 74
    lateral stabilizing structures, 89
    left osteoarthritic knee, 75
    ligament structure parameters, 73
    "pie crust technique", 89
    right osteoarthritic knee, 73, 74
    sliding lateral femoral condyle osteotomy, 89
    tibial tubercle osteotomy, 74
Varus knee deformity
    alignment and stability, 88
    angulations, 70
    balancing, 71
    collateral ligament, 88
    left osteoarthritic knee, 70, 71
    medial structures, 86–88
Varus valgus constrained (VVC) implants,
    170, 188–189
Visual analogue scale (VAS), 104, 139

W
Whiteside line, 92
Whole body vibration (WBV), 229
Wii Fit™ motion controlled video game system,
    232–233

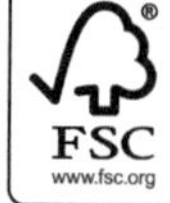

MIX
Papier aus verantwortungsvollen Quellen
Paper from responsible sources
FSC® C105338

If you have any concerns about our products,
you can contact us on
ProductSafety@springernature.com

In case Publisher is established outside the EU,
the EU authorized representative is:
Springer Nature Customer Service Center GmbH
Europaplatz 3, 69115 Heidelberg, Germany

Printed by Libri Plureos GmbH
in Hamburg, Germany